Placebo Effects Through the Lens of Translational Research

T0176439

Placebo Effects Through the Lens of Translational Research

Edited by

Luana Colloca, Jason Noel, Patricia D. Franklin,
and Chamindi Seneviratne

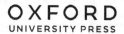

OXFORD
UNIVERSITY PRESS

OXFORD
UNIVERSITY PRESS

Oxford University Press is a department of the University of Oxford. It furthers
the University's objective of excellence in research, scholarship, and education
by publishing worldwide. Oxford is a registered trade mark of Oxford University
Press in the UK and certain other countries.

Published in the United States of America by Oxford University Press
198 Madison Avenue, New York, NY 10016, United States of America.

© Oxford University Press 2023

© Some rights reserved. This is an open access publication, available online and distributed under the terms of
the Creative Commons Attribution-Non Commercial-No Derivatives 4.0 International licence (CC BY-NC-ND
4.0), a copy of which is available at http://creativecommons.org/licenses/by-nc-nd/4.0/. Enquiries concerning use
outside the scope of the licence terms should be sent to the Rights Department, Oxford University Press.

All rights reserved. No part of this publication may be reproduced, stored in
a retrieval system, or transmitted, in any form or by any means, without the
prior permission in writing of Oxford University Press, or as expressly permitted
by law, by license, or under terms agreed with the appropriate reproduction
rights organization. Inquiries concerning reproduction outside the scope of the
above should be sent to the Rights Department, Oxford University Press, at the
address above.

You must not circulate this work in any other form
and you must impose this same condition on any acquirer.

Library of Congress Cataloging-in-Publication Data
[Names: Colloca, Luana, editor. | Noel, Jason, editor. |
Franklin, Patricia D., editor. | Seneviratne, Chamindi, editor.]
Title: Placebo effects through the lens of translational research
[edited by] Luana Colloca, Jason Noel, Patricia D. Franklin, and Chamindi Seneviratne.
Description: New York, NY : Oxford University Press, [2023] |
Includes bibliographical references and index.
Identifiers: LCCN 2023032622 (print) | LCCN 2023032623 (ebook) |
ISBN 9780197645444 (paperback) | ISBN 9780197645451 (epub) |
ISBN 9780197645475 (online)
Subjects: MESH: Placebo Effect | Placebos—therapeutic use |
Translational Research, Biomedical
Classification: LCC R733 (print) | LCC R733 (ebook) | NLM WB 330 |
DDC 615.5—dc23/eng/20230727
LC record available at https://lccn.loc.gov/2023032622
LC ebook record available at https://lccn.loc.gov/2023032623

DOI: 10.1093/med/9780197645444.001.0001

This material is not intended to be, and should not be considered, a substitute for medical or other professional
advice. Treatment for the conditions described in this material is highly dependent on the individual
circumstances. And, while this material is designed to offer accurate information with respect to the subject
matter covered and to be current as of the time it was written, research and knowledge about medical and health
issues is constantly evolving and dose schedules for medications are being revised continually, with new side
effects recognized and accounted for regularly. Readers must therefore always check the product information
and clinical procedures with the most up-to-date published product information and data sheets provided by
the manufacturers and the most recent codes of conduct and safety regulation. The publisher and the authors
make no representations or warranties to readers, express or implied, as to the accuracy or completeness of this
material. Without limiting the foregoing, the publisher and the authors make no representations or warranties as
to the accuracy or efficacy of the drug dosages mentioned in the material. The authors and the publisher do not
accept, and expressly disclaim, any responsibility for any liability, loss, or risk that may be claimed or incurred as a
consequence of the use and/or application of any of the contents of this material.

Printed by Marquis Book Printing, Canada

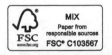

Contents

Editor's Biography

Dr. Luana Colloca is an Mpower distinguished professor at University of Maryland, Baltimore. She holds an MD from University Magna Graecia of Catanzaro and a PhD in Neuroscience from the University of Turin School of Medicine, Italy. She completed her post-doctoral training at the Brain Imaging Center at the Karolinska Institute, Sweden, and currently serves as a Professor of Pain and Translational Symptom Science and the Director of the Placebo Beyond Opinions (PBO) Center at the University of Maryland, Baltimore School of Nursing. Dr. Colloca is an internationally recognized expert in studying the biological mechanisms of placebo effects, with a multi-faceted approach encompassing pharmacological, genetic, and behavioral aspects. Her groundbreaking research has significantly advanced the understanding of how placebo effects are formed, nociception and clinical pain modulation and has led to the development of innovative strategies to optimize therapeutic outcomes in clinical practice. She has published in top-ranked international journals and her research has been featured on The National Geographic, The New Scientist, Science daily, The New Yorker, Nature, The Guardian, The Wall Street Journal, News and World Reports and USA Today.

Dr. Jason Noel is a faculty member at the University of Maryland School of Pharmacy. He holds a Bachelor's of Science and a Doctor of Pharmacy degree from Rutgers University and has completed a residency in Psychiatric Pharmacy Practice at the University of Maryland School of Pharmacy. He has also attained a Master's degree in Public Administration from the University of Baltimore. With expertise in various areas of psychiatric pharmacy practice, including intellectual/developmental disabilities, acute psychiatry, and long-term care, Dr. Noel brings a wealth of experience to his role. He is an accomplished clinical educator, teaching in multiple programs, such as the Pharm.D., advance practice nursing, and physician assistant programs at UMB. Dr. Noel also has over a decade of experience in administering ACPE-accredited continuing education programs at the School of Pharmacy. His research focuses on optimizing integrated treatment and contextual effects for psychiatric and behavioral disorders in individuals with developmental disabilities. Dr. Noel is board certified by the Board of Pharmaceutical Specialties in Psychiatric Pharmacy.

Dr. Patricia D Franklin has enjoyed a successful nursing career spanning practice, program management, academia, and professional development. With experience in primary care practice, she has served on professional association, government, and coalition boards and committees, including holding the position of president in a national professional association. Dr. Franklin's transition to the non-profit sector was marked by her management of a multi-year, multi-site grant from the John A. Hartford Foundation (JAHF), which grew from a $2 million to a $26 million award within a decade. As a faculty member at the University of Maryland School of Nursing, she taught health policy, health systems, and leadership in graduate programs. Dr. Franklin also served as the Director of the Office of Professional Education (OPE), where she developed professional continuing education programs and established an interprofessional CE consortium involving colleagues from various disciplines. She notably led a five year state-awarded grant worth $2.5 million to build nurse leadership capacity in Maryland, designing and running the School's inaugural Leadership Institute. Dr. Franklin retired from the School of Nursing in 2019 but continues to contribute as a consultant.

Dr. Chamindi Seneviratne is a faculty member at the Institute for Genomic Sciences (IGS), University of Maryland School of Medicine. She holds an MD degree, and completed her post-doctoral research training in neurobiochemistry at the University of Texas at San Antonio, and molecular genomics at the University of Virginia. She has nearly two decades of expertise in studying molecular genomic underpinnings in substance misuse, and how we can utilize genomics to improve treatment responses, particularly focusing on alcohol misuse. She has served as a principal investigator or co-investigator on multiple National Institutes of Health (NIH)-funded research projects on substance use disorders. Current research in Dr. Seneviratne's lab at the IGS is dedicated to contributing to the growing understanding of the role of pharmacogenomics of investigational medications and the placebo responses in individuals with alcohol and other substance use disorders to develop personalized approaches to improving treatment outcomes.

Acknowledgments

Placebo Effects Through the Lens of Translational Research is the result of a synergic collaboration of researchers from over 10 countries, and it encompasses several interdisciplinary specialties.

We wish to thank all the contributing authors for their contributions and interest in researching distinct mechanisms and translational aspects of placebo effects. We also wish to thank the funding agencies that support the different authors and their research. In particular, we thank the funding agencies for this book which include the National Institute on Alcohol Abuse and Alcoholism (1R13AA028424), the German collaborative research center "Treatment Expectation" TRR289, the Samueli Foundation and the Society for Interdisciplinary Placebo Studies, an international association whose goal is to understand placebo and nocebo effects and their translation into healthcare and related fields.

We wish to thank Jane Kirschling, Bruce Jarrell and Erika Friedman who supported us in a variety of ways to launch the Placebo Beyond Opinions (PBO) Center which aims to advance unbiased knowledge of the mechanisms and translational aspects of placebo (and nocebo) effects across disciplines. Finally, we thank our families and friends for their continuous support and unconditional love.

Introduction

Luana Colloca, Jason Noel, Patricia D. Franklin,
and Chamindi Seneviratne

The challenge of improving health outcomes for individuals and populations remains daunting. Fortunately, collaboration among multiple disciplines accelerates our appreciation of innate and external determinants of health for individuals and populations. Interprofessional research, education, and practice also strengthens our capacity to design, disseminate, and deliver effective strategies and policies to prevent and treat diseases, and improve health. It is therefore encouraging when research describes an effective therapeutic strategy that translates to clinical practice across disciplines, especially one that can enhance treatment efficacy without detrimental side effects. An example of such research is the placebo phenomenon.[1]

This book sheds light on the translation of current mechanistic research on placebo effects to develop comprehensive and adequate strategies for better symptom management and treatment in clinical practices.

The history of the placebo stretches back to ancient times and is often associated with unsavory stories of scams and maltreatments. However, its past also reveals, what has long been suspected and then proven through research, that the placebo effect is a phenomenon grounded in neurobiological, behavioral, and psychological sciences. Further, the placebo effect is moderated by the same factors that determine health trajectories and outcomes. These include individual's expectations, experiences, psychosocial and cultural backgrounds, and temporal events that affect the response to both sham and active drugs, and other nonpharmacological treatments. Similarly, research describes factors that amplify and diminish the nocebo effect in influencing therapeutic interventions.

The Society for Interdisciplinary Placebo Studies (SIPS) "is an international association of scholars who share the goal of understanding the placebo effect in medical treatment, psychotherapy, and complementary and alternative treatment" (https://placebosociety.org/about-sips). In 2018 and 2020, a group of experts who organized and participated in the first SIPS, invitational conference published a report on results of the meeting and its survey. Goals of the meetings were to develop consensus and recommendations about evidence-based and ethical use of placebo and nocebo effects for clinical practice. One particular area of agreement among this group was "the importance of informing patients about placebo and nocebo effects and training health professionals in patient-clinician communication to maximize placebo and minimize nocebo effects" (p. 52).[2] Later on the group further recognized that "research is needed on how to optimally tailor information to specific clinical conditions and patients' needs, and on developing standardized disclosure training modules for clinicians" (p. 50).[2]

This book continues the development of evidence-based use of placebo. Specifically, we identified three core aspects to bridge state-of-the-art concepts with day-to-day clinical practice. First, lessons from mechanistic placebo research indicate neurobiological bases underlying placebo effects. Second, placebo research can improve the design of clinical trials to advance drug development. Third, placebo effects can be exploited in daily clinical practice to optimize patient-clinician communication and relationships and clinical outcomes.

Lessons from mechanistic placebo research indicate a neurobiological basis of placebo effects

Often it has been said that the history of prescientific Medicine is the history of the placebo effect.[3-5] However, the revolution within the placebo research occurred when objective measurements and neuropsychological mechanisms were tied to this area of research. Contrasting the role of expectancy versus conditioning, Voudouris and colleagues introduced the study of placebo effects in human laboratory settings.[6,7] The pioneering design involved instruction, conditioning, and test phases. Participants were informed that a placebo would have either relieved or increased painful stimulations. During the conditioning phase of these studies, the intensity of the painful stimulations was surreptitiously manipulated contingently with the application of the placebo cream to strength the experience of analgesia (or reduction of the painful stimulations). The test phase included same-intensity painful stimulations, and each reduction from the control condition was operationally defined as a *placebo effect*.

Since these studies, many researchers have used verbal suggestions and conditioning to explore behavioral and biological responses to placebos for nociception and pain.[8-13] Other conditions such as taste,[14] immune responses,[15] cough,[16] and motion-induced nausea[17,18] have been investigated.

Notably, Voudouris and colleagues' design,[6,7] which included within-subjects repeated stimulations with and without the placebo conditions, had the greatest impact on the science of placebo because it paved the way for neuro-imaging studies on placebo effects, including high-resolution electroenceph-alography (EEG),[9] Positron Emission Tomography (PET),[19] and functional Magnetic Resonance Imaging (fMRI),[20] which was not possible with pharma-cological conditioning studies.[21,22]

The first PET study on placebo analgesia using oxygen-15 water (H_2O^{15}) suggested the activation of the rostral anterior cingulate cortex (rACC) and the orbitofrontal cortex. The authors suggested that placebo analgesia acts on similar neuronal mechanisms of opioid-induced pain reduction be-cause they found increased functional connectivity between the rACC and the brainstem in both the opioid and placebo conditions compared with no-treatment group. Endogenous opioids play a central role in placebo analgesia as evidenced by studies with a μ–opioid receptor-selective radiotracer [^{11}C] carfentanil.[23] Recently, pharmacological and spinal fMRI studies[24,25] showed that placebo analgesia is associated with activation of descending modulation systems that can change the experience of pain and nociception signaling.

Placebo science can improve the design of clinical trials to advance drug development

Placebos were introduced as controls in clinical trials and became the main-stay of modern Medicine. A trial commissioned by Louis XVI in 1784 tested the "animal magnetism"—a hypothetical invisible force that Franklin Mesmer thought had healing properties.[26] Franklin and Lavoisier exposed patients to "mesmerized" objects or untreated objects (i.e., placebos) without informing them to which object they were being exposed to. Responses to the objects were entirely unrelated to whether or not the object had been mesmerized. They concluded that mesmerized objects had no effect and, thus, no scien-tific basis.

The advent of the double-blind placebo-controlled trial advanced scien-tific methods, and in 1900, the phenomenon of the placebo was revamped by Beecher.[27] Data from the placebo groups of 15 studies related to pain, seasick-ness, cough, and anxiety showed that placebos led to a significant improve-ment in symptoms. While Beecher's methodology was later criticized,[28] his research sparked interest in the potential healing power of placebo effects across conditions. *Placebo effects* refer to a beneficial effect produced by a pla-cebo drug or treatment or a manipulation of the participant's belief, which cannot be attributed to the properties of the placebo/manipulation itself and is, therefore, due to the cascade of neurobiological changes related to expectancy, prior therapeutic experiences, observation of benefits in others, contextual and treatment cues, and interpersonal interactions.[29]

A no-treatment control group is ultimately necessary to dissociate placebo effects from the placebo responses. Thus, clinical trials that only include the new-treatment group, the active control group, and a placebo group but not a no-treatment group, capture various nonspecific effects driven by the natural history, regression to the mean, false positive and negative errors, and biases that can confound findings.

In clinical trials, it is important to rule out placebo responses, and this requires and adequate study design.[30,31] Different clinical trial designs have been suggested to identify placebo responses.[1,32] Most clinical trials use the placebo-controlled design. However, other designs such as the balanced-placebo design,[33] the double-blind versus deceptive design,[34] the open-hidden treatment administration (also called overt-covert treatment administration),[35–37] open-label placebo design,[38,39] sequential parallel comparison,[40] and enriched enrollment with randomized withdrawal design,[41] among others, have been designed to identify placebo responses (for details, see Chapter 5.4).

Additionally, placebo effects can be controlled by measuring expectations[42] (Chapters 1.2 and 5.4). It is possible to measure anticipated outcomes, desire of benefits, allocation guess, perception of benefits, and patients' direct experiences. Distinct scales for measuring expectations[43] have been proposed, including set of validated questions or visual analogue scales.[44] Other aspects to be taken into consideration are the measure's sensitivity, outcome perception (e.g., teens and parents value different outcomes), and outcome choice (e.g., use of pain disability versus pain intensity).[1] Finally, knowledge about Patient-Centered Outcome Research would also need to be incorporated into what constitutes good evidence for validating a new treatment or intervention, especially for the decision makers (e.g., stakeholders, policy makers).[45] Optimally, all parties should collaborate to design, implement, and disseminate the study in a manner that ensures translation to patients and caregivers, and stakeholders.[46]

Placebo effects can be exploited in daily clinical practice to optimize patient-clinician communication, relationships, and clinical outcomes

Placebo effects exist and operate in daily clinical practice when treatments as usual are administered and without using traditional placebos (e.g., saline solution, micro cellulose tablets and pills, and sham surgeries). Indeed, placebo effects derive from the psychosocial context and/or therapeutic encounters around any treatments. Patient-clinician relationships and communication along with medical history and past therapeutic experiences can affect any clinical outcomes and therefore contribute to ameliorating the intrinsic action of treatments. Similarly, negative contents as part of the routine patient-clinician communication and prior unsuccessful treatments can affect outcomes in the routine of clinical practices. As with their nocebo counterpart, placebo responses interact with therapeutic contexts and the patient's mindsets. The placebo phenomenon is demonstrated with approaches that shed light on the impact of informing patients about the administration of a treatment, such as an infusion of morphine for postoperative pain, with a significantly more rapid improvement of postoperative pain as compared to when the treatment is given through an infusion pump without informing the patient.

Research on placebo (and nocebo) effects draws attention to the potentially important ways in which possible therapeutic effects are disclosed to patients in routine clinical care. It is becoming evident that placebo effects can modulate the outcome of a given therapy in a positive way. Importantly, placebo effects can operate in the absence of any placebo. A careful balance must exist between communicating truthful information and ensuring a positive therapeutic context while respecting the patient's autonomy with the delivery of nondeceptive information. Tailoring information is necessary to account for what patients know about their condition during the era of digital Medicine. Clinical notes and patient-based approaches should be developed with attention to equity, inclusiveness, and diversity. Clinicians in all disciplines will benefit from learning about the science of placebo, the disclosure process, ethical requirements to tailor the information delivery toward an optimization of patients' needs, and, ultimately, placebo effects. Clinicians' efforts should be devoted to optimizing realistic expectations and the most effective communication as part of the therapeutic journey.

A blueprint of the book

This book consists of six Sections that outline cutting-edge themes in research related to placebo effects.

Section 1 introduces the reader to the concepts of healing, expectations, future perspectives, and cultural influences. The author of Chapter 1.1 describes clinical practices and behaviors that use placebo mechanisms for optimization of healing and discusses the implications of placebo research for delivering a person-cantered clinical decision-making process. The chapter also summarizes tools to enhance placebo-based healing in routine practice, recognize placebo mechanisms occurring in clinical practice, implement healing rituals in patient care, and access the HOPE Note Toolkit for ethically optimizing placebo-based healing in clinicians own practice.

The authors of Chapter 1.2 discusses how expectations should be defined and measured. The chapter also discuss conceptualizations and new frameworks related to treatment expectations, and it clarifies when and how expectations contribute—not only to placebo effects, but also to treatment effects in general.

Chapter 1.3 discusses the current state of placebo research as a first step to justifying placebo-based clinical interventions. First and foremost, there is a need for training healthcare clinicians and the broader healthcare workforce to deliberately and effectively leverage the psychological and social forces underlying placebo effects to improve patient satisfaction and health outcomes. In particular, interventions focused on empowering patients to establish a more adaptive mindset as they progress through treatment are encouraged.

Finally, Chapter 1.4 discusses how mindsets, meanings, and expectations are rooted in individual cultural beliefs, norms, values, worldviews, and experiences. Among others, contextual factors such as spiritual and religious beliefs may inform coping and other health behaviors that are important for eliciting treatment (and placebo) responses. To maximize healing, cultural factors would also need to be considered to fully understand individuals' dynamic treatment and outcomes expectations.

Section 2 of this book focuses on biomarkers and precision medicine. Most research on mechanisms of placebo effects has been conducted in laboratory settings. Such studies identified learning mechanisms that can explain observed effects, and provided evidence that placebo effects are associated with nociception, with reproducible patterns of brain activity. Yet, over the years, placebo effects have been seen as unstable over time and across contexts; the occurrence and/or magnitude of a participant's placebo effect in one setting does not generalize to other settings, suggesting that placebo effects are mostly driven by immediate, context-specific factors and thus remain unpredictable and therefore difficult to implement in real-life settings.[47,48]

Chapter 2.1 challenges these commonly held beliefs and describes how placebo effects in chronic pain can be predicted by genetics, brain characteristics, and language use. If replicated, these results hint to clinically relevant and biologically driven placebo effects that can be not only well-understood but also implemented in clinical treatment of chronic pain and beyond. Behavioral and brain mapping have been used to identify neurobiological mechanisms of placebo effects.

To identify molecular pathways of placebo effects, recent studies have investigated genomic and pharmacological effects on response to placebo treatments in experimental and clinical trial settings. Chapter 2.2 discusses genomic and pharmacological responses in irritable bowel syndrome, pain, depression, inflammatory disease, and COVID diseases among others.

Chapter 2.3 elaborates on significant variations in neurobiological regulation in alcohol use/misuse and alcohol use disorder and chronic pain related to a person's genetic background. The dynamic nature of neurobiological dysregulations highlights a need for research conducted to identify genes whose expression alterations drive molecular-level changes underlying responses to placebos and other treatments.

Genetics and omics are thought to contribute to understanding placebo effects, and the overall set of proteins that can be expressed by genome, cells, tissues, or organisms at a given time must be considered.[49,50] Especially promising are plasma proteomics in combination with advanced computational tools to identify potential biomarkers that enable the prediction and monitoring responses to placebos and other treatments in the context of clinical trials. Chapter 2.4 discusses methods of plasma proteomics and illustrates their implementation to the study of laboratory-induced nausea.

There is a multiplicity of mechanisms of placebo effects across different medical conditions and body systems.[51] Section 3 of this book, presents new examples of placebo effects in conditions related to sleep, (paradoxical) cough, immune system, sport and exercise, migraine, and COVID-19, for example.

Chapter 3.1 describes interactions between sleep and the opioid system, as well as positive affect and the occurrence and consolidation of placebo effects and expectations.

Chapter 3.2 describes studies showing that placebo treatments can reduce cough by 40% in trials, and this large placebo effect confounds the outcome of clinical trials. There is some doubt about the pharmacological efficacy of over-the-counter cough medicines because they contain over 100 ingredients that enhance the viscosity, taste, color, smell, and sensory effect of the medicine and enhance placebo effects.

One of the most sophisticated conditions for placebo effects is immunomodulation. Chapter 3.3 provides an overview of behaviorally conditioned placebo responses, discussing them in the context of organ transplantation or inflammatory autoimmune diseases. Continuous treatment with immunomodulatory drugs is an inevitable prerequisite for many clinical conditions. Thus, the prospect to harness conditioned immune responses is a promising adjuvant treatment to current immunopharmacological regimens, with the goal of minimizing the overall required drug dosages.

Placebo effects apply not only to medicine but also to daily life. An example is the separation between placebo effects in sport and placebo effects in exercise. Chapter 3.4 expands upon enhanced performance in sport and improved psychological and affective responses to exercise. The reduction of drug use by athletes in sport and the enhancement of mental health in exercisers are two relevant fields where placebo research and its applications can play an important role.

Chapter 3.5 summarizes recent evidence on placebo arms and reactions to placebos (so-called nocebo responses[52,53]) in clinical trials for treating migraine with pharmaceutical agents. It presents how nocebo responses might affect drug safety, tolerability profiles, and adherence to treatments for migraine treatments, along with patients' preference and decision-making.

Finally, placebo and nocebo concepts have been noted during the global COVID-19 pandemic, which has proven to be an unprecedented disruptor of our way of life since its inception in early 2020. COVID-19 brought personal fear about health and well-being, suspicions of scientific credibility, and resentment over individual rights in terms of access and choice of treatment and prevention. Chapter 3.6 explores the current understanding of COVID-19 pathogenesis and implications of placebo and nocebo effects on clinical expression of the illness, as well as the efficacy and toxicity of its treatments and vaccine acceptance and tolerability.

Section 4 describes the issue of placebo effects in mental health. Mental health therapeutics and antidepressants in particular are routinely prescribed and administered worldwide.[54,55] Yet their efficacies represent global health challenges. There is considerable debate about the potential differences in efficacy of placebo versus mental health therapeutics.[56,57] Also, development of new drugs becomes difficult because of placebo responses, which tend to grow over time.[58] Chapter 4.1 discusses several factors, such as expectancy and interactions with the physician, that contribute to placebo responses. Specifically, the authors propose that expectancies related to treatment efficacy and side effects could be manipulated to optimize clinical outcomes and reduce side effects.

Chapter 4.2 discusses that most tangible way to shape expectations is to contextualize, whenever possible, informed consent and frame treatment information without dismissing the ethical implications of manipulating expectancies in the context of clinical trials. There is growing evidence that expectations during treatments and/or interventions can affect performance assessments.

Chapter 4.3 considers participants' expectations in cognitive training and the extent that they affect the results of cognitive training interventions, as well as potential strategies for how they could be minimized or alternatively harnessed to maximize the effectiveness of interventions.

Chapter 4.4 discusses the perception of expectations and strategies and how they can be shaped by the use of psychedelics.[59,60] The chapter also discusses the evolution of communication strategies and the shift from the dogma that deception is needed for placebos to work. The chapter describes the use of open-label placebos and how their use can be incorporated into psychotherapy. It proposes that open-label placebos work as a form of psycho-therapy by promoting a transparent engagement of patients in the therapeutic processes.

New trends in utilization of placebos (i.e., open-label[61] and dose-extending placebos), therapeutic manipulations of expectations, and communication strategies (e.g., informed consents and side-effects disclosure) open up a new perspective for ethical evaluation and considerations. The landscape of pla-cebo mechanistic research, placebo in clinical trials and practices, is evolving, and classical ethical frameworks are often inadequate to capture the full com-plexity of evidence-based approaches and ethical use of placebos and patient-centered approaches. Section 5 presents several considerations related to the use of placebos in clinical practice.

Chapter 5.1 considers biopsychological models to healing and ethics of pla-cebo effects. Chapter 5.2 raises concerns about the lack of research aimed at implementing the science of placebo into clinical practice for patient benefit. Chapter 5.3 expands upon this aspect by introducing the concept of contex-tual factors and empathetic patient-doctor relationships.

Finally, Chapter 5.4 discusses how nuances of social-cultural and personal-historical contexts influence therapeutic outcomes. Additionally, the chapter discusses the necessity of integrating a person-cantered perspective into a regulatory perspective, with implications for the interpretation of results from randomized placebo-controlled clinical trials and consideration of what "good evidence" of a therapeutic effect is, in order to move the new results from placebo research forward to clinical practice.

Implementing research on placebos and nocebos into clinical practice presents challenges but also exciting new opportunities. Section 6 illustrates how health care continues to evolve with patient-oriented approaches in clinical practice to clinical notes, equity, and digital therapeutics.[62] Chapter 6.1 describes a person-based approach to develop a digital intervention for primary care practitioners based on findings from placebo research as an example of research that is patient-oriented, engaging, and translational. Chapter 6.2 describes the effect of transparent communication between health care providers and patients, in for example, open notes in medical charts that document active and past medical history, acute and chronic diseases, testing results, treatments, and more. Chapter 6.2 proposes that clinical notes are likely to facilitate placebo and nocebo effects with distinct nuances among minorities, raising concerns about equity.

Chapter 6.3 describes the emergence of digital therapeutics, a field that is rapidly expanding and holds promise for the future of healthcare. However, the authors argue that much of the research evaluating new approaches needs to be guided by more appropriate methodological considerations regarding controls and designs that help define *efficacy*, *effectiveness*, and *patients' needs and acceptability*. Chapter 6.4 builds upon collective decades of experience in digital therapeutics related to placebo research to describe the effect of immersive virtual reality in Medicine, Education, and other contexts.

Overall, *Placebo Effects Through the Lens of Translational Research* appraises the most recent scientific advances and implications of placebo research for healthcare systems, clinicians, patients, and caregivers. The reader shall gain new and insightful knowledge related to placebo research from scholars from several countries and with a large range of multidisciplinary competences.

References

1. Colloca L, Barsky AJ. Placebo and nocebo effects. *New England Journal of Medicine*. 2020;382(6):554–561.
2. Evers AWM, Colloca L, Blease C, et al. Implications of placebo and nocebo effects for clinical practice: Expert consensus. *Psychotherapy and Psychosomatics*. 2018;87(4):204–210.
3. Shapiro AK, Shapiro E. *The Powerful Placebo: From Ancient Priest to Modern Physician*. John Hopkins University Press; 1997.
4. Moerman DE. Physiology and symbols: The anthropological implications of the placebo effect. In: Romanucci-Ross L, Moerman DE, Tancredi LR, eds. *The Anthropology of Medicine: From Culture to Method*. 3rd ed. Bergin & Garvey; 1997.

5. Wolf S. Effects of suggestion and conditioning on the action of chemical agents in human subjects: The pharmacology of placebos. *Journal of Clinical Investigation.* 1950;29(1):100–109.

6. Voudouris NJ, Peck CL, Coleman G. Conditioned placebo responses. *Journal of Personality and Social Psychology.* 1985;48(1):47–53.

7. Voudouris NJ, Peck CL, Coleman G. The role of conditioning and verbal expectancy in the placebo response. *Pain.* 1990;43(1):121–128.

8. Colloca L, Petrovic P, Wager TD, Ingvar M, Benedetti F. How the number of learning trials affects placebo and nocebo responses. *Pain.* 2010;151(2):430–439.

9. Wager TD, Matre D, Casey KL. Placebo effects in laser-evoked pain potentials. *Brain, Behavior, and Immunity.* 2006;20(3):219–230.

10. Montgomery GH, Kirsch I. Classical conditioning and the placebo effect. *Pain.* 1997;72(1-2):107–113.

11. Colloca L, Benedetti F. How prior experience shapes placebo analgesia. *Pain.* 2006;124(1–2):126–133.

12. Colloca L, Sigaudo M, Benedetti F. The role of learning in nocebo and placebo effects. *Pain.* 2008;136(1–2):211–218.

13. Au Yeung ST, Colagiuri B, Lovibond PF, Colloca L. Partial reinforcement, extinction, and placebo analgesia. *Pain.* 2014;155(6):1110–1117.

14. Zunhammer M, Goltz G, Schweifel M, Stuck BA, Bingel U. Savor the flavor: A randomized double-blind study assessing taste-enhanced placebo analgesia in healthy volunteers. *Clinical and Translational Science.* 2022;15(11):2709–2719.

15. Kirchhof J, Petrakova L, Brinkhoff A, et al. Learned immunosuppressive placebo responses in renal transplant patients. *Proceedings of the National Academy of Sciences of the U S A.* 2018;115(16):4223–4227.

16. Leech J, Mazzone SB, Farrell MJ. The effect of placebo conditioning on capsaicin-evoked urge to cough. *Chest.* 2012;142(4):951–957.

17. Horing B, Weimer K, Schrade D, et al. Reduction of motion sickness with an enhanced placebo instruction: An experimental study with healthy participants. *Psychosomatic Medicine.* 2013;75(5):497–504.

18. Quinn VF, MacDougall HG, Colagiuri B. Galvanic vestibular stimulation: A new model of placebo-induced nausea. *Journal of Psychosomatic Research.* 2015;78(5):484–488.

19. Petrovic P, Kalso E, Petersson KM, Ingvar M. Placebo and opioid analgesia: Imaging a shared neuronal network. *Science.* 2002;295(5560):1737–1740.

20. Wager TD, Rilling JK, Smith EE, et al. Placebo-induced changes in FMRI in the anticipation and experience of pain. *Science.* 2004;303(5661):1162–1167.

21. Fields HL, Levine JD. Biology of placebo analgesia. *American Journal of Medicine.* 1981;70(4):745–746.

22. Levine JD, Gordon NC, Fields HL. The mechanism of placebo analgesia. *Lancet.* 1978;2(8091):654–657.

23. Zubieta JK, Bueller JA, Jackson LR, et al. Placebo effects mediated by endogenous opioid activity on mu-opioid receptors. *Journal of Neuroscience.* 2005;25(34):7754–7762.

24. Eippert F, Finsterbusch J, Bingel U, Buchel C. Direct evidence for spinal cord involvement in placebo analgesia. *Science.* 2009;326(5951):404.

25. Eippert F, Bingel U, Schoell ED, et al. Activation of the opioidergic descending pain control system underlies placebo analgesia. *Neuron.* 2009;63(4):533–543.

26. Kaptchuk TJ. Placebo controls, exorcisms, and the devil. *Lancet.* 2009;374(9697):1234–1235.

27. Beecher HK. The powerful placebo. *Journal of the American Medical Association.* 1955;159:1602–1606.

28. Kienle GS, Kiene H. The powerful placebo effect: Fact of fiction? *Journal of Clinical Epidemiology.* 1997;50(20):1311–1318.

29. Colloca L. The Placebo effect in pain therapies. *Annual Review of Pharmacology and Toxicology*. 2019;59:191–211.
30. Hohenschurz-Schmidt D, Draper-Rodi J, Vase L. Dissimilar control interventions in clinical trials undermine interpretability. *JAMA Psychiatry*. 2022;79(3):271–272.
31. Hohenschurz-Schmidt D, Draper-Rodi J, Vase L, et al. Blinding and sham control methods in trials of physical, psychological, and self-management interventions for pain (article II): A meta-analysis relating methods to trial results. *Pain*. 2023;164(3):469–484.
32. Colloca L, Benedetti F. Placebos and painkillers: Is mind as real as matter? *Nature Reviews Neuroscience*. 2005;6(7):545–552.
33. Ross S, Krugman AD, Lyerly SB, Clyde, J D. Drugs and placebos: A model design. *Psychological Reports*. 1962;10(2):383–392.
34. Kirsch I, Weixel LJ. Double-blind versus deceptive administration of a placebo. *Behavioral Neuroscience*. 1988;102(2):319–323.
35. Colloca L, Lopiano L, Lanotte M, Benedetti F. Overt versus covert treatment for pain, anxiety, and Parkinson's disease. *Lancet Neurology*. 2004;3(11):679–684.
36. Benedetti F, Maggi G, Lopiano L, et al. Open versus hidden medical treatments: The patient's knowledge about a therapy affects the therapy outcome. *Prevention & Treatment*. 2003;6:n.p.
37. Benedetti F, Colloca L, Lanotte M, Bergamasco B, Torre E, Lopiano L. Autonomic and emotional responses to open and hidden stimulations of the human subthalamic region. *Brain Research Bulletin*. 2004;63(3):203–211.
38. Park LC, Covi L. Nonblind placebo trial: An exploration of neurotic patients' responses to placebo when its inert content is disclosed. *Archives of General Psychiatry.*. 1965;12:36–45.
39. Kaptchuk TJ, Friedlander E, Kelley JM, et al. Placebos without deception: A randomized controlled trial in irritable bowel syndrome. *PLoS ONE*. 2010;5(12):e15591.
40. Fava M, Evins AE, Dorer DJ, Schoenfeld DA. The problem of the placebo response in clinical trials for psychiatric disorders: Culprits, possible remedies, and a novel study design approach. *Psychotherapy and Psychosomatics*. 2003;72(3):115–127.
41. Staud R, Price DD. Role of placebo factors in clinical trials with special focus on enrichment designs. *Pain*. 2008;139(2):479–480.
42. Rosenkjaer S, Lunde SJ, Kirsch I, Vase L. Expectations: How and when do they contribute to placebo analgesia? *Frontiers in Psychiatry*. 2022;13:817179.
43. Younger J, Gandhi V, Hubbard E, Mackey S. Development of the Stanford Expectations of Treatment Scale (SETS): A tool for measuring patient outcome expectancy in clinical trials. *Clinical Trials*. 2012;9(6):767–776.
44. Colloca L, Akintola T, Haycock NR, et al. Prior therapeutic experiences, not expectation ratings, predict placebo effects: An experimental study in chronic pain and healthy participants. *Psychotherapy and Psychosomatics*. 2020;89(6):371–378.
45. Sheridan S, Schrandt S, Forsythe L, Hilliard TS, Paez KA. The PCORI engagement rubric: Promising practices for partnering in research. *Annals of Family Medicine*. 2017;15(2):165–170.
46. Schanberg LE, Mullins CD. If patients are the true north, patient-centeredness should guide research. *Nature Reviews Rheumatology*. 2019;15(1):5–6.
47. Hrobjartsson A, Gotzsche PC. Is the placebo powerless? Update of a systematic review with 52 new randomized trials comparing placebo with no treatment. *Journal of Internal Medicine*. 2004;256(2):91–100.
48. Hrobjartsson A, Gotzsche PC. Is the placebo powerless? An analysis of clinical trials comparing placebo with no treatment. *New England Journal of Medicine*. 2001;344(21):1594–1602.
49. Colagiuri B, Schenk LA, Kessler MD, Dorsey SG, Colloca L. The placebo effect: From concepts to genes. *Neuroscience*. 2015;307:171–190.

50. Hall KT, Loscalzo J, Kaptchuk TJ. Genetics and the placebo effect: the placebome. *Trends in Molecular Medicine*. 2015;21(5):285–294.

51. Benedetti F. *Placebo Effects*. Oxford University Press; 2014.

52. Colloca L. Nocebo effects can make you feel pain. *Science*. 2017;358(6359):44.

53. Colloca L, Miller FG. The nocebo effect and its relevance for clinical practice. *Psychosomatic Medicine*. 2011;73(7):598–603.

54. Cipriani A, Salanti G, Furukawa TA, et al. Antidepressants might work for people with major depression: Where do we go from here? *Lancet Psychiatry*. 2018;5(6):461–463.

55. Cipriani A, Salanti G, Furukawa TA, Turner E, Ioannidis JPA, Geddes JR. Network meta-analysis of antidepressants—Authors' reply. *Lancet*. 2018;392(10152):1012–1013.

56. Kirsch I, Jakobsen JC. Network meta-analysis of antidepressants. *Lancet*. 2018; 392(10152):1010.

57. Moncrieff J, Kirsch I. Efficacy of antidepressants in adults. *British Medical Journal*. 2005;331(7509):155–157.

58. Jones BDM, Razza LB, Weissman CR, et al. Magnitude of the placebo response across treatment modalities used for treatment-resistant depression in adults: A systematic review and meta-analysis. *JAMA Network Open*. 2021;4(9):e2125531.

59. Butler M, Jelen L, Rucker J. Expectancy in placebo-controlled trials of psychedelics: If so, so what? *Psychopharmacology (Berl)*. 2022;239(10):3047–3055.

60. Gukasyan N, Nayak SM. Psychedelics, placebo effects, and set and setting: Insights from common factors theory of psychotherapy. *Transcultural Psychiatry*. 2022;59(5):652–664.

61. Benedetti F, Shaibani A, Arduino C, Thoen W. Open-label nondeceptive placebo analgesia is blocked by the opioid antagonist naloxone. *Pain*. 2023;164(5):984–990.

62. Honzel E, Murthi S, Brawn-Cinani B, et al. Virtual reality, music, and pain: Developing the premise for an interdisciplinary approach to pain management. *Pain*. 2019; 160(9):1909–1919.

1

PLACEBO EFFECTS

An introduction

This Section explores placebo concepts and their implications for clinical practice. Four primary objectives are pursued: examining core placebo concepts and their practical manifestations, discussing clinical practices for optimizing healing through placebo mechanisms, exploring the significance of placebo research in person-centered clinical decision-making, and summarizing tools to enhance placebo-based healing in routine practice.

Chapter one explains how healthcare providers can gain insights into recognizing placebo mechanisms within their practice and learning to incorporate healing words and rituals that leverage placebo mechanisms.

Expectations play a crucial role in placebo effects, and Chapter two presents approaches for conceptualizing and assessing expectations. New frameworks shed light on conscious and unconscious aspects of treatment expectations, improving our understanding of placebo and treatment effects. Evidence is presented to showcase training of healthcare to effectively leverage psychological and social forces underlying the placebo effect and empower patients to establish adaptive mindsets during treatment.

The influence of cultural beliefs, norms, values, worldview, and experiences on the meaning of illness, treatment context, and expectations is explored in Chapters 4.2 and 4.3. Cultural factors heavily impact treatment responses, including preferences for treatment elements, marketing strategies, and rituals. It emphasizes the importance of training healthcare providers, leveraging patient expectations, and considering cultural factors to enhance treatment outcomes.

1.1

From placebo research to healing

Wayne B. Jonas

Introduction

The placebo is the sleeping giant of health care. By that I mean it has a major influence over research, practice, and payment decisions, yet is rarely acknowledged or accommodated. It influences every aspect of practice and plays no favorites; being equally devastating to ancient healing claims, complementary medicine, and mainstream health care.[1] The placebo effect is often the Achilles heel of many of those claims, demonstrating that the cause of healing is not what investigators, health care providers, and patients often think. It is not devastating to healing itself, but rather, what it destroys is our theories of what's working, what produces that healing. Theories come and go. Healing, however, once the mechanisms of placebo are understood, can be enhanced or diminished with that information for any treatment.

The concept of the placebo effect is very old. Plato, for example, described the treatment of headache, where he said, "the thing was a certain leaf, but there was a charm to go with the remedy, and if one uttered the charm at the same moment of its application, the remedy made one perfectly well; but without the charm, there was no efficacy in the leaf."[2] What Plato was referring to as "the charm" we would call *the ritual* today. "The thing" is the drug, and the context is the area in which the drug and the ritual come together. Thus, context must be carefully examined to optimize healing when using any "thing." Plato's statement is an example of how to elicit placebo responses. This chapter will show how research on modern "charms" are put together with treatments to elicit placebo effects for healing.

Background and history

While the placebo has been discussed for hundreds of years, and formal research was conducted on this phenomenon since the time of Benjamin

Franklin with his investigation of mesmerism, the more recent era of placebo research began in 1995 with the first US National Institutes of Health (NIH) conference on placebo that same year.

In April of 1995, the NIH Office of Alternative Medicine and the Office of Behavioral and Social Science Research held a conference called *Placebo and Complementary Medicine*, where investigators illustrated how ubiquitous and large placebo effects were in behavioral and complementary medical approaches.[3] Five years later, NIH held another conference sponsored by the National Center for Complementary and Alternative Medicine (NCCAM), the National Institute of Drug Abuse (NIDA), and the National Institute of Alcohol Abuse and Alcoholism (NIAAA) on November 11, 2000, called *The Science of the Placebo*, elucidating what we knew about underlying mechanisms of placebo effects.[4]

Then, in November 2009, an international conference was held at Lake Sternberg, Germany. The conference, titled *Psychological Mediators and Clinical Relevance of Placebo Effects*, was supported by the Samueli Foundation and the Theophrastus Foundations. This conference formed the basis of a special issue in the Philosophical Transactions of the Royal Society several years later.[5] Two years later, on November 17, 2011, the conference *The Placebo Effect: Mechanisms and Methodology* was held again at NIH and, again, sponsored by NIDA, NIAAA, and the NCCAM. Then in 2012, two conferences, cosponsored by the Samueli Foundation and the NIH, including NCCAM and NIDA were held. The first was held January 16 and 17, 2012, and was called *Using Placebo Responses in Clinical Practice*, and then a second was held at the Uniform Services University, called *Placebo and Performance: Implications for Program Practice and Policy*.

These more recent scholarly activities on the mechanisms of placebo led, ultimately, to the formation of the Society of Interdisciplinary Placebo Studies, which has now held three international conferences: the first in Leiden, Netherlands (April 2–4, 2017); the second also in Leiden (July 7–9, 2019), and then the third in Baltimore, Maryland (2021). These meetings have illustrated the tremendous growth in our understanding of placebo and its underlying mechanisms.

Placebo mechanisms and Medicine

In the rest of this chapter, I will focus on three mechanisms of the placebo effect derived from this research and illustrate their implications and use in Medicine. The first mechanism is expectation, or the power of belief; the second is the effect of social learning. I will show how ritual manipulates both expectation and social meaning, which in turn influences treatment. Then I will explore a third mechanism of placebo effects called conditioning, which illustrates the power of the body to learn and heal in very specific ways.

Let me begin with a clinical case to illustrate the first two mechanisms mentioned. I'll call the patient Joe (not his real name, but a real case). Joe was a patient who came to see me after having retired from the Navy with 30 years of service. His back had started to hurt after a motor vehicle accident 15 years before he saw me. The pain was musculoskeletal, and he received many treatments, including nonsteroidal anti-inflammatory drugs, psychotropics, opioids, injections, and surgery. Joe also had other health conditions, including hypertension, high cholesterol, and being overweight. He had retired 4 years earlier and wanted to play more golf and to see his grandchildren. But his chronic back pain, despite all the interventions, including surgery, still prevented him from these activities.

Joe had access to complete health care services including the availability of all specialties, drugs, and procedures. He had many medical visits during which most of his medical professionals used an approach known as SOAP. SOAP stands for subjective (what the patient describes), objective, (what you observe and test), assessment, (the diagnosis and the code for the diagnosis), and plan (the treatment that meets the assessment). Over the years Joe was asked repeatedly What's the matter?, after which he would describe his pain and then get a medical diagnosis and a treatment plan. The treatments themselves focused on "the thing," as Plato would say, the pills and the procedures, the needles and the knives. Joe's SOAP notes over the years gave him the diagnosis of degenerative disease of the spine with narrowing at L4-S1. He had x-rays, CT scans, MRI scans, physical therapy, chiropractic treatments, electrical stimulation, two surgeries with disc fusion, injection with steroids, and was placed on nonsteroidals and opioids. When he finally saw me, he was off opioids. To get off opioids, Joe had been to the behavioral medicine clinic, where he was diagnosed with depression and started on another drug, an antidepressant. Joe's "team" (and I put *team* in quotes because they, in fact, didn't work as a team) included his primary care physician, physical therapist, pain specialist, chiropractor, surgeon, behavioral medicine specialist, and pharmacologist. Joe's treatments were as varied as his specialists and had included over the years, analgesics, nonsteroidal anti-inflammatories, muscle relaxants, antidepressants, injections, instructions to bed rest, instructions increase activity, exercises, physical therapy, traction, manipulation, supplements, and surgery.

"Is it all placebo, doc?"

When Joe came to see me, he was, rightfully so, quite skeptical of anything I had to offer. He had heard that I used alternative approaches such as acupuncture. His wife was Korean, and she had urged him to get acupuncture treatments, which she said worked very well in her family for pain. So, he came to ask me about acupuncture. His question to me was simple and straightforward. "Doc, is acupuncture all a placebo effect?" In other words, he was asking me if acupuncture was real and based on evidence, or was it a sham, with similar effects to a placebo. To answer him, I had to delve into the evidence for not only acupuncture but the other treatments he was offered and treated with.

As with many patients, I was trying to identify the best research to answer four questions that help in clinical decision-making: The first question, Is the treatment better than a placebo? The second question, Is it better than no treatment at all? The third question, Is it better than or equal to proven treatments? And the fourth question, "What are the adverse effects and the costs of the intervention?" Putting on this evidence-based Medicine hat, I looked at all of the treatments Joe had received using a spreadsheet to determine what had the best evidence for efficacy. Along the left side of the sheet was a vertical list of all the treatments he had, and across the top were the four questions for which I was seeking answers. Of all the treatments he'd had, there was only one intervention that was proven better than placebo and better than no treatment. That was nonsteroidal anti-inflammatory drugs. He had been using those for many years. For any of the other treatments the evidence was unknown or unclear, or in some cases, the evidence had shown that treatments were harmful for back pain, such as traction and bedrest. When I looked at acupuncture, it appeared that acupuncture was better than no treatment and usually as good as other treatments, but the evidence was not clear whether it was better than placebo.

To illustrate this, let me summarize a large, randomized study published in the *Annals of Internal Medicine* that was released in 2006.[6] It was a high-quality, three-arm study looking at chronic pain. Patients were randomly assigned to receive traditional Chinese acupuncture, in which active points had needles inserted. The second arm was sham acupuncture, in which needles were inserted superficially into nonactive points, according to Chinese acupuncture theory. And the third arm was the best conventional therapy available at the time, most of which Joe had already had. The authors of this study looked at pain scores at 13 weeks and again at 26 weeks, which showed clear results. Traditional acupuncture was almost twice as effective as standard therapy. However, sham acupuncture was also almost twice as effective and the difference between traditional acupuncture and sham acu-puncture was not statistically significant. So here I was faced with a type of evidence that many clinicians and patients find. I call it the placebo paradox. Here a treatment works better than no treatment. It is as good as or even better than proven treatment and standard care, but it is no better than its own pla-cebo. So based on this research, I would have to tell Joe that acupuncture is no better than placebo. Yet is that the best information to offer him, given the fact that if properly delivered, acupuncture might give him significant pain relief? Acupuncture was likely to help Joe even if it was mostly due to the "charm" of the acupuncture ritual. Was the answer "it's all placebo" in the best interest of Joe's healing?

Comparative evidence

To better understand the best approach for Joe, I explored in more detail the evidence for the other main treatments he had previously received. The proven therapy in my evidence chart were the nonsteroidal anti-inflammatory drugs. A review of these drugs by the Cochrane Collaboration indicated that the quality of evidence for the efficacy of nonsteroidal drugs over placebos was quite low.[7] In addition, the effect sizes were also quite small. On a pain scale of 1–100, improvement, on average, was 7 points. In other words, nonsteroidal medications did have an effect on pain that could be proven—they were better than placebo—but the effects size was small. Side effects were also significant, especially when the drugs were taken for long periods.

The second area I looked at was surgery. Joe had had two surgeries on his back. To better assess whether surgery was better than placebo, we did a meta-analysis and systematic review of placebo surgeries for chronic pain, including chronic low back pain, as compared to sham surgeries. We found seven studies, totaling 445 patients, which were randomly assigned to either back surgery or sham back surgery. The effect size of sham surgeries was 73% as large as the real surgeries, which was not statistically significant.[8] However, the overall effect size was over 90%. In other words, surgery produced a large effect, but it was no better than placebo, just like acupuncture.

In more recent studies, we saw that acupuncture indeed was better than its own placebo when analyzed using individual patient data from over 29 randomized control trials with close to 18,000 patients. This study published in the *Journal of American Medical Association* in 2014 by Andrew Vickers demonstrated that compared with sham acupuncture and no acupuncture controls, the average response rates were 30% when doing nothing, 42.5% for sham acupuncture, and 50% for actual acupuncture, which was statistically significant over no acupuncture and sham acupuncture.[9] Thus, I had evidence that acupuncture was not all placebo, and its effect size was moderate—bigger than nonsteroidal drugs but smaller than surgery.

This evidence, however, created a dilemma when trying to decide what the optimal healing was for Joe. Should I use evidence-based Medicine? Or should I use person-centered care that would incorporate the effect of placebo effects and the context of treatment? If the treatment ("the thing") produces a relatively large effect size and has a small meaning effect ("the charm"), then it can be easily demonstrated by science and becomes good "evidence-based medicine." This then gets incorporated into guidelines, which become the standard of care and reimbursed by insurance. If, however, the specific effect of a treatment ("the thing") is small, but the meaning effect ("the charm") is large, this could result in significantly better healing even while not being able to be proven to be better than a placebo and be called evidence-based. In my experience, most patients, if you ask them, prefer the larger healing rate even though that contradicts what scientists will say works and regulators will pay for.

In the case that I just illustrated, we see the inappropriate application of two mechanisms of placebo effects that contribute to the chronification or continued aggravation of Joe's pain. One mechanism involved the reinforcement of unconscious expectations through social learning as meaning, which was delivered by authorities over multiple visits and communicated to Joe via the message that he was not just failing the treatments, but he himself was a failed patient. This is essentially the delivery of nocebo effect and was influenced by multiple factors, including the way the treatments and the side effects were described, Joe's prior experiences, and the cultural expectations and assumptions of what the science says will and will not work. These lead to the enhancement of nocebo responses. What happened with Joe over the years (and is routine in medical practice) was the unconscious expectation that he was a failure in all therapy. He'd learned this through experience.

Now Joe had come to me to ask about "trying" acupuncture (another "thing"). How we delivered the "charm" with acupuncture to Joe would be crucial to his healing. Klaus Linde, in an article published in the journal *Pain* several years ago, illustrated this in an acupuncture study, the therapy that Joe was seeking.[10] Throughout treatment, those with high expectations had higher efficacy rates than those with lower expectations. This was seen regardless of how and when the questions on expectation were asked. In other words, the impact of Joe's expectations and the social learning that reinforced those expectations would largely determine the benefit he gets from acupuncture and have a major influence on his overall healing. Thus, if we are to utilize the mechanisms of expectation and social learning to help heal Joe, we need to explicitly bring in appropriate context and ritual (the "charm") with the acupuncture (the "thing") and deliver them together. The importance of properly using these mechanisms for patients like Joe applies across all therapies, not just acupuncture.[11]

Clinical tools for use of placebo effects

What Joe needed was for us to set up the reverse of what had happened to him over the years. We needed his team to deliver consistent experiences, expectations, and social learning components for healing. To do this, we needed to consistently reinforce high expectations throughout his healing journey. I have developed a set of tools for bringing these dimensions of healing together called the HOPE Note Toolkit. HOPE stands for healing-oriented practices and environments, and it begins by first asking patients what matters to them in their own life (invoking meaning), and then explores the patients' personal determinants of healing through four dimensions: mental and spiritual factors, social and emotional dimensions, behavior and lifestyle, and the body and external environment.

Let's look at how this was applied for Joe. Part of what mattered to Joe was medication management. He'd been placed on multiple medications by many providers, and he wanted to have clear directions on what to use. So, I and the pharmacologist on our team helped him sort through those. As we explored what mattered most deeply to Joe, he discovered that what he wanted to do was to get in a car, drive 5 to 6 hours down to where his grandchildren lived, and then to get down on the floor and be able to play with them. This was a deeper motivating factor, and it provided the core meaning for Joe's therapy.

To incorporate this goal for Joe we decided to take him over to physical therapy with specific instructions to work on his core muscles to get him up and down off the floor. We paired this with acupuncture so that the acupuncture was done right before the physical therapy and mitigated the pain that he knew this regiment would produce. After several sessions of this, Joe was beginning to feel stronger, although his pain was still there. After about 4 months, he called me up and explained that he'd driven down to see his grandchildren and had been able to get down on the floor to play with them. Joe was now motivated to continue his stretching, strength building, and acupuncture. Eventually, he reduced his medications and improved his pain and function. Joe's team worked together to reinforce his expectation through social learning. The same meaningful message was delivered by the physician helping to coordinate the care, the pharmacologist working with his drugs, the behaviorist and health coach supporting habit change, and the acupuncturist and physical therapist working in concert. They all worked to reinforce the message that his body could experience recovery and healing.

Joe was a patient who had been repeatedly failed by all treatments. This reinforced his chronic disease by repeatedly delivering a nocebo effect. To reverse this process, proper communication and ritual training was a skill all team members needed to use. An example of such training has been described by Dr. Steve Bierman, who combines placebo research with hypnotic techniques for reframing individuals' beliefs and expectations.[12] The goal is to prevent them from being what he calls "cursed" by the medical profession, usually inadvertently with negative or nocebo suggestions, and to deliver positive expectations and directions to the body for healing.[13]

Ethical issues in use of placebo effects

Given that we must properly use the mechanisms of placebo effects in Medicine, is the use of placebo research knowledge ethical? Is the use of what are labeled "unproven" treatments acceptable if they're used openly with rituals, so-called open placebo treatment? Who is influenced more by placebo, the patient or the provider? Ultimately, we want to know how we can use this knowledge to diminish harm and enhance healing in practice. Ultimately, clinicians want to know how they can use it in their own practice.

The first question of whether it is ethically feasible to use placebos in practice boils down largely to the issue of deception.[14] Being deceptive would make placebo use unethical; however, it's been demonstrated repeatedly that one does not need to deceive the patient to obtain a placebo effect. There are many studies of so-called open-label placebos in which patients are told that they're being given an inert treatment, but that if they go through the ritual and meaning (the "charm") it is likely to produce a positive effect. These studies have demonstrated in multiple conditions that open-label placebo is as effective as blinded placebo.[15] Thus, placebo effects can be delivered without deception. This is how optimal healing has probably always been delivered. If you look back over the general use of placebos by clinicians, studies report that the majority of physicians often use a treatment that they know is biologically ineffective.[16] Whereas in Henry Beecher's time, the use of sugar pills as placebos was considered ethical, it is not today. However, other types of inert substances are routinely prescribed, including antibiotics for viral infections, sedatives when they are not indicated, vitamins and minerals, over-the-counter analgesics, and others. Clinicians know that the evidence does not support these, yet they also know the "charm" of the ritual of treatment delivery is important.

We should be asking if it is unethical *not* to use placebo effects in practice. If the way in which we deliver information and a treatment would harm a patient if done negatively or help a patient if done positively, and if the authority and the trust in the doctor-patient relationship is a powerful context for producing such effects, then it is unethical to not maximize placebo responses. This is no different than how we use other treatments—making the right decisions and the right actions for the right reasons at the right time. Dr. David Rakel brilliantly illustrates that the clinical encounter itself, as embodied by the physician in relation to the patient and the culture, is a powerful tool for healing.[17] How then can we as clinicians and clinician-scientists integrate placebos into practice? How can we put together both meaning and medicine, the context of healing and the content of healing? The thing and the charm.

Optimizing placebo effects

There are now over 15 behaviors that can enhance placebo effects in clinical practice as supported by data-based research.[18,19] I would like to pick out six of those that are the most powerful and are simple steps that one can use in practice. These steps and the evidence behind them are summarized in a recent guide produced for clinicians and patients.[20]

The first is to inform the patient about what they can expect and the use of positive images when informing them. Patients who are better informed about their treatment and who receive positive messages about what to expect, heal more, and so let the patient know the intention of the treatments. The second is to determine which treatments your patient believes in. As with Joe, this means talking to the patient about their condition and treatment beliefs and recommending safe approaches that are aligned with those beliefs. Likewise, make sure you believe in them too, so that yours and the patient's beliefs align. Third, listen, provide empathy and understanding during the encounter. Listening to the patient enhances the therapeutic effect. Fourth, follow up and repeat the treatment. Reinforce the therapeutic interaction by following up with patients through reminders, such as text messages, phone calls from staff, or more frequent office visits. This taps into the mechanisms of conditioning and reinforce expectancy. Fifth, incorporate reassurance, relaxation, suggestion, and anxiety-reducing methods into the interaction. An expression of caring along with authority can induce relaxation, a technique from hypnosis for embedding instructions for healing into the person. Deliver the message with specific language. Use statements that contain phrases like what "you, the patient, can expect" rather than negative language that often accompanies discussing statistics or risk factors. Finally, use a benign agent (a "thing"), such as a pill, needle, laser, or knife. Be sure the treatment is not harmful or expensive and can be easily used, to reinforce an experience of healing. Change the treatment when needed. Plato said the charm had to go along with the thing, but we also know that the thing helps enhance the charm.

Integrating placebo effects into practice

To put these together into routine practice, I refer you to the HOPE Note Toolkit that I illustrated with my patient, Joe. The HOPE Toolkit has three components: the Personal Health Inventory, the HOPE Note, and the Personalized Healing Plan. The Family Medicine Education Consortium and the Samueli Foundation completed a 16-clinic learning collaborative exploring how these tools can be integrated into routine practice. See the summary and case reports on the use of these tools.[21-22] For clinicians dealing with patients in chronic pain and with opioid misuse, there is a free Continuing Medical Education course from Tufts University School of Medicine, where you can learn about these tools and their applications to patients with chronic pain.[23]

The time has come for research and information about placebo effects to be used more systematically in practice. Standard competencies for appropriate communication, ritual, and meaning-making in practice to reduce nocebo and enhance the healing of treatments need to become part of every provider's training. As Plato said, "Without charm, there is no efficacy." Bring charm into your practice through an understanding and use of the science of placebo effects.

References

1. Jonas W. *How Healing Works: Get Well and Stay Well Using Your Hidden Power to Heal.* Lorena Jones Books; 2018:16.
2. Plato. *Plato in Twelve Volumes.* Vol. 8. Lamb, W, trans. Harvard University Press;1955.

3. National Institutes of Health Office of Alternative Medicine Placebo Working Group. Placebo effects and research in alternative and conventional medicine. *Court of Chief Judicial Magistrate.* 1996;2:141–148. https://doi.org/10.1007/BF02969672

4. de Craen AJM. The science of the placebo: Toward an interdisciplinary research agenda. *British Medical Journal.* 2002;324(7351):1460. http://doi:10.1136/bmj.324.7351.1460

5. Meissner K, Kohls N, Colloca L. Introduction to placebo effects in medicine: Mechanisms and clinical implications. *Philosophical Transactions of the Royal Society B: Biological Sciences.* 2011;366(1572):1783–1789. http://doi:10.1098/rstb.2010.0414

6. Scharf HP, Mansmann U, Streitberger K, et al. Acupuncture and knee osteoarthritis: A three-armed randomized trial. *Annals of Internal Medicine.* 2006;145(1):12–20. http://doi:10.7326/0003-4819-145-1-200607040-00005

7. Enthoven WTM, Roelofs PDDM, Deyo RA, van Tulder MW, Koes BW. Non-steroidal anti-inflammatory drugs for chronic low back pain. *Cochrane Database of Systematic Reviews.* 2016;2(8):CD012087. http://doi:10.1002/14651858.CD012087

8. Jonas WB, Crawford C, Colloca L, et al. Are invasive procedures effective for chronic pain? A systematic review. *Pain Medications.* 2019;20(7):1281–1293. http://doi:10.1093/pm/pny154

9. Vickers AJ, Linde K. Acupuncture for chronic pain. *JAMA.* 2014;311(9):955–956. http://doi:10.1001/jama.2013.285478

10. Linde K, Witt CM, Streng A, et al. The impact of patient expectations on outcomes in four randomized controlled trials of acupuncture in patients with chronic pain. *Pain.* 2007;128(3):264–271. http://doi:10.1016/j.pain.2006.12.006

11. Bialosky JE, Bishop MD, Cleland JA. Individual expectation: An overlooked, but pertinent, factor in the treatment of individuals experiencing musculoskeletal pain. *Physical Therapy.* 2010;90(9):1345–1355. http://doi:10.2522/ptj.20090306

12. Bierman S. *HEALING—Beyond Pills & Potions: Core Principles for Helpers & Healers.* Gyro Press International; 2020.

13. Miller FG, Colloca L, Kaptchuk TJ. The placebo effect: Illness and interpersonal healing. *Perspectives in Biology and Medicine.* 2009;52(4):518–39. http:// doi:10.1353/ pbm.0.0115

14. Colloca L, Howick J. Placebos without deception: Outcomes, mechanisms, and ethics. *International Review of Neurobiology.* 2018;138:219–240. http://doi:10.1016/bs.irn.2018.01.005

15. von Wernsdorff M, Loef M, Tuschen-Caffier B, Schmidt S. Effects of open-label placebos in clinical trials: A systematic review and meta-analysis. *Scientific Reports.* 2021;11(1):3855. http://doi:10.1038/s41598-021-83148-6

16. Tilburt JC, Emanuel EJ, Kaptchuk TJ, Curlin FA, Miller FG. Prescribing "placebo treatments": Results of national survey of US internists and rheumatologists. British Medical Journal. 2008;337:a1938. http://doi:10.1136/bmj.a1938

17. Rakel D. The salutogenesis-oriented session: Creating space and time for healing in primary care. *Explore.* 2008;4:42–7.

18. Walach H, Jonas WB. Placebo research: The evidence base for harnessing self-healing capacities. *Journal of Alternative and Complementary Medicine.* 2004;10(Suppl):S109.

19. Jonas WB. Reframing placebo in research and practice. *Philosophical Transactions of the Royal Society B: Biological Sciences.* 2011;366(1572):1896–1904. http://doi:10.1098/rstb.2010.0405

20. Jonas WB. *Placebo Guide.* 2020. Accessed September 23, 2022. https://drwaynejonas.com/resource/placebo/

21. The Family Medicine Education Consortium – Samueli Foundation. *The Susan Samueli Integrative Health Institute Catalyzes Inter-professional Collaboration: Integrative Health Learning Collaborative Case Study.* The Samueli Foundation; 2022 Mar. [cited 2022 June 2]. Available from: https://healingworksfoundation.org/wp-content/uploads/2022/03/Irvine-Samueli-Case-Study.pdf

22. The Family Medicine Education Consortium – Samueli Foundation. *University of Cincinnati Adds More Integrative Health to Group Visits: Integrative Health Learning Collaborative Case Study.* The Samueli Foundation; 2022 Mar. [cited 2022 June 2]. Available from: https://healingworksfoundation.org/wp-content/uploads/2022/03/UCincinnati-Case-Study.pdf

23. Center for Innovation in Family Medicine. *Integrative Approaches to Chronic Pain Management Course [Internet].* 2019 [cited 2022 Jun 2]. Available from: https://healing worksfoundation.org/cme/

1.2

Expectations

What do we know and where do we need to go?

Sigrid Juhl Lunde, Irving Kirsch, Ulrike Bingel, Christian Büchel, and Lene Vase

Introduction

Expectations are inextricably linked with placebo effects. An expert group has defined *placebo effects* as, "effects that occur in clinical or laboratory medical contexts, respectively, after administration of an inert treatment or as part of active treatments, due to mechanisms such as expectancies of the patient."[1] The important contribution of expectations is exemplified and substantiated by findings demonstrating that positive expectations can enhance the effect of the potent opioid remifentanil, while negative expectations can almost abolish the analgesic effect.[2] Yet, when looking across placebo mechanism studies, not all results support a key role for expectations. In some studies, expected pain levels contribute to placebo analgesia effects to a high extent,[3,4] whereas other studies show no substantial association between expected and perceived pain levels.[5,6] In addition to heterogeneity in results, studies differ greatly in their approaches for measuring expectations. Despite a consensus the definition of *placebo effects*, there is no consensus on exactly how to define *expectations*. Individual-level data on expectation and placebo effects suggest, however, that we may have to revisit the general concept of *expectation* and how we measure it.

What do we know? Stating the discrepancy based on theoretical and empirical work

Expectation can be conceptualized as a belief or prediction about the future. Importantly, this prediction holds two separate components that require two different ways of measuring expectations.[7,8] One component is a subjective probability that something will happen. Studies may assess this probability by asking participants, "How certain are you that you will feel less pain?" Another component is a predicted magnitude of the expected event. This may be assessed by asking participants, "How much pain do you think you will feel?"

Although expectancies do not need to be in conscious awareness to affect our experience, asking our patients and participants about the probability and predicted magnitude of an expected event does imply that such things are introspectable, meaning that both measures require a consciously accessible belief about the future event.[7,9,10] In a treatment setting, this belief can be induced and affected by several contextual factors, such as the clinical setting, previous experiences, suggestions about the treatment, and the clinician-patient relationship.[11] Adding to this, placebo mechanism studies have used verbal suggestions, conditioning, and social observation to induce expectations—with different magnitudes of effects in clinical populations.[12] Using verbal suggestions, patients and participants may be informed that "The agent that you have just received is known to powerfully reduce pain in some patients."[13] The delivery of this information has been associated with medium-to-large effects on patients' pain levels.[12] In studies using conditioning procedures, on the other hand, a placebo treatment is typically paired with reduced pain stimulation—unbeknownst to the patient or participant— to facilitate pain relief when the placebo treatment is administered in subsequent test situations. The combination of conditioning and verbal suggestions has been associated with medium effects on patients' pain levels.[12] Finally, using social observation (e.g., of pain relief) has been associated with small effects on patients' pain levels.[12]

Even though these procedures are assumed to induce expectations, many of the studies using verbal suggestions, conditioning, or social observation do not actually *assess* the patients' or participants' levels of expectations. Further, in studies that do assess expectations, these measures are often used without further defining the concept of *expectation* or how expectations are applied in the studies. To exemplify this, some studies use expectations as a primary outcome measure, whereas other studies include measures of expectations as a manipulation check of whether study procedures succeeded in inducing expectations.[14] The question remains, however, as to whether these measures capture the complexity of expectations.

In a study on conditioned placebo analgesia in healthy participants, a manipulation check showed that participants had high expectations toward the efficacy of an analgesic treatment (i.e., rating their expectations verbally from "no pain relief" to "complete pain relief").[15] Accordingly, conditioning procedures were successful in inducing expectations, and results showed small, but significant, placebo analgesia effects. Surprisingly, however, there was no correlation between the participants' expectations and the actual placebo analgesia effect.

In another study on healthy participants, both treatment expectations and placebo analgesia effects were found to be modulated by prior experience.[16] Here, participants were given either positive or negative analgesic treatment experiences across 2 consecutive test days before being introduced to a new treatment using a different route of administration. Although the first treatment experiences induced positive and negative treatment expectations, respectively, the change in treatment context changed the participants' expectations. At the same time, however, results showed that this change in expectation was *not* reflected in the analgesic response. Rather, this response was driven by the participants' prior treatment experience, with no correlation between treatment expectations and treatment outcome.

Together, these results suggest that verbally assessed expectations may not correspond to what we see across findings on placebo effects. Although study procedures such as verbal suggestions, conditioning, and social observation, succeed in inducing expectations, we may fail to tap into these expectations adequately when measuring them.

Where do we need to go? New frameworks and directions for future research

A recent framework suggested that treatment expectation may be defined as the prediction of treatment-related health outcomes, that is, the subjective probability of a health-relevant event occurrence such as pain relief (see Figure 1.2.1).[17] These expectations are determined by interindividual differences and prior information available to the individual to predict health outcomes.

"Prior information" includes experience we have from previous treatment, information we receive about the specific treatment, and observational learning and contextual factors embedded in the treatment setting. Within this framework, prior information is fed back to predict future treatment outcomes. Importantly, predictions relate to both positive and negative treatment outcomes, including adverse events.[18] Further, they may have explicit or implicit components and conscious awareness to varying degrees, as illustrated by the study showing carry-over effects from previous treatment experiences.[16] Accordingly, our treatment expectations may enhance

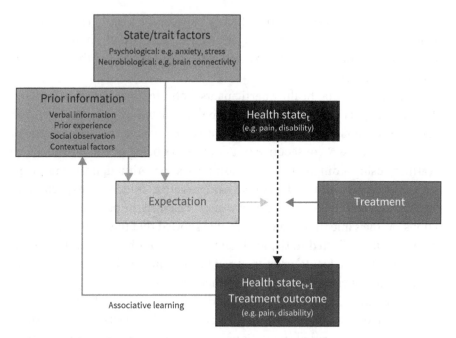

Figure 1.2.1 A new framework for treatment expectation.
Reprinted from Bingel.[17]

or diminish our treatment outcome. The framework highlights why it may be pivotal to consider the role and complexity of these treatment expectations, including factors such as the individual's experiences from previous treatments and present emotional state, to optimize patients' current treatment experiences.[17]

Another theoretical framework that elaborates how previous experiences contribute to current experiences is Bayesian integration. This framework models how our expectations and sensory information are integrated to form a percept (e.g., our experience of something painful, but also our experience of an effective treatment). Using the Bayesian framework, this will estimate the probability of perceived pain levels taking prior knowledge into account.[19]

Various studies have tested this conceptualization experimentally in relation to acute pain.[20,21] For instance, one study has tested the precision of expectation in healthy participants exposed to heat pain.[22] Here, verbal suggestions and conditioning procedures were used to create constant or variable expectation, and formal Bayesian integration mathematically predicted different placebo effects based on this precision. Placebo effects were more pronounced in participants with more precise, constant treatment expectations and correlated positively with the relative precision of the prior expectation. Accordingly, high precision of expectations led to stronger placebo effects that were less driven by sensory information—in agreement with the Bayesian model. Although this study did not measure expectations explicitly using verbal ratings, results substantiate the importance of implicit expectations and predictions. In agreement with studies showing that nonconscious cues can trigger pain modulation and placebo effects,[23] the relation between conscious and nonconscious components in placebo analgesia effects—and appropriate ways of measuring these aspects—should be further investigated.

One line of research that taps into nonconscious aspects of placebo effects is open-label placebo (OLP) studies.[24] These studies address the intrinsic paradox that patients receiving inactive treatments experience symptom relief even when they know that it is a placebo. Expectations are typically not measured systematically in OLP studies.[25,26] Yet, the few studies that have assessed expectations among patients and healthy participants receiving OLPs have found no association between treatment expectations at the start of the study and later treatment effects (after 3 weeks of OLP treatment).[27,28] However, the provision of a rationale indicating how OLPs can produce benefits has been shown to be a central component to their effects.[29] Future research should elaborate on the role of explicit and implicit expectations and investigate the gaps—and bridges—between different components of expectations and adequate ways of assessing their role in both classical experimental placebo trials and OLP studies.

Adding to these considerations on how to understand and measure expectations, more studies should investigate the temporal component and dynamic evolvement of expectations. Expectations may change over time and across different treatment settings based on, for example, information given about the expected treatment outcome or timing of these effects.[17,30,31] For instance, giving participants specific information on the expected onset of a treatment effect has been found to influence the time course of a placebo effect by, in one study, delaying the onset of the effect.[30] Further, when measured at different time points, expected pain levels have been found to predict perceived pain levels to a high extent—even when taking a gradual learning effect into account.[32] Accordingly, expectation is not a static construct, and studies should not only consider *how* but also *when* and *how often* they assess patients' and participants' treatment expectations.

Hoping for the best, but expecting the worst

Another question appears when investigating the role of expectations, Do findings from experimental studies translate to clinical settings with patients that may have experienced numerous previous treatments and—possibly—lack of treatment effects?

In taking the framework of treatment expectations (Figure 1.2.1) into account, it seems reasonable that patients with chronic diseases adjust their predictions continuously throughout the course of their treatment history. Further, placebo analgesia studies in patients with chronic pain suggest that we may have to access more than just the patients' expected outcome. Findings have shown that both expected pain relief and desire for pain relief contribute significantly to placebo analgesia effects in patients—with an emphasis on the interaction between the two.[33,34] For instance, in patients with irritable bowel syndrome, expected pain levels and desire for pain relief were found to explain 81% of the variance in pain ratings when patients received rectal lidocaine.[33]

Desire is conceptually orthogonal to expectation: we may expect something that we want—or want *not*—to happen. *Hope*, on the other hand, may be conceptualized as a desire for an expected outcome—although not necessarily probable.[35] To illustrate this, a patient with chronic pain may have a strong desire that a new treatment will take away his pain, although previous treatments have not succeeded in providing adequate pain relief. At the same time, however, he may still expect the new treatment to fail—taking prior information into account. Particularly, the phenomenon of nocebo effects indicates that expectations can shape experience even when they are the opposite of our hopes and desires.[36]

Thus, it may be important to consider how prior information—including previous treatment experiences—influences and interacts with patients' expectations, desires, and hopes to predict health outcomes. In order for us to know more about their clinical relevance, we need to be able to take these constructs apart and look at them both separately and combined—assessing *both* the magnitude and the subjective probability of the expected outcome.

References

1. Evers AWM, Colloca L, Blease C, et al. Implications of placebo and nocebo effects for clinical practice: Expert consensus. *Psychotherapy and Psychosomatics.* 2018;87(4):204–210. https://doi:10.1159/000490354
2. Bingel U, Wanigasekera V, Wiech K, et al. The effect of treatment expectation on drug efficacy: Imaging the analgesic benefit of the opioid remifentanil. *Science Translational Medicine.* 2011;3(70):70ra14. https://doi:10.1126/scitranslmed.3001244
3. Elsenbruch S, Roderigo T, Enck P, Benson S. Can a brief relaxation exercise modulate placebo or nocebo effects in a visceral pain model? *Frontiers in Psychiatry.* 2019;10:144. https://doi:10.3389/fpsyt.2019.00144

4. Schmitz J, Müller M, Stork J, et al. Positive treatment expectancies reduce clinical pain and perceived limitations in movement ability despite increased experimental pain: A randomized controlled trial on sham opioid infusion in patients with chronic back pain. *Psychotherapy and Psychosomatics.* 2019;88(4):203–214. https://doi:10.1159/000501385

5. Colloca L, Akintola T, Haycock NR, et al. Prior therapeutic experiences, not expectation ratings, predict placebo effects: An experimental study in chronic pain and healthy participants. *Psychotherapy and Psychosomatics.* 2020;89(6):371–378. https://doi:10.1159/000507400

6. Bąbel P, Bajcar EA, Adamczyk W, et al. Classical conditioning without verbal suggestions elicits placebo analgesia and nocebo hyperalgesia. *PLoS One.* 2017;12(7):e0181856. https://doi:10.1371/journal.pone.0181856

7. Kirsch I. Response expectancy as a determinant of experience and behavior. *American Psychologist.* 1985;40(11):1189–1202. https://doi:10.1037/0003-066X.40.11.1189

8. Kirsch I, Weixel LJ. Double-blind versus deceptive administration of a placebo. *Behavioral Neuroscience.* 1988;102(2):319–323. https://doi:10.1037//0735-7044.102.2.319

9. Kirsch I, Lynn SJ. Automaticity in clinical psychology. *American Psychologist.* 1999;54(7):504–515. https://doi:10.1037//0003-066x.54.7.504

10. Kirsch I. *Changing Expectations: A Key to Effective Psychotherapy.* Pacific Grove, CA: Brooks/Cole. Reviewed by JR Council. *American Journal of Clinical Hypnosis.* 1991;34(2):138–140. https://doi:10.1080/00029157.1991.10402974

11. Wager TD, Atlas LY. The neuroscience of placebo effects: Connecting context, learning and health. *Nature Reviews Neuroscience.* 2015;16(7):403–418. https://doi:10.1038/nrn3976

12. Peerdeman KJ, van Laarhoven AI, Keij SM, et al. Relieving patients' pain with expectation interventions: A meta-analysis. *Pain.* 2016;157(6):1179–1191. https://doi:10.1097/j.pain.0000000000000540

13. Price DD, Craggs J, Verne GN, Perlstein WM, Robinson ME. Placebo analgesia is accompanied by large reductions in pain-related brain activity in irritable bowel syndrome patients. *Pain.* 2007;127(1-2):63–72. https://doi:10.1016/j.pain.2006.08.001

14. Schmitz J, Müller M, Stork J, et al. Positive treatment expectancies reduce clinical pain and perceived limitations in movement ability despite increased experimental pain: A randomized controlled trial on sham opioid infusion in patients with chronic back pain. *Psychotherapy and Psychosomatics.* 2019;88(4):203–214. doi:10.1159/000501385

15. Zunhammer M, Gerardi M, Bingel U. The effect of dopamine on conditioned placebo analgesia in healthy individuals: A double-blind randomized trial. *Psychopharmacology.* 2018;235(9):2587–2595. https://doi:10.1007/s00213-018-4951-3

16. Zunhammer M, Ploner M, Engelbrecht C, Bock J, Kessner SS, Bingel U. The effects of treatment failure generalize across different routes of drug administration. *Science Translational Medicine.* 2017;9(393):eaal2999. https://doi:10.1126/scitranslmed.aal2999

17. Bingel U. Placebo 2.0: The impact of expectations on analgesic treatment outcome. *Pain.* 2020;161(Suppl 1):S48–S56. https://doi:10.1097/j.pain.0000000000001981

18. Kessner S, Wiech K, Forkmann K, Ploner M, Bingel U. The effect of treatment history on therapeutic outcome: An experimental approach. *JAMA Internal Medicine.* 2013;173(15):1468–1469. https://doi:10.1001/jamainternmed.2013.6705

19. Büchel C, Geuter S, Sprenger C, Eippert F. Placebo analgesia: A predictive coding perspective. *Neuron.* 2014;81(6):1223–1239. https://doi:10.1016/j.neuron.2014.02.042

20. Geuter S, Boll S, Eippert F, Büchel C. Functional dissociation of stimulus intensity encoding and predictive coding of pain in the insula. *eLife.* 2017;6:e24770 https://doi:10.7554/eLife.24770

21. Strube A, Rose M, Fazeli S, Büchel C. The temporal and spectral characteristics of expectations and prediction errors in pain and thermoception. *eLife.* 2021;10:e62809 https://doi:10.7554/eLife.62809

22. Grahl A, Onat S, Büchel C. The periaqueductal gray and Bayesian integration in placebo analgesia. *eLife*. 2018;7:e32930. https://doi:10.7554/eLife.32930

23. Jensen KB, Kaptchuk TJ, Kirsch I, et al. Nonconscious activation of placebo and nocebo pain responses. *Proceedings of the National Academy of Sciences of the United States of America*. 2012;109(39):15959–15964. https://doi:10.1073/pnas.1202056109

24. Kaptchuk TJ. Open-label placebo: Reflections on a research agenda. *Perspectives in Biology and Medicine*. 2018;61(3):311–334. https://doi:10.1353/pbm.2018.0045

25. Carvalho C, Caetano JM, Cunha L, Rebouta P, Kaptchuk TJ, Kirsch I. Open-label placebo treatment in chronic low back pain: A randomized controlled trial. *Pain*. 2016;157(12):2766–2772. https://doi:10.1097/j.pain.0000000000000700

26. Kaptchuk TJ, Friedlander E, Kelley JM, et al. Placebos without deception: A randomized controlled trial in irritable bowel syndrome. *PLoS ONE*. 2010;5(12):e15591. https://doi:10.1371/journal.pone.0015591

27. Kleine-Borgmann J, Schmidt K, Billinger M, Forkmann K, Wiech K, Bingel U. Effects of open-label placebos on test performance and psychological well-being in healthy medical students: A randomized controlled trial. *Scientific Reports*. 2021;11(1):2130. https://doi:10.1038/s41598-021-81502-2

28. Kleine-Borgmann J, Schmidt K, Hellmann A, Bingel U. Effects of open-label placebo on pain, functional disability, and spine mobility in patients with chronic back pain: A randomized controlled trial. *Pain*. 2019;160(12):2891–2897. https://doi:10.1097/j.pain.0000000000001683

29. Locher C, Frey Nascimento A, Kirsch I, Kossowsky J, Meyer A, Gaab J. Is the rationale more important than deception? A randomized controlled trial of open-label placebo analgesia. *Pain*. 2017;158(12):2320–2328. https://doi:10.1097/j.pain.0000000000001012

30. Camerone EM, Piedimonte A, Testa M, et al. The effect of temporal information on placebo analgesia and nocebo hyperalgesia. *Psychosomatic Medicine*. 2021;83(1):43–50. https://doi:10.1097/psy.0000000000000882

31. Camerone EM, Wiech K, Benedetti F, et al. "External timing" of placebo analgesia in an experimental model of sustained pain. *European Journal of Pain*. 2021;25(6):1303–1315. https://doi:10.1002/ejp.1752

32. Lunde SJ, Vuust P, Garza-Villarreal EA, Kirsch I, Møller A, Vase L. Music-induced analgesia in healthy participants is associated with expected pain levels but not opioid or dopamine-dependent mechanisms. *Frontiers in Pain Research. (Lausanne)*. 2022;3:734999. https://doi:10.3389/fpain.2022.734999

33. Vase L, Robinson ME, Verne NG, Price DD. The contributions of suggestion, desire, and expectation to placebo effects in irritable bowel syndrome patients. *Pain*. 2003;105(1):17–25. https://doi:10.1016/s0304-3959(03)00073-3

34. Price DD, Finniss DG, Benedetti F. A comprehensive review of the placebo effect: Recent advances and current thought. *Annual Review of Psychology*. 2008;59:565–590. https://doi:10.1146/annurev.psych.59.113006.095941

35. Leung KK, Silvius JL, Pimlott N, Dalziel W, Drummond N. Why health expectations and hopes are different: The development of a conceptual model. *Health Expectations*. 2009;12(4):347–360. https://doi:10.1111/j.1369-7625.2009.00570.x

36. Benedetti F, Lanotte M, Lopiano L, Colloca L. When words are painful: Unraveling the mechanisms of the nocebo effect. *Neuroscience*. 2007;147(2):260–271. https://doi:10.1016/j.neuroscience.2007.02.020

1.3

New translational opportunities for placebo research

Ben Alter, Kari Leibowitz, Alia Crum, and Marta Peciña

Introduction

Placebo interventions play an important role as a control in randomized placebo-controlled clinical trials. Yet mounting evidence, emerging from the field of placebo analgesia research, posits that placebos are far from being controls or inert substances.[1] Instead, placebos, commonly understood as the response to social learning, expectancy, conditioning mechanisms, and patient-doctor interactions, have proven to radically affect treatment efficacy through the engagement of neural circuits and neurotransmitter systems that result in clinical improvement across many symptoms and disorders.

Over the last 2 decades, neuroscientists have used neuroimaging, genetics, neuroendocrinology, and other tools to understand placebo effects.[2] A large body of literature using these tools demonstrates the biological tractability of this phenomenon (Figure 1.3.1), which opens the possibility of modulating these molecular and neural circuits to enhance health outcomes in clinical practice.[3] However, despite significant progress in the field of placebo research, very few studies report empirical investigations of placebos in routine clinical practice.[4] In this chapter, we will review the biological mechanisms implicated in placebo effects and use this evidence to justify large-scale changes in the training of healthcare providers and clinical staff to ensure that placebo effects are safely and effectively empowered.

Biological evidence for the development of placebo-based clinical interventions

Classical theories have consistently argued that placebo effects result from positive expectancies regarding the beneficial effects of a drug and classical

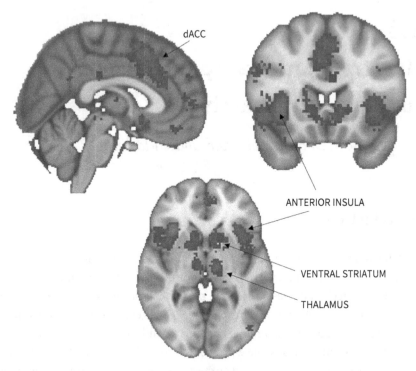

Figure 1.3.1 Maps depicting the term-based meta-analyses (332 studies, uniformity test) from Neurosynth when using the term *placebo*.[3]

conditioning, where the paring of a neutral stimulus (i.e., the placebo pill), with an unconditioned stimulus (i.e., the active drug) results in conditioned responses or placebo effects.[2] This effect also depends on the psychosocial context surrounding treatment, including patient-provider interactions.[5] These conceptual theories have then been incorporated into trial-by-trial manipulations of both expectancies of pain relief and the pain sensory experience, rapidly advancing our understanding of the neural and molecular mechanisms of placebo analgesia. These neuroimaging studies have demonstrated placebo-induced activation in several cortical areas[6,7] as well as the descending pain modulating system reaching down to the spinal cord.[8,9] Collectively, these neuroimaging studies have provided evidence for the involvement of brain regions linked to nociceptive processing, including early pain-gating mechanisms, decision-making, cognitive appraisal, reward/motivation, emotional regulation, and other forms of learning and social processing.[5]

Beyond the neural tractability of placebo effects, molecular neuroimaging and pharmacological studies have contributed to our understanding of the molecular mechanisms implicated in placebo effects. In the first study to show the biological underpinnings of placebo analgesia, patients received the μ-opioid receptor antagonist naloxone or placebo after undergoing wisdom tooth extraction.[10] In this study, patients who received naloxone reported higher postsurgical pain than those who received placebo, suggesting that naloxone blocked placebo effects. This landmark study was followed by a plethora of studies confirming the role of μ-opioid neurotransmission in placebo effects.[6,11-13] Beyond the opioid system, many relevant peptides and neurotransmitter systems have been implicated in placebo effects, including dopamine,[14] the endocannabinoid system,[15,16] vasopressin,[17] and serotonin[18] signaling pathways. In addition, robust evidence has linked placebo effects to the immune system.[19] Further, along with advances in knowledge about the neurotransmitters and neural pathways, high-throughput analysis technologies and large-scale omics data of genes, RNA, and proteins have provided additional opportunities to investigate the molecular targets of placebo effects.[20]

While the utility of these biomarkers is still under investigation, it is plausible to think that these biomarkers could be used during drug development, for example, to identify placebo responders and exclude them from randomized control trials (RCTs) and maximize assay sensitivity, replacing commonly used placebo lead-in phases. Alternatively, this information could be used to account for expectancy and learning mechanisms across the different arms of an RCT, reducing noise and improving overall signal detection. These approaches, while practically possible, are yet to be fully developed and tested.

The extent to which these neural and molecular targets can be modulated to improve treatment outcomes has been explored much less. There is much to be learned about the ways in which this information could be used in routine clinical practice or used to train the next generation of clinicians and health care providers. This chapter provides two examples of how to accomplish these goals: using open-label placebo interventions and shaping patient mindsets.

Placebo-based clinical interventions

Open-label placebo interventions
Effectively translating placebo research to clinical practice is a significant challenge. Extracting component mechanisms of placebo effects on social, psychological, and neurobiological levels is one approach to this problem.

As outlined above, the patient-provider interaction represents a key area to applying placebo-based interventions and improving clinical outcomes. This section will focus on additional examples of placebo-based clinical applications, including open-label placebos for symptom management and translating placebo research findings to improve medical diagnosis and pharmacologic treatment selection.

An open-label placebo (OLP), which is sometimes referred to as "honest" placebo, has received increased attention in both the lay press and clinical research with both fierce advocates and vocal critics.[21-23] An OLP intervention consists of a medical interaction during which patients are prescribed and administered placebo, typically for symptom management such as pain, fatigue, or itch. OLP is "open-label" and "honest" because patients are aware of being administered placebos and they provide informed consent, which includes the knowledge that the pills recommended or given in research-related trials are inert. This placebo-based intervention attempts to capture many aspects of placebo responses observed in a blinded randomized clinical trial. However, details of how patients are "unblinded" during the informed consent process and how OLP interventions are administered are likely to affect the translational success of OLP.

Before a detailed discussion of OLPs, an important consideration is whether OLPs meet ethical standards for medical care. For example, the American Medical Association's code of medical ethics suggests that it is ethically acceptable.[24] However, the opinion is broadly written, focusing on other uses of placebos in clinical practice. For example, a placebo may be used in an "N-of-1" trial as a way of determining the efficacy of active medication for a single patient, which is a promising concept but not in widespread clinical practice.[25] Importantly, OLPs are not specifically mentioned in the AMA medical ethics opinion. Given the fundamental differences between N-of-1 trials in which a pharmacologically active treatment is given at some point during the trial and OLPs, which lack a "pharmacologically active" treatment, the assessment of OLPs by the AMA may not apply. Therefore, additional consideration of the ethical merits of OLPs have been undertaken by several leading researchers, finding that OLPs meet ethical standards, but more clinical research about efficacy is needed before OLPs are used in clinical practice.[26] Importantly, studies support the notion that patients would also find OLPs acceptable.[27] However, it is worth ongoing consideration of the ethics of OLPs, since provision of informed consent is crucial and potential harms of OLP therapy in a clinical setting could include unintended violation of autonomy through unappreciated power imbalances favoring the provider and/or undetected undue influence by the provider. Additionally, other ethical principles, including social justice,[28] must be addressed in the future, ideally including patient input in future clinical research.

Overall, the results from OLP randomized controlled trials are promising. A recent meta-analysis summarizes the use of OLPs in outpatient settings for different indications, providing evidence of robust effects.[23] Eleven OLP randomized controlled trials were included investigating effects on chronic low back pain, migraine, cancer-related fatigue, irritable bowel syndrome, major depressive disorder, activity deficit hyperactivity disorder, and allergic rhinitis. When compared to "treatment-as-usual" or "no treatment," OLP use had a significant positive effect on primary outcomes with the standardized mean difference across all symptoms being 0.72 (95% confidence intervals: 0.39–1.5). Although this meta-analysis is promising, notable weaknesses that were identified in it included the relatively small study sizes and moderate risk of bias. As previously discussed,[29] studies within each clinical population are needed to rigorously assess OLP efficacy.

One important area of future research is to resolve the specifics of OLP administration, such as what specific information should be conveyed to patients as part of the initial medical encounter. Across current studies, details of this medical counseling varied.[23] After consent, most studies involve some amount of verbal instruction. The majority of studies used structured scripts that highlight several points: (1) placebos contain no active medication; (2) placebo effects can be powerful; (3) conditioning mediates some of placebo effects (with phrases such as "like Pavlov's dogs that salivated when they heard the bell"); (4) a positive attitude may help but is not necessary; and (5) a participant needs to take the placebo consistently. One study used news media related to prior OLP results as part of the informed consent process. This news report suggested that OLP effects were surprisingly effective and did not require an initial belief that OLPs would work.

The variation in OLP administration raises questions about what the key component parts are in OLP medical interaction. The role of expectations in the use of OLPs is interesting and unresolved. In a study of allergic rhinitis, extended information accompanying an OLP, including positive suggestions to engender positive treatment expectations, did not affect the primary outcome but instead improved overall well-being.[30] The clinical context of OLPs may also be important. In a study of postoperative pain, OLP counseling started preoperatively in the outpatient setting and continued with placebo pill administration during hospitalization and 2 weeks after discharge from the hospital, and it produced significant effects throughout large contextual changes, including inpatient and outpatient environments and after recovery from anesthesia.[31] With increasing popularity of telemedicine, in which medical encounters are conducted through the telephone or videoconference, aspects of OLP could be done from a patient's home for patient convenience and cost reduction of OLP therapy itself. However, remote administration of OLPs via a videoconferencing encounter and mail delivery of placebos did not produce significant improvement in allergic rhinitis symptoms, potentially because of the virtual patient-provider interaction,[32] possibly owing to a lack of appropriate control conditions. This raises important future questions not only about OLP but about the benefits of telemedicine versus traditional "in-person" medical encounters for symptom management (see Chapter 6.3).

As identified in mechanistic studies, conditioned responses are likely to be involved in OLP use. Several studies have capitalized on this by incorporating conditioning in the OLP administration. For example, after counseling participants about what OLPs are, patients are instructed to take a placebo pill at the same time as they take the active medication. This contingent pairing of a placebo pill with active medication forms an association between the placebo and a medication effect, and when the pairing stops, the placebo takes on the targeted medication effect. Typically, active medication is continued as needed in this phase, prompting a description of "dose-extension" of this particular OLP paradigm. In a clinical trial, combining OLPs with a conditioning component was found to improve postoperative pain and reduce the use of opioid analgesics.[31] Similar results were observed in a small group of patients recovering from spinal cord injury.[33] Studies have applied the application of a conditioned or "dose-extending" OLP to the treatment of opioid-use disorder.[34] The relative importance of contingent pairing in a robust OLP effect is unknown, and pragmatic trials comparing OLP use with and without conditioning could be helpful in resolving this question. Up until now, the active medication used for conditioning in published OLP studies has been opioid agonists. In mechanistic studies, nonsteroidal anti-inflammatory drugs have been used to condition placebo analgesia,[35] suggesting that conditioned OLP could be broadened to involve other active medications. This may be particularly relevant if endogenous opioidergic pathways are altered in certain patient populations (e.g., patients with opioid tolerance), in which case nonopioid conditioning may provide a mechanistically distinct pathway to achieve conditioned OLP effects.[15] Overall, OLPs show promise as a unique treatment to reduce symptom severity in several conditions, particularly in pain management. Moreover, OLP use could reduce the use of other medications, such as opioids, which themselves carry risks. Additional clinical trials to determine the specifics of OLP administration and to reproduce results currently in the literature will aid in translating OLP use to clinical practice.

Apart from placebo-based interventions, knowledge gained from the study of placebo effects has the potential to improve clinical outcomes. For example, placebo analgesia shares some neurobiological features with other endogenous pain inhibitory processes thought to impact pain and its treatment.[36] These processes are reflected in lab-based quantitative sensory tests, including "conditioned pain modulation," in which painful stimulation of a remote body site decreases pain at the primary test site,[37] and "offset analgesia," in which fulfilled predictions of pain relief from slight decreases in a noxious stimulus robustly decreased reported pain intensity.[38] Quantitative sensory testing measures assessing pain inhibition may provide additional information for pain diagnosis or guide treatment selection, personalizing the management of chronic pain.[39,40] Much work remains to be done to translate this into clinical practice. Understanding the endogenous pain inhibitory system in the context of placebo analgesia promises to accelerate this clinical application.

In summary, placebo-based interventions show promise for clinical translation. Additional research is needed, specifically clarifying details of OLP administration and further elucidating placebo mechanisms. For OLP use, continued evaluation of its ethical validity will be important. Currently, placebos are being marketed and sold for symptom management,[22] based on the clinical trials reviewed above. A cursory examination of customer feedback includes ethically dubious uses of placebo pills by relatives of patients without the patients' consent (Figure 1.3.2). Although certainly unintended by the scientists performing these studies, this highlights the importance of large-scale, multisite clinical trials that measure not only the potential benefits of placebo-based interventions but also their potential harms.

Training clinical healthcare teams to leverage placebo mechanisms in practice

Most researchers—and practitioners—primarily consider placebo effects in the context of the RCT, during which drugs or treatments in development are compared against placebos. The purpose of this comparison is to separate any improvements that may be due to placebo effects to see if the drug or treatment in question has a significant benefit beyond the robust, and often underestimated, placebo effects. While this is a highly useful procedure for developing new drugs and treatments, it has left us with a misguided view of placebo effects. Placebo effects are often seen as mysterious—amorphous, nonspecific effects that must be subtracted from active medications and treatments.

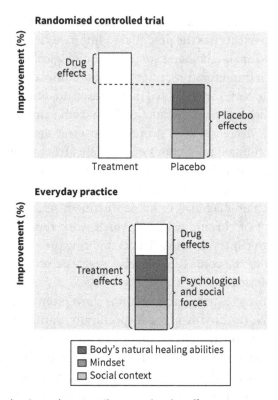

Figure 1.3.2 Mechanisms that contribute to placebo effects.

Yet in the practice of Medicine, these placebo effects are not separated: they remain active and at play. Any beneficial effects of treatment are a result of a combination of the active components of treatment and the benefits of placebo effects.[41] Further, placebo effects are not mysterious, amorphous, or nonspecific effects. Research into placebo effects over the past several decades has revealed that placebo effects are specific and measurable and can be explained and understood. As described above, several known mechanisms contribute to placebo effects. These mechanisms include patient's expectations around treatment, conditioned responses to stimuli in the healthcare encounter, and the body's natural healing abilities (e.g., the immune, opioid, and endocrine systems) (these natural bodily healing systems may also be responsible for regression to the mean when it comes to symptom reduction (Figure 1.3.2).[41-45] When we see placebo effects for what they really are, social and psychological forces that catalyze healing in the body, we can also see that it is possible to harness the same mechanisms that lead to placebo effects alongside active medication and treatment. No deception, sugar pills, or sham procedures are necessary to leverage mechanisms like patient expectations deliberately and consistently in healthcare. One promising avenue we can use for harnessing these placebo forces lies in shaping patient mindsets in the healthcare encounter. *Mindsets* are core beliefs or assumptions about the nature and working of things in the world. Mindsets orient us to one particular focus of ambiguous and complex realities. In doing so, mindsets help us create meaning, predict what is likely to happen next, and motivate our behavior. A growing body of research indicates that mindsets powerfully influence our experience and can positively or negatively impact health, performance, and well-being.[46-49]

Mindsets represent one particularly promising avenue for harnessing placebo effects in clinical practice. Many studies suggest that placebo effects work, in part, by shaping patient expectations about treatment. When patients believe that a treatment is likely to work for them, that treatment is more effective.[50,51] When medication is administered via IV outside of patients' awareness, that treatment is less effective.[52,53] And when side effects are emphasized, patients experience these side effects more often.[54,55] Thus, shaping patient mindsets about treatment—such as by instilling the mindset that treatment is likely to benefit the patient and not cause harm or side effects—is one way to nondeceptively leverage placebo effects alongside active medications and treatments. And emerging research is revealing other mindsets that may be particularly influential in a healthcare context. For example, patients may have the mindset that an illness is a catastrophe, or they may have the mindset that it is manageable or even is an opportunity to make positive life changes.[56] When they are sick or in pain, patients may hold the mindset that their body has failed them, or they may see their bodies as capable of handling their illness.[56] These mindsets don't mean that patients like, enjoy, or are happy about their illness: patients can see their illness as manageable (or even as an opportunity) and their body as capable without liking their illness or being happy to experience it.

Patient-provider interactions are an opportunity to shape patient mindsets to improve treatment outcomes. Research suggests that a warm, trusting, and positive patient-provider encounter can enhance placebo effects.[57-62] And the doctor-patient relationship itself represents another potential mindset in the clinical encounter: the mindset that the patient is in good hands with a care team that is both competent (e.g., "gets it" in terms of Medicine) and warm (e.g., "gets them" as people with goals, needs, and concerns).[63] When interacting with patients, providers can deliberately harness the mechanisms that lead to placebo effects by shaping patient mindsets.

In order to harness placebo effects nondeceptively, alongside active medications in clinical treatment, we (Leibowitz & Crum) developed a program to train healthcare teams to recognize and shape patient mindsets in clinical practice.[62] This training, which we call Medicine Plus Mindset, (a) informs primary care teams about the power of patient mindsets in shaping treatment outcomes, (b) provides care teams with a language and framework to identify which patient mindsets may be at play (i.e., patients' mindsets about illness, treatment, their body, and the provider/care team), and (c) equips care teams with skills and techniques to effectively shape patients' mindsets to improve health outcomes. The training is designed for all members of the care team: not just physicians, but also medical assistants, nurse practitioners, and clinic staff, since all members of the care team have the opportunity to shape mindsets, set expectations, and contribute to patient perceptions of the clinic—all factors known to boost placebo effects. The training opens with an overview of research on the power of placebo effects, and then outlines much of what we've described here: that the forces that contribute to placebo effects can be explained, understood, and harnessed deliberately, and that shaping key patient mindsets in practice is one avenue for doing so.

The main goal of the Medicine Plus Mindset training is to provide increased motivation for care teams to engage with the psychological and social forces that contribute to placebo effects. By highlighting the centrality and necessity of these forces in practicing effective healthcare, the Medicine Plus Mindset training seeks to transform the medical view of the mechanisms that lead to placebo effects from being seen as peripheral or superfluous to being seen as valuable and critical in healthcare. This is one current initiative to bring the power of placebo effects into clinical practice.

In an initial assessment, Medicine Plus Mindset training was delivered to all five of Stanford University's Primary Care clinics. While the full results of this implementation are reported elsewhere, initial data suggest that this training was extremely well received, with participants rating the training as highly useful and enjoyable, themselves as highly committed to using what they learned from the training in clinical practice, and indicating that they would be highly likely to recommend the training to a colleague. The encouraging positive reception of this training suggests that care teams are open to learning how to harness the forces that lead to placebo effects nondeceptively in clinical practice, without the use of sham treatments or sugar pills.

Conclusions

Supported by over 4 decades of clinical neuroscience research, placebo-based interventions show promise for clinical translation. As highlighted above, we identified a growing body of research indicating that interventions such as OLPs and mindset training can powerfully influence our experience and can positively impact health, performance, and well-being, opening new opportunities for patient treatments and the training of future healthcare providers. Ultimately, the medical field should evolve to ensure that placebo effects are safely and effectively empowered.

References

1. Kaptchuk TJ, Miller FG. Open label placebo: Can honestly prescribed placebos evoke meaningful therapeutic benefits? *British Medical Journal.* 2018;363:k3889. http://doi:10.1136/bmj.k3889

2. Wager TD, Atlas LY. The neuroscience of placebo effects: Connecting context, learning and health. *Nature Reviews Neuroscience.* 2015;16(7):403–418. http://doi:10.1038/nrn3976

3. Yarkoni T, Poldrack RA, Nichols TE, Van Essen DC, Wager TD. Large-scale automated synthesis of human functional neuroimaging data. *Nature Methods.* 2011;8(8):665–670. doi:10.1038/nmeth.1635.

4. Colloca L, Barsky AJ. Placebo and nocebo effects. *New England Journal of Medicine.* 2020;382(6):554–561. doi:10.1056/NEJMra1907805.

5. Atlas LY. A social affective neuroscience lens on placebo analgesia. *Trends in Cognitive Sciences.* 2021;25(11):992–1005. http://doi:10.1016/j.tics.2021.07.016

6. Petrovic P, Kalso E, Petersson KM, Ingvar M. Placebo and opioid analgesia: Imaging a shared neuronal network. *Science (New York, N.Y.).* 2002;295(5560):1737–1740. doi:10.1126/science.1067176.

7. Wager TD, Rilling JK, Smith EE, Sokolik A, Casey KL, Davidson RJ, Kosslyn SM, Rose RM, Cohen JD. Placebo-induced changes in fMRI in the anticipation and experience of pain. *Science.* 2004;303(5661):1162–1167. doi:10.1126/science.1093065.

8. Eippert F, Finsterbusch J, Bingel U, Büchel C. Direct evidence for spinal cord involvement in placebo analgesia. *Science (New York, N.Y.).* 2009;326(5951):404. http://doi:10.1126/science.1180142

9. Geuter S, Büchel C. Facilitation of pain in the human spinal cord by nocebo treatment. *Journal of Neuroscience.* 2013;33(34):13784–13790. http://doi:10.1523/JNEUROSCI.2191-13.2013

10. Levine JD, Gordon, NC, Fields HL. The mechanism of placebo analgesia. *Lancet.* 1978;312(8091):654–657. http://doi:10.1016/S0140-6736(78)92762-9

11. Zubieta J-K, Bueller JA, Jackson LR, Scott DJ, Xu Y, Koeppe RA, Nichols TE, Stohler CS. Placebo effects mediated by endogenous opioid activity on opioid receptors. *Journal of Neuroscience.* 2005;25(34):7754–7762. doi:10.1523/JNEUROSCI.0439-05.2005.

12. Peciña M, Azhar H, Love TM, Lu T, Fredrickson BL, Stohler CS, Zubieta JK. Personality trait predictors of placebo analgesia and neurobiological correlates. *Neuropsychopharmacology.* 2013;38(4):639–646. doi:10.1038/npp.2012.227.

13. Pecina M, Love T, Stohler CS, Goldman D, Zubieta JK. Effects of the Mu opioid receptor polymorphism (OPRM1 A118G) on pain regulation, placebo effects and associated personality trait measures. *Neuropsychopharmacology.* 2015;40(4):957–965. http://doi:10.1038/npp.2014.272

14. de la Fuente-Fernández R, Ruth TJ, Sossi V, Schulzer M, Calne DB, Stoessl AJ. Expectation and dopamine release: Mechanism of the placebo effect in Parkinson's disease. *Science.* 2001;293(5532):1164–1166. doi:10.1126/science.1060937.

15. Benedetti F, Amanzio M, Rosato R, Blanchard C. Nonopioid placebo analgesia is mediated by CB1 cannabinoid receptors. *Nature Medicine.* 2011;17(10):1228–1230. doi:10.1038/nm.2435.

16. Pecina M, Martínez-Jauand M, Hodgkinson C, Stohler CS, Goldman D, Zubieta JK. FAAH selectively influences placebo effects. *Molecular Psychiatry.* 2014;19(3):385–391. http://doi:10.1038/mp.2013.124

17. Colloca L, Pine DS, Ernst M, Miller FG, Grillon C. Vasopressin boosts placebo analgesic effects in women: A randomized trial. *Biological Psychiatry.* 2016;79(10):794–802. doi:10.1016/j.biopsych.2015.07.019.

18. Furmark T, Appel L, Henningsson S, Ahs F, Faria V, Linnman C, Pissiota A, Frans O, Bani M, Bettica P, Pich EM, Jacobsson E, Wahlstedt K, Oreland L, Långström B, Eriksson E, Fredrikson M. A link between serotonin-related gene polymorphisms, amygdala activity, and placebo-induced relief from social anxiety. *Journal of Neuroscience.* 2008;28(49):13066–13074. doi:10.1523/JNEUROSCI.2534-08.2008.

19. Hadamitzky M, Sondermann W, Benson S, Schedlowski M. Placebo effects in the immune system. *International Review of Neurobiology.* 2018;138:39–59. doi:10.1016/bs.irn.2018.01.001.

20. Hall KT, Loscalzo J, Kaptchuk T. Pharmacogenomics and the placebo response. *ACS Chemical Neuroscience.* 2018;9(4):633–635. http://doi:10.1021/acschemneuro.8b00078

21. Kaptchuk TJ, Miller FG. Open label placebo: Can honestly prescribed placebos evoke meaningful therapeutic benefits? *British Medical Journal.* 2018;363:k3889. http://doi:10.1136/bmj.k3889

22. Maher CG, Traeger AC, Abdel Shaheed C, O'Keeffe M. Placebos in clinical care: A suggestion beyond the evidence. *Medical Journal of Australia.* 2021;19;215(6):252–253.e1. doi:10.5694/mja2.51230.

23. von Wernsdorff M, Loef M, Tuschen-Caffier B, Schmidt S. Effects of open-label placebos in clinical trials: A systematic review and meta-analysis. *Scientific Reports.* 2021;11(1):3855. doi:10.1038/s41598-021-83148-6. Erratum in: Sci Rep. 2021 Aug 25;11(1):17436.

24. American Medical Association. *Opinion 2.1.4 Use of Placebo in Clinical Practice, Code of Medical Ethics.* 2022. Accessed May 17, 2023. https://www.ama-assn.org/delivering-care/ethics/use-placebo-clinical-practice

25. Guyatt G, Sackett D, Adachi J, Roberts R, Chong J, Rosenbloom D, Keller J. A clinician's guide for conducting randomized trials in individual patients. *Canadian Medical Association Journal.* 1988;139(6):497–503.

26. Evers AWM, Colloca L, Blease C, Annoni M, Atlas LY, Benedetti F, Bingel U, Büchel C, Carvalho C, Colagiuri B, Crum AJ, Enck P, Gaab J, Geers AL, Howick J, Jensen KB, Kirsch I, Meissner K, Napadow V, Peerdeman KJ, Raz A, Rief W, Vase L, Wager TD, Wampold BE, Weimer K, Wiech K, Kaptchuk T. Implications of placebo and nocebo effects for clinical practice: Expert consensus. *Psychotherapy and Psychosomatics.* 2018;87(4):204–210. doi:10.1159/000490354.

27. Haas JW, Rief W, Doering BK. Open-label placebo treatment: Outcome expectations and general acceptance in the lay population. *International Journal of Behavioral Medicine.* 2021;28(4):444–454. http://doi:10.1007/s12529-020-09933-1

28. Specker Sullivan L. More than consent for ethical open-label placebo research. *Journal of Medical Ethics.* 2020; p. medethics-2019-105893. http://doi:10.1136/medethics-2019-105893

29. Colloca L, Howick J. Placebos without deception: Outcomes, mechanisms, and ethics. *International Review of Neurobiology.* 2018;138:219–240. http://doi:10.1016/bs.irn.2018.01.005

30. Schaefer M, Sahin T, Berstecher B. Why do open-label placebos work? A randomized controlled trial of an open-label placebo induction with and without extended information about the placebo effect in allergic rhinitis. *PLoS ONE.* 2018;13(3):e0192758. http://doi:10.1371/journal.pone.0192758

31. Flowers KM, Patton ME, Hruschak VJ, Fields KG, Schwartz E, Zeballos J, Kang JD, Edwards RR, Kaptchuk TJ, Schreiber KL. Conditioned open-label placebo for opioid reduction after spine surgery: A randomized controlled trial. *Pain.* 2021;162(6):1828–1839. doi:10.1097/j.pain.0000000000002185.

32. Kube T, Hofmann VE, Glombiewski JA, Kirsch I. Providing open-label placebos remotely: A randomized controlled trial in allergic rhinitis. *PLoS One.* 2021;16(3):e0248367. doi:10.1371/journal.pone.0248367. Erratum in: PLoS One. 2021 Jun 2;16(6):e0252850.

33. Morales-Quezada L, Mesia-Toledo I, Estudillo-Guerra A, O'Connor KC, Schneider JC, Sohn DJ, Crandell DM, Kaptchuk T, Zafonte R. Conditioning open-label placebo: A pilot pharmacobehavioral approach for opioid dose reduction and pain control. *Pain Reports.* 2020;5(4):e828. doi:10.1097/PR9.0000000000000828.

34. Belcher AM, Cole TO, Massey E, Billing AS, Wagner M, Wooten W, Epstein DH, Hoag SW, Wickwire EM, Greenblatt AD, Colloca L, Rotrosen J, Magder L, Weintraub E, Wish ED, Kaptchuk TJ. Effectiveness of conditioned open-label placebo with methadone in treatment of opioid use disorder: A Randomized Clinical Trial. *JAMA Network Open.* 2023;6(4):e237099. doi:10.1001/jamanetworkopen.2023.7099.

35. Amanzio M, Benedetti F. Neuropharmacological dissection of placebo analgesia: Expectation-activated opioid systems versus conditioning-activated specific subsystems. *Journal of Neuroscience.* 1999;19:484–494.

36. Schafer SM, Geuter S, Wager TD. Mechanisms of placebo analgesia: A dual-process model informed by insights from cross-species comparisons. *Progress in Neurobiology.* 2018;160:101–122. http://doi:10.1016/j.pneurobio.2017.10.008

37. Nir R-R, Yarnitsky D. Conditioned pain modulation. *Current Opinion in Supportive and Palliative Care.* 2015;9:131–137. http://doi:10.1097/SPC.0000000000000126

38. Alter BJ, Aung MS, Strigo IA, Fields HL. Onset hyperalgesia and offset analgesia: Transient increases or decreases of noxious thermal stimulus intensity robustly modulate subsequent perceived pain intensity. *PLoS ONE.* 2020;15(12):e0231124. doi:10.1371/journal.pone.0231124.

39. Fernandes C, Pidal-Miranda M, Samartin-Veiga N, Carrillo-de-la-Peña MT. Conditioned pain modulation as a biomarker of chronic pain: A systematic review of its concurrent validity. *Pain.* 2019;160(12):2679–2690. doi:10.1097/j.pain.0000000000001664.

40. Petersen KK, Vaegter HB, Stubhaug A, Wolff A, Scammell BE, Arendt-Nielsen L, Larsen DB. The predictive value of quantitative sensory testing: A systematic review on chronic postoperative pain and the analgesic effect of pharmacological therapies in patients with chronic pain. *Pain.* 2021;162(1):31–44. doi:10.1097/j.pain.0000000000002019.

41. Crum AJ, Leibowitz KA, Verghese A. Making mindset matter. *British Medical Journal.* 2017;356:j674. doi:10.1136/bmj.j674. Erratum in: *BMJ.* 2017 Nov 15;359:j5308.

42. Benedetti F. How the doctor's words affect the patient's brain. *Evaluation & the Health Professions.* 2002;25(4):369–386. http://doi:10.1177/0163278702238051

43. Benedetti F, Pollo A, Lopiano L, Lanotte M, Vighetti S, Rainero I. Conscious expectation and unconscious conditioning in analgesic, motor, and hormonal placebo/nocebo responses. *Journal of Neuroscience.* 2003; 23(10):4315–4323. doi:10.1523/JNEUROSCI.23-10-04315.2003.

44. Price DD, Finniss DG, Benedetti F. A comprehensive review of the placebo effect: Recent advances and current thought. *Annual Review of Psychology*. 2008;59:565–590.

45. Crum A, Zuckerman B. Changing mindsets to enhance treatment effectiveness. *JAMA*. 2017;317(20):2063–2064. doi:10.1001/jama.2017.4545.

46. Dweck CS. *Mindset: The New Psychology of Success*. Random House; 2006.

47. Crum AJ, Langer EJ. Mind-set matters. *Psychological Science*. 2007;18(2):165–171. http://doi:10.1111/j.1467-9280.2007.01867.x

48. Zion SR, Schapira L, Crum AJ. Targeting mindsets, not just tumors. *Trends in Cancer*. 2019;(10):573–576. doi:10.1016/j.trecan.2019.08.001.

49. Canning EA, Murphy MC, Emerson KTU, Chatman JA, Dweck CS, Kray LJ. Cultures of genius at work: Organizational mindsets predict cultural norms, trust, and commitment. *Personality and Social Psychology Bulletin*. 2020;46(4):626–642. doi:10.1177/0146167219872473.

50. Benedetti F, Piedimonte A, Frisaldi E. How do placebos work? *European Journal of Psychotraumatology*. 2018;9(Suppl 3):1533370. http://doi:10.1080/20008198.2018.1533370

51. Darnall BD, Colloca L. Optimizing placebo and minimizing nocebo to reduce pain, catastrophizing, and opioid use: A review of the Science and an Evidence-Informed Clinical Toolkit. *International Review of Neurobiology*. 2018;139:129–157. doi:10.1016/bs.irn.2018.07.022. Epub 2018 Aug 6.

52. Benedetti F, Maggi G, Lopiano L, Lanotte M, Rainero I, Vighetti S, Pollo A. Open versus hidden medical treatments: The patient's knowledge about a therapy affects the therapy outcome. *Prevention & Treatment*. 2003;6(1):1a. http://doi:10.1037/1522-3736.6.1.61a

53. Colloca L, Lopiano L, Lanotte M, Benedetti F. Overt versus covert treatment for pain, anxiety, and Parkinson's disease. *Lancet Neurology*. 2004;3(11):679–684. doi:10.1016/S1474-4422(04)00908-1.

54. Van Laarhoven AIM, Vogelaar ML, Wilder-Smith OH, van Riel PLCM, van de Kerkhof PCM, Kraaimaat FW, Evers AWM. Induction of nocebo and placebo effects on itch and pain by verbal suggestions. *Pain*. 2011;152(7):1486–1494. doi:10.1016/j.pain.2011.01.043. Epub 2011 Feb 24.

55. Colloca L, Finniss DG. Nocebo effects, patient-clinician communication, and therapeutic outcomes. *JAMA*. 2012;307(6):567–568. http://doi:10.1001/jama.2012.115

56. Zion SR, Schapira L, Crum AJ. Targeting mindsets, not just tumors. *Trends Cancer*. 2019 Oct;5(10):573–576. doi:10.1016/j.trecan.2019.08.001.

57. Kaptchuk TJ, Kelley JM, Conboy LA, Davis RB, Kerr CE, Jacobson EE, Kirsch I, Schyner RN, Nam BH, Nguyen LT, Park M, Rivers AL, McManus C, Kokkotou E, Drossman DA, Goldman P, Lembo AJ. Components of placebo effect: Randomised controlled trial in patients with irritable bowel syndrome. *British Medical Journal*. 2008;336(7651):999–1003. doi:10.1136/bmj.39524.439618.25.

58. Kelley JM, Lembo AJ, Ablon JS, Villanueva JJ, Conboy LA, Levy R, Marci CD, Kerr CE, Kirsch I, Jacobson EE, Riess H, Kaptchuk TJ. Patient and practitioner influences on the placebo effect in irritable bowel syndrome. *Psychosomatic Medicine*. 2009;71(7):789–797. doi:10.1097/PSY.0b013e3181acee12.

59. Benedetti F. Placebo and the new physiology of the doctor-patient relationship. *Physiological Reviews*. 2013;93(3):1207–1246. doi:10.1152/physrev.00043.2012.

60. Blasini M, Peiris N, Wright T, Colloca L. The role of patient–practitioner relationships in placebo and nocebo phenomena. *International Review of Neurobiology*. 2018;139:211–231. doi:10.1016/bs.irn.2018.07.033. Epub 2018 Aug 9.

61. Costanzo C, Verghese A. The physical examination as ritual: Social Sciences and embodiment in the context of the physical examination. *Medical Clinics of North America*. 2018;102(3): 425–431. doi:10.1016/j.mcna.2017.12.004.

62. Leibowitz KA, Hardebeck EJ, Goyer JP, Crum AJ. Physician assurance reduces patient symptoms in US adults: An experimental study. *Journal of General Internal Medicine.* 2018;33(12):2051–2052. doi:10.1007/s11606-018-4627-z.
63. Howe LC, Leibowitz KA, Crum AJ. When your doctor "gets it" and "gets you": The critical role of competence and warmth in the patient-provider interaction. *Frontiers in Psychiatry.* 2019 Jul 4;10:475. doi:10.3389/fpsyt.2019.00475.

1.4

Cultural influences on placebo and nocebo effects

Rachel L. Cundiff-O'Sullivan, Desai Oula, Roni Shafir, and Luana Colloca

Introduction

Let us imagine a scenario in which a young scientist receives a unique opportunity to test the analgesic power of placebos with the Sinhalese peoples of North Sentinel Island, one of the last remaining uncontacted tribes in the world. Wearing her white coat, the scientist assesses participants' pain tolerance with and without providing them with a strong pain reliever pill (in fact a placebo). After addressing the Sinhaleses' confusion as to how they should take the pill, she assesses their pain and, to her surprise, finds no placebo effects. She wonders What made the Sinhalese people not susceptible to the well-known placebo effects?

The isolated Sentinelese do not have the same context and understanding of the therapeutic meaning of the small, round object as that of the young scientist, trained within a Western biomedical system. In modern biomedical systems, pills are usually associated with an expectation of relief or improvement in conditions. This expectation is shaped by the shared acceptance of pills as common biomedical treatments, previous self-experience with taking pills, and learning from social interactions that pills are accepted and effective treatments. In other words, our culture influences the meaning and expectation we place on the action of taking a pill. This meaning and expectation, significant components underlying placebo and nocebo effects, are rooted in culture.

Culture includes beliefs, behaviors, jargon, norms, worldview, and values shared by members of a group, which can be defined by ethnicity, occupation, or geographical location, to name a few.[1] Although some criticize the use of the term *culture* as being too broad in categorizing people based on generalizations that do not apply to each individual in the group,[2] it is undeniable that these shared beliefs and experiences significantly influence our understanding of health and illness. In this chapter, we discuss only some of the many factors that relate to one's cultural beliefs and how these in turn can influence a person's responsiveness to placebos and nocebos.

Social norms, aesthetic preferences, and placebos in the media and marketing

Underlying culture are social norms, preferences, and daily experiences that can have a significant impact on the way health, illness, and treatments are conceptualized, understood, and accepted. Different cultures have ascribed different meanings to the elements that surround the treatment context,[3] changing the meaning of the symbols and rituals of healthcare that play into the placebo and nocebo responses.

Aesthetics

Different emotions can be attributed to colors[3,4] based on meanings derived from rites and rituals, visual perceptions, and historical influences that differ among cultures.[4] For example, Chinese people often prefer colors that are considered fresh, clean, or modern in treatment contexts.[3] White Americans perceive white capsules as analgesic, whereas Black/African Americans perceive black capsules as analgesic.[4]

However, there are similarities across cultures with regards to the meaning of colors. For example, blue is often seen as sedative, while[3,4] red and green are universally associated with danger and safety, respectively.[4] Stimulant medications tend to be marketed and perceived as more effective when warm colors (reds, oranges, yellows) are used, whereas cool colors (blues, greens, purples) are used for sedative medications.[3–6] In one experiment, those that took pink placebo pills felt more stimulating effects, whereas those that took blue placebo pills felt more sedating effects, suggesting that color not only influences perception but can shape placebo effects as well.[5,6] In a study of participants from the United States, China, and Colombia, white pills were considered the most effective in treating headache.[6] Color not only influences the physical treatment but also the surroundings, as one study found that blue hospital walls decreased anxiety in a virtual setting.[6]

The size of oral medications also influences treatment expectations. Larger capsules are considered more potent than smaller capsules, but for Black individuals, this relationship is reversed.[4,6] Both large and very small tablets are thought to be more potent than aspirin-sized tablets.[7] These visual cues draw on socially observed norms and preferences, experiences, and other learned associations to inform what patients expect, thereby shaping placebo and nocebo responses.

Administration

The context where treatments are administered can also influence patients' perceptions and expectations of treatment. Generally, the greater number of doses involved in a treatment regimen, the more intense and potent the treatment is perceived to be.[3,5,6] In a systematic review of 79 studies, healing rates were higher at 4-weeks post abdominal surgery for patients who received treatment four times a day as compared to twice a day.[6]

The setting may improve treatment responses depending on how similarly it meets patients' expectations. A Chinese American seeking acupuncture may be more likely to prefer a Chinese practitioner who is continuing a family tradition in a setting that fits the traditional aesthetic of ancient Chinese medical practices, whereas a White or European American seeking acupuncture may more likely choose a certified professional in a sterilized setting fitting the traditional aesthetic of Western biomedical hospitals.[8] Placebo effects are likely to occur in a setting that aligns with patients' medical belief systems.

The route of administration or type of treatment is another important factor shaping treatment expectations. More elaborate, detailed, time-consuming, fashionable, or dangerous treatments are perceived as being more effective.[9] In the United States, capsules and injections are perceived as stronger than tablets,[3,7] and treatments using lasers are perceived as even more effective.[5] However, some of these studies are dated, and it is likely that the novelty of these treatments when examined influenced these associations.[6] Indeed, later studies found that capsules and oval tablets were only preferred for antibiotic treatments, whereas round tablets were preferred for almost all other types of treatments.[6] The symptoms being treated can also influence which treatment types are viewed as most effective: for pain, injections were viewed as better, whereas topical medications were viewed as better for itch.[6]

Treatments utilizing technology or devices are considered more effective than oral treatments (e.g., pills and tables),[9–11] and, in general, patients view invasive procedures (e.g., surgery) as the most effective kind of treatments.[12] The more invasive the method, the stronger the expectation of positive outcomes, leading to larger placebo effects.[6,11] For instance, one meta-analysis on placebo use in migraine prophylaxis found that more invasive treatments were perceived to be more beneficial.[11] The authors suggested that the extensive ritual of surgery, in addition to increased clinical attention, likely underlies the greater expectation of symptom relief.[11] These differing characteristics of the treatment can influence its meaning, which in turn affects expected outcomes and placebo and nocebo responses.

Marketing

How treatments are marketed can heavily shape perceptions and expectations. Brand-name active tablets were found to be more effective than brand-name-labeled placebo tablets, which were better than generic-labeled active and placebo tablets.[5,7] In another study, headache relief was lowest when the pills were labeled as a placebo and greater when pills were labeled as active or uncertain (i.e., could be active or placebo).[13] Treatments with names that are popular or familiar will be viewed as more likely than treatments with generic or unfamiliar names to improve symptoms.[6,7] Generic-labeled medications may even induce nocebo effects, with some studies reporting that participants experience more side effects with generic-labeled than active-labeled placebo pills.[6] Lack of knowledge and misperceptions about biosimilars (i.e., non-brand-name biologic medications) have also resulted in significant nocebo responses.[14]

In countries like the United States, where technological advancement is highly valued, "newer" is often considered "better,"[1] so as new drugs are introduced to the public with heavy marketing campaigns, healthcare providers and the general population become excited for the newer treatments, and older treatments become less effective.[7] Reciprocally, countries like China, Britain, and Austria, where tradition is of high value, "newer" can mean "untested," so traditional treatments that have been used by millions of people for thousands of years tend to be preferred.[1,8,15] In this case, the use of newer treatments may induce nocebo responses because of fear or uncertainty of side effects. However, in their meta-analysis of tricyclic and SSRI antidepressants, Walsh and colleagues found that both active and placebo response rates have increased since going on the market.[16] The perception that pills are effective treatments for depression changed as antidepressants became more prevalent in society, thereby actually altering their effectiveness.[7] As attitudes change and understanding evolves over time, so too do opinions and expectations.[17]

The condition to which a drug is marketed may lead to differing rates of placebo responses, both between and within cultures. In a study comparing

Brazilian, Danish, and German participants in clinical trials, German participants exhibited the highest placebo rate for treating ulcers but the lowest in treating hypertension.[5,7] Moerman noted that this may be because Germans are particularly concerned about having low blood pressure, so treating hypertension is of low priority.[5] Similarly, the belief among the Hmong people that epilepsy is attributable to possession by a powerful spirit rather than desynchronized neuronal firing makes them less anxious about treating this condition.[1] In both these examples, when patients receive treatment for conditions they are less concerned about, they will not respond strongly to placebos. Without the desire to produce valued treatment outcomes, expectations are inhibited, limiting the occurrence of placebo effects.

The cost of medication also influences expectations of treatment effectiveness. Typically, price is correlated with perceived quality of a product,[6] so treatment response is usually greater when a patient believes the drug is more expensive.[18] Marketing a treatment at a higher cost (or simply nondiscounted) can increase placebo effects, and marketing a treatment at a lower or discounted cost can increase nocebo responses.[6] One study assigned healthy male participants to two groups who were given two identical inert creams but, one was described as an expensive analgesic and the other as a low-priced analgesic. The study found that a greater reduction of pain intensity was reported with use of the "expensive" cream.[19] However, treatments that are too expensive would likely eliminate placebo effects if, for instance, patients are not financially able to receive the entire treatment at once.[8]

Media

There is no doubt that the opinions of others can significantly sway perceptions of illness and expectations of treatment, including perception and acceptance of placebos.[20] Many media reports of randomized, placebo-controlled clinical trials use the placebo response rate to determine whether the results are credible or not.[18] These media reports are often used to decide what treatments are safe and effective and what treatments should be avoided, which can lead to potential nocebo responses if the study is misrepresented. In a widely publicized study on statin tolerance,[21] the pattern of side effects that causes many people to abandon statin use was nearly identical for both active and placebo arms. The authors suggested that patients are primed for nocebo effects from family and friends, media and the internet, and side effects listed in the drug leaflets, leading to the high rate of nonpharmacological side effects.[21]

Media reports contribute to the popular idea that placebos are equivalent to sham, fake, or deceptive practices.[18] In qualitative interviews, Thompson, Ritenbaugh, and Nichter reported that most patients viewed placebos as harmless or useless substances of which one should be skeptical.[18] On the one hand, if placebos are seen as harmless to try, the optimism and willingness to try them can itself create positive expectations or induce a (conditioned) response. On the other hand, the skepticism and belief that a particular treatment will not have any effect can make it much less likely for placebo effects to be elicited. Overall, how placebos are reported in media can weigh heavily in illness perception and treatment outcomes. An example of this phenomenon is the influence of media on perception of Covid-19 symptoms and reactogenicity of the vaccine (see Chapter 3.6).

Spirituality: coping and rituals

Spiritual and religious subcultures guide their believers' worldview and establish what values are of greatest importance to people's lives, which can be a major component underlying their medical beliefs and placebo responsiveness. While spirituality broadly encompasses the beliefs, practices, and experiences concerning the meaning of life and transcendence, religion is the sociocultural dimension, giving a framework for the interpretation of spirituality by providing rituals and other explanatory models for understanding the world.[22,23] Spirituality is strongly interconnected with the illness and healing experiences, offering a means of expression through rituals and symbols, and mobilizing social support to validate suffering and aid in the return to health—all of which also influence placebo and nocebo effects.[22]

Coping, social support, and avoidance of health risks

Studies on spirituality have generally found more support for a positive effect on health outcomes.[23] One large study on health and religiosity in over 4,000 Americans found that those who identified as being religious also tended to report better overall health and happiness.[24] Having the belief that suffering is temporary or necessary to ultimately achieve some transcendental states (such as going to heaven or achieving nirvana)[25] can improve coping and decrease anxiety related to distressing illness experiences.[23] Those that are highly spiritual were found to be better able to reinterpret the perception and meaning of pain and its associated distress as temporary.[22] This mechanism of coping may guide patients' health behaviors and affect their likelihood to respond to a placebo. Indeed, Hyland et al. found that spirituality was predictive of placebo effects, independent of expectancy.[26]

One component of coping that may contribute to better health is increased social support and engagement through religious participation.[22] Colloca and Benedetti were among the first to experimentally demonstrate that observing positive responses to a treatment through social learning induced large placebo effects to a similar degree as first-hand experience.[27] Strong social networks are known to be beneficial for health,[24] so it follows that social learning within a social network can have a particularly important role in placebo and nocebo effects. Theoretically, this may make religious and spiritual people more likely to respond to a placebo, but it has not been verified whether it is because religious and spiritual people have stronger social networks than nonreligious or nonspiritual people do or if it is due to their religious beliefs and spirituality per se.[20]

A second mechanism that many believe underlies the positive relationship between spirituality and improved health is the avoidance of health risks because of specific spiritual and religious teachings.[22] Religious beliefs can influence a variety of health-related behaviors like dietary preferences, such as a Jewish person keeping kosher; restrictions on types of medical treatments allowed, such as a Jehovah's witness refusing all blood products; or who can examine a patient, such as the avoidance of contact with the opposite sex in Islamic traditions.[25] These rules and behaviors help conceptualize health and illness within the framework of spiritual beliefs, providing purpose and meaning that can be utilized to boost placebo effects. However, some people may feel that illness is a consequence of sacrilegious behavior or other infraction committed against their God(s), like breaking the rules of their religion. This could result in adverse health outcomes and nocebo effects, particularly if the faith component is not addressed in conjunction with the biomedical component.[1]

External locus of control

Those endorsing an external locus of control (ELOC) (i.e., a belief that powerful others, chance, or fate have more control over life events than one's own actions) generally report poorer health behaviors and decreased self-efficacy.[23,28,29] Although the relationship between ELOC and spirituality and religiosity is disputed,[23,28] the evidence suggests that those who believe in a higher power tend to have greater ELOC,[23] yet the specific belief that God(s) are in control is associated with positive health outcomes.[23,29] In a sample of predominantly Catholic Christians in Australia, ELOC was associated with poorer overall health, but specific God locus of control was associated with better health.[29]

In their systematic review, Horing et al. found that ELOC was a consistent predictor of placebo responsiveness.[30] This may be because those who have the predominant view that chance or powerful others, like God(s), have control over life events may be more attuned and reliant on external or social cues to help inform their expectations of treatment outcomes. Alternatively, those with stronger faith that a deity will take care of them may act with the understanding that their own actions have little consequence: "It's in God's hands."[1] With their self-efficacy diminished, these patients may exhibit no or dampened placebo effects.

Negative effects of spirituality

Despite typically positive associations between spirituality and health, there are numerous ways in which spiritual and religious beliefs can negatively affect health behaviors and perceptions. In fact, in a review of 91 studies on spirituality and health, 47 showed a negative relationship.[22] Some spiritual experiences can cause distress, feelings of crisis, or other negative physiological and psychological effects.[22]

For example, some Latin American and African tribal cultures believe that bewitching leads to rapid voodoo death; similarly, some aboriginal Australian cultures believe that pointing a bone at a person results in their quick death.[31] Anthropologist Walter B. Cannon in 1942 noted that death from these types of ritual or symbolic phenomena were likely due to heightened emotional stress and chronic activation of the sympathetic nervous system.[31] Today, it is accepted that chronic stress can alter a variety of biological processes.[32] Therefore, intensely stressful spiritual beliefs can lead to powerful nocebo effects that can affect mortality, potentially through biological mechanisms of chronic stress.

As another example, in a large-scale study on spiritual beliefs and health, Chinese Americans diagnosed with lymphatic cancer that were born in Chinese astrological "earth years," who are thought to be susceptible to diseases involving lumps, nodules, or tumors, died an average of 4 years earlier than White Americans and Chinese Americans born in non-earth years.[5] The age at death strongly correlated with the strength of commitment to Chinese cultural beliefs.[5] Their astrological beliefs likely led those born in earth years to experience more nocebo effects, which could have negatively affected their health behavior.[10] Distressing spiritual and religious beliefs can thus have a negative influences on the perception of health and expectations of illness, making nocebo effects more likely to occur.

Rituals and traditional modes of healing

The belief that germs cause disease is not shared across cultures. Many believe that illness is due to spirit possession, voodoo, soul loss or theft, a breach of taboo, or punishment from some deity.[1,24] The effectiveness of many "traditional" healing rituals that address these other causes are attributed to placebo effects.[8,10,18] It is a combination of patient responsiveness to the ritual, the relationship with the healer, trust in the healer's mastery and abilities, and the sheer belief that the ritual will result in relief—all components of placebo effects—that produces the beneficial outcomes, despite a lack of understanding of the underlying physiology.[9,18] However, many have argued that it is not just the belief that the ritual will work, but that the physical act of *doing* the ritual is critical.[9,18,33]

In many cultures and throughout history, religious leaders were the main healthcare providers.[25] Spirituality and healing were inseparable. The secularization of modern Western biomedicine has made it difficult for those operating within that belief system to utilize these other modalities of healing,[8,24] even if shown to have powerful effects. The lack of an understood biological mechanism has historically led Western societies to write-off traditional modes of healing as primitive, irrational, or based on merely the suggestibility of the participants in the ritual.[15]

However, Western biomedicine is not without its own rituals.[5,9,10,34] Many propose that simply seeking care or receiving a diagnosis are important forms of ritual healing.[5,9,10,34] Welch goes as far as comparing the process of seeking medical care within the Western biomedical framework to a "pilgrimage" of healing.[9] A patient goes to a "temple of healing" (a hospital), where their identity is transformed from citizen to "pilgrim" (patient), donning a "new name" (medical record number) and removing the "identifiers from the outside world" (changing into a gown).[9] A "temple priest" (doctor), wearing "robes" (white coat) ask the pilgrim to "confess" (discuss their health concern) and assesses them using "sacred instruments" (stethoscope).[9] They consult with "sacred texts" (test results) to procure a diagnosis, devising a healing regimen often including a "sacrament" (pill) or ointment "to be anointed" in order to return from medical pilgrim back to healthy citizen.[9] Welch also describes how surgery may be viewed as "being born again," as the pilgrim undergoes surgery when sick and wakes up from anesthesia healed.[9] The understanding that symbols form the bedrock of medical practice in *all* cultures is of vital importance, as these symbols can be leveraged to maximize the likelihood of placebo effects.

Language, the patient-provider interaction, and historical distrust

The goal of the provider is to instill hope and confidence, promote self-efficacy, and provide education to adjust the patient's expectations and improve treatment response.[5,10,34] To this end, placebos were used by physicians for centuries to give patients hope when no other treatments were available.[18,33,35] The art of Medicine lies in the provider's ability to engage with the patient in a positive manner, demonstrating care and maintaining trust.[8,10,12]

Verbal and nonverbal language

The way in which an illness is described can differ by culture, which influences not only the types of treatments sought but also the response to treatments.[1] Importantly, the practitioner's language has a powerful influence on patient's placebo effects. Their words can communicate, implicitly or explicitly, cultural biases and beliefs which will alter the patient's expectations.[34] Brody noted elements of verbal instructions that providers can implement to optimize healing: providing an understandable and satisfying explanation of the illness, demonstrating care and concern about the patient's distress, promising control over symptoms, and giving hope.[36] Even a short explanation of treatment mechanism of action can significantly improve treatment response.[7,34] Equally important is to avoid overemphasizing negative information while maintaining honesty to help reduce potential nocebo effects.[34]

Nonverbal language is also of vital importance, as nearly 55% of a message is said to derive from body language.[34] To demonstrate this, Gracely and colleagues randomized dental patients to receive placebo, naloxone, or fentanyl prior to a dental procedure.[37] Some of the participating clinicians were told that because of a "problem" with the study, they could no longer administer fentanyl. Half of these clinicians were later told that the "problem" had been fixed, so fentanyl could be administered again. Those treated by clinicians who thought fentanyl could not be administered did not experience any pain relief with fentanyl, but those who were treated by clinicians who knew fentanyl could be administered experienced pain relief even with placebo. The biases of the clinician, not explicitly discussed with the patient, were conveyed through their body language, which influenced the patients' placebo effects. Different cultures have different ways of expressing nonverbal communication, which can cause confusion or friction between the patient and the provider when the styles of nonverbal communication do not match. For example, US physicians were more accurate at decoding the facial expressions of Caucasian than South Asian patients, and as a result, South Asian patients were less likely to be satisfied with their physician and adhere to their prescribed treatments.[38] The language used by the provider, both verbal and nonverbal, can validate or invalidate patients' suffering[10,15,34] and give them the opportunity to "make meaning" out of the clinical experience,[7] significantly affecting the trust in the provider, treatment expectations, and, ultimately, placebo and nocebo responses.

Trust as the principal element of the interaction

To some degree, placebo effects are present in every healthcare encounter.[5,12,18,34] The interaction with the patient must be warm, friendly, empathetic, nonjudgmental, and supportive, conveyed by active listening, receptiveness and responsiveness to concerns, and showing care through body language and facial expressions.[34] Barrett et al. listed a series of actions a provider can take to maximize placebo effects, including empowering the patient with encouragement and education, learning about the patient's values and belief system, and creating a ritual to facilitate and shape the meaning and expectations of the healthcare encounter.[35]

A critical element of this interaction is maintaining trust.[18,34,35] Trust in the physician's ability and judgment can shape a patient's expectations and their response to any treatments. If, for example, a physician were to be overenthusiastic about a treatment and this positive expectancy was not confirmed, the treatment may end up eliciting a nocebo effect, and the patient will lose trust in the physician.[18] This distrust would color every encounter thereafter, enhancing the likelihood of developing further nocebo effects with other treatments.

There may be systematic differences in the way the patient and provider interact within the broader healthcare system that might account for varying rates of placebo responses in different countries.[5,34] Therefore, from the patient's perspective, finding a "good fit" with a healthcare provider who addresses concerns while acknowledging and respecting cultural values and beliefs is vital.[18] For example, the rural Sinhalese in Sri Lanka feel that the habit and authority of their practitioner is more important than developing a warm and empathetic relationship.[18] How well the provider "plays the role" of healer according to the patient's belief system will affect the trust in the provider's capabilities, resulting in enhanced placebo effects.

Distrust of medical authority

In some cultures, healers are viewed with reverence, and patients do as they are told without question because of trust and respect in the healer's expertise. In others, there is a deep, historical distrust of medical authority, and patients who seek care from within "the system" are often skeptical of the healer's expertise or honesty.[1]

For example, practitioners in South Asia may spend little time with their patients, but there is a high degree of trust in their medical authority, so this does not adversely affect the patient-provider relationship.[15] Conversely, in places like the United States, the short, business-like interaction can decrease patients' confidence in the physician's competence and reinforce negative perceptions of the healthcare system.[34] The pattern of use of complementary and alternative medicines (CAMs) in the United States reflects this distrust. It was mainly devout Christians who utilized CAMs first because of a mistrust of secular institutions.[15] Even today, there is a sentiment that CAMs are less biased by commercial interests, so this distrust of medical authority still underlies much of its use today.[15]

Historical discrimination is a major component underlying distrust in medical authority.[39-41] In the United States, the racial trauma inflicted on Black/African Americans has led to a deep-seated distrust of institutions established by the White majority.[39-41] Exploitation of Black/African Americans has led to experimentation like the forced sterilization and testing of anesthetics on Black women, the Tuskegee Syphilis Study, and a study done in the 1990s in Black/African American boys that included multiple ethical violations, including withholding water and administering drugs thought to increase aggressiveness.[39,41] Such abuses of power have left many racial minorities to be "primed" to find discrimination in clinical encounters.[1,39] Even when physicians mean well, their words, tone, or behaviors could be perceived as prejudicial,[1] which will result in significant damage to the relationship, a decline in trust or respect of the physician, and, ultimately, enhanced likelihood of nocebo effects.

Sustained racial disparities in healthcare continue to reinforce that the medical institution should not be trusted.[41] For example, the persistent belief that African Americans experience pain differently than White Americans do has led to consistent under prescribing of pain-relieving medications.[41] Studies have found that physicians rate African American patients as less effective communicators,[41] and patients of racial minorities are given less empathy, attention, and information than White patients are given.[39–41] These elements of the patient-provider relationship are important in maximizing the placebo phenomenon. At best, this leaves racial minorities with less opportunity to benefit from placebos; at worst, it supports continued disparities and increased nocebo effects.[40] Okusogu et al. reported that Black/African Americans showed smaller placebo effects than Whites did, but interestingly, the race and sex of the experimenter influenced responsiveness to placebo, such that concordance between the experimenter's and participant's race resulted in improved placebo effects.[42] This may suggest that implicit biases on both the provider and patient's sides can have an influence on placebo and nocebo effects.

Although most of the current literature focuses on the mistrust among Black/African Americans, medical injustices have occurred to other marginalized racial and ethnic communities, both within the United States and internationally. While much work needs to be done to remedy the effects of racial discrimination and biases in Medicine, thoughtful dialogue, discussion, and action can significantly improve expectations to optimize healing and placebo effects and minimize nocebo effects.

In summary, culture encompasses many components that help form our beliefs, values, worldview, and understanding of our experiences. This chapter has given an overview of only some of the elements that can influence perceptions and expectations of illness and treatment including placebo and nocebo outcomes.

Acknowledgments

This work is supported by National Center for Complementary and Integrative Health (NCCIH) (R01 AT011347-01A1 and R01AT01033, LC). The funding agencies have no role in the study. The views expressed here are the authors own and do not reflect the position or policy of the National Institutes of Health or any other part of the federal government.

References

1. Galanti G-A. *Basic Concepts. Caring for Patients from Different Cultures.* 5th ed. University of Pennsylvania Press; 2014.
2. Fuentes A. What is culture? In *Why We Believe:* Evolution and the *Human Way* of Being. Yale University Press; 2019:77–96.
3. Ventriglio A, Magnifico G, Borraccino L, Rinaldi A, Bellomo A. Placebo and cultural responses. *Nordic Journal of Psychiatry.* 2018;72(Suppl 1):S33–S35. http://doi:10.1080/08039488.2018.1525637
4. Bhugra D, Ventriglio A, Till A, Malhi G. Colour, culture and placebo response. *Indian Journal of Social Psychiatry.* 2015;61(6):615–617. http://doi:10.1177/0020764015591492
5. Moerman DE. Cultural variations in the placebo effect: Ulcers, anxiety, and blood pressure. *Medical Anthropology Quarterly.* 2000;14(1):51–72.
6. Meissner K, Linde K. Are blue pills better than green? How treatment features modulate placebo effects. *International Review of Neurobiology.* 2018;139:357–378. http://doi:10.1016/bs.irn.2018.07.014
7. Moerman DE, Harrington A. Making space for the placebo effect in pain medicine. *Seminars in Pain Medicine.* 2005;3(1):2–6. http://doi:10.1016/j.spmd.2005.02.008
8. Micozzi MS. Culture, anthropology, and the return of "Complementary Medicine." *Medical Anthropology Quarterly.* 2002;16(4):398–403.
9. Welch JS. Ritual in Western medicine and its role in placebo healing. *Journal of Religion and Health.* 2003;42(1):21–33.
10. Miller FG, Colloca L, Kaptchuk TJ. The placebo effect: Illness and interpersonal healing. *Perspectives in Biology and Medicine.* 2009;52(4):518–39. http://doi:10.1353/pbm.0.0115
11. Meissner K, Fassler M, Rucker G, et al. Differential effectiveness of placebo treatments: A systematic review of migraine prophylaxis. *JAMA Internal Medicine.* 2013;173(21):1941–1951. http://doi:10.1001/jamainternmed.2013.10391
12. Moerman DE, Jonas WB. Deconstructing the placebo effect and finding the meaning response. *Annals of Internal Medicine.* 2002;136(6):471–476.
13. Kam-Hansen S, Jakubowski M, Kelley JM, et al. Altered placebo and drug labeling changes the outcome of episodic migraine attacks. *Science Translational Medicine.* 2014;6(218):218ra5. http://doi:10.1126/scitranslmed.3006175
14. Colloca L, Panaccione R, Murphy TK. The clinical implications of nocebo effects for biosimilar therapy. *Frontiers in Pharmacology.* 2019;10:1372. http://doi:10.3389/fphar.2019.01372
15. Kirmayer LJ. Medicines of the Imagination: Cultural phenomenology, medical pluralism, and the persistence of mind-body dualism. In: Naraindas H, Quack J, Sax WS, eds. *Asymmetrical Conversations: Contestations, Circumventions, and the Blurring of Therapeutic Boundaries.* Berghahn Books; 2014:26–55.
16. Walsh TB, Seidman SN, Sysko R, Gould M. Placebo response in studies of major depression: Variable, substantial, and growing. *JAMA.* 2002;287(14):1840–1847.
17. Tuttle AH, Tohyama S, Ramsay T, et al. Increasing placebo responses over time in U.S. clinical trials of neuropathic pain. *Pain.* 2015;156(12):2616–2626. http://doi:10.1097/j.pain.0000000000000333
18. Thompson JJ, Ritenbaugh C, Nichter M. Reconsidering the placebo response from a broad anthropological perspective. *Culture, Medicine, and Psychiatry.* 2009;33(1):112–152. http://doi:10.1007/s11013-008-9122-2
19. Geuter S, Eippert F, Hindi Attar C, Buchel C. Cortical and subcortical responses to high and low effective placebo treatments. *Neuroimage.* 2013;67:227–236. http://doi:10.1016/j.neuroimage.2012.11.029

20. Enck P, Klosterhalfen S, Weimer K. Unsolved, forgotten, and ignored features of the placebo response in medicine. *Clinical Therapeutics*. 2017;39(3):458–468. http://doi:10.1016/j.clinthera.2016.11.016

21. Howard JP, Wood FA, Finegold JA, et al. Side effect patterns in a crossover trial of statin, placebo, and no treatment. *Journal of the American College of Cardiology*. 2021;78(12):1210–1222. http://doi:10.1016/j.jacc.2021.07.022

22. Kohls N, Sauer S, Offenbacher M, Giordano J. Spirituality: An overlooked predictor of placebo effects? *Philosophical Transactions of the Royal Society B: Biological Sciences*. 2011;366(1572):1838–1848. http://doi:10.1098/rstb.2010.0389

23. Timmins F, Martin C. Spirituality and locus of control—A rapid literature review. *Spirituality in Clinical Practice*. 2019;6(2):83–99. http://doi:10.1037/scp0000192

24. Lindenfors P. Divine placebo: Health and the evolution of religion. *Human Ecology*. 2019;47(2):157–163. http://doi:10.1007/s10745-019-0066-7

25. Swihart DL, Yarrarapu SNS, Martin RL. Cultural religious competence in clinical practice. 2022 Nov 14. In: StatPearls [Internet]. Treasure Island (FL): StatPearls Publishing; 2023 Jan–.

26. Hyland ME. Motivation and placebos: Do different mechanisms occur in different contexts? *Philosophical Transactions of the Royal Society B: Biological Sciences*. 2011;366(1572):1828–1837. http://doi:10.1098/rstb.2010.0391

27. Colloca L, Benedetti F. Placebo analgesia induced by social observational learning. *Pain*. 2009;144(1–2):28–34. http://doi:10.1016/j.pain.2009.01.033

28. Boyd JM, Wilcox S. Examining the relationship between health locus of control and God locus of health control: Is God an internal or external source? *Journal of Health Psychology*. 2020;25(7):931–940. http://doi:10.1177/1359105317739099

29. Ryan ME, Francis AJ. Locus of control beliefs mediate the relationship between religious functioning and psychological health. *Journal of Religion and Health*. 2012;51(3):774–785. http://doi:10.1007/s10943-010-9386-z

30. Horing B, Weimer K, Muth ER, Enck P. Prediction of placebo responses: A systematic review of the literature. *Frontiers in Pharmacology*. 2014;5:1079. http://doi:10.3389/fpsyg.2014.01079

31. Hahn RA, Kleinman A. Belief as pathogen, belief as medicine: "Voodoo death" and the "placebo phenomenon" in anthropological perspective. *Medical Anthropology Quarterly*. 1983;14(4):3–19.

32. McEwen BS. Neurobiological and systemic effects of chronic stress. *Chronic Stress (Thousand Oaks)*. 2017;1:2470547017692328. http://doi:10.1177/2470547017692328

33. Ostenfeld-Rosenthal AM. Energy healing and the placebo effect: An anthropological perspective on the placebo effect. *Anthropology and Medicine*. 2012;19(3):327–38. http://doi:10.1080/13648470.2011.646943

34. Blasini M, Peiris N, Wright T, Colloca L. The role of patient-practitioner relationships in placebo and nocebo phenomena. *International Review of Neurobiology*. 2018;139:211–231. http://doi:10.1016/bs.irn.2018.07.033

35. Barrett B, Muller D, Rakel D, Rabago D, Marchand L, Scheder JC. Placebo, meaning, and health. *Perspectives in Biology and Medicine*. 2006;49(2):178–198. http://doi:10.1353/pbm.2006.0019

36. Brody H. The lie that heals: The ethics of giving placebos. *Annals of Internal Medicine*. 1982;97:112–118.

37. Gracely RH, Dubner R, Deeter WR, Wolskee PJ. Clinicians' expectations influence placebo analgesia. *Lancet*. 1985;1(8419):43. doi:10.1016/s0140-6736(85)90984-5

38. Coelho KR, Galan C. Physician cross-cultural nonverbal communication skills, patient satisfaction and health outcomes in the physician-patient relationship. *International Journal of Family Medicine*. 2012;2012:376907. http:// doi:10.1155/2012/376907

39. Scharff DP, Mathews KJ, Jackson P, Hoffsuemmer J, Martin E, Edwards D. More than Tuskegee: Understanding mistrust about research participation. *Journal of Health Care for the Poor and Underserved*. 2010;21(3):879–97. http://doi:10.1353/hpu.0.0323

40. Friesen P, Blease C. Placebo effects and racial and ethnic health disparities: An unjust and underexplored connection. *Journal of Medical Ethics and History of Medicine*. 2018;44(11):774–781. http://doi:10.1136/medethics-2018-104811

41. Strand NH, Mariano ER, Goree JH, et al. Racism in pain medicine: We can and should do more. *Mayo Clinic Proceedings*. 2021;96(6):1394–1400. http://doi:10.1016/j.mayocp.2021.02.030

42. Okusogu C, Wang Y, Akintola T, et al. Placebo hypoalgesia: Racial differences. *Pain*. 2020;161(8):1872–1883. http://doi:10.1097/j.pain.0000000000001876

2

PLACEBOS AND THEIR PREDICTABILITY

Placebo effects, mainly studied in lab settings with painful stimuli, involve learning mechanisms and brain activity patterns associated with sensorial and affective modulatory systems. However, these effects are context-specific and unpredictable, driven by immediate expectations and contextual factors. Recent research challenges this view, showing that placebo effects in chronic pain patients can be predicted by genetics, brain signatures, and language use, potentially aiding treatment.

Behavioral, genetic and neuroimaging studies offer insights into placebo factors but overlook the molecular changes. To explore these pathways, recent investigations explore genomic and pharmacological effects on placebo responses in trials. Genetic and neurological correlations of placebo responses are examined in various diseases like irritable bowel syndrome, pain, depression, inflammation, and other symptoms.

The interaction between genetics and environment plays a role in neurobiological dysregulation in chronic disorders, affecting responses to treatments, including placebos. Research focuses on identifying genes underlying placebo responses in drug and alcohol use disorders, highlighting similarities with chronic pain. Understanding their relationship is crucial for effective treatment and prevention.

The human proteome, encompassing proteins expressed by the genome, plays a vital role in biological pathways. Omics and proteomics, combined with computational tools, shows promise in identifying biomarkers to predict and monitor placebo responses in clinical trials.

This Section introduces open questions and challenges in discovering predictors of placebo responsiveness.

2.1

Predictability of placebo responses and their clinical implications

Paulo Branco, Etienne Vachon-Presseau, Kathryn T. Hall,
Tor D. Wager, and A. Vania Apkarian

Introduction

An extensive body of literature establishes the mechanisms that may underlie placebo effects at several levels of analysis, including psychological (e.g., expectations and learning) and brain (e.g., frontal-brainstem pathways, opioids, and other neurochemicals). Multiple learning mechanisms have been demonstrated to underlie placebo effects, and an extended brain circuitry associated with the phenomenon. Excellent reviews cover these topics,[1] and we will not address them here. The bulk of this research has been and continues to be performed in healthy subjects and in artificial, but well-controlled, laboratory settings. However, in the field of pain, placebo procedures remain most relevant in clinical trials. The great strength of randomized clinical trial (RCT) designs is that, if properly conducted, a significant active treatment vs. control effect (e.g., drug vs. placebo) generally allows one to infer a causal relationship between the successful treatment and the condition under study. From this viewpoint, it is not surprising that most clinical trials for treating acute and chronic pain continue to fail. Placebo treatment arms are almost universally used in such studies, and overall responses driven by placebos ("placebo responses") are often several times larger than the incremental active treatment effect. Two opposing interpretations can be derived from such observations: (1) the study is not well controlled, and various nuisance variables drive placebo responses and thus obscure the real biological treatment effects, or (2) the active arm has no, or minimal, causal benefit on the condition being studied.

Over the last decade, pain trialists have championed the concept that if one could minimize placebo responses, then RCTs would yield more significant active treatment effects. This interpretation essentially blames placebo responses magnitude for negative clinical trials. In this same period, improvements in placebo arms have grown larger, while drug effects remain stable, resulting in a shrinking drug versus placebo difference.[2] This increase parallels improvements in the quality of RCTs, the amount of time spent with patients, and the number of study visits. These observations give further impetus to the concept that placebo responses need to be controlled to increase the chances of positive RCTs. These issues are particularly relevant to chronic pain, where pharmacological treatments have not made any serious progress over the last 20 years or so, although preclinical studies continue to identify many potential druggable targets.

There is irrefutable evidence that chronic pain is a large unmet medical need urgently requiring novel nonaddictive therapies, as it diminishes quality of everyday life in about 20% of the world population, with a staggering annual healthcare cost of more than $600 billion just in the United States.[3] Often, chronic pain persists for a lifetime and commonly leads to depression,[4] insomnia, depressed immune function, changes in eating patterns,[5,6] substance abuse,[4] impaired cognitive function,[7] and costs to families and caregivers.[8]

Chronic pain patients are commonly treated with opioids, and thus remain a primary contributor to the ongoing opioid epidemic—particularly in the United States[9]—which has only worsened in the Covid-19 pandemic era. Available treatments for chronic pain do not cure the condition, and the majority of patients remain dissatisfied. For example, although nonsteroidal anti-inflammatory drugs (NSAIDs) are widely prescribed and used by the public, a Cochrane review of 65 clinical trials (11,237 total patients) found they are only modestly better than placebos for chronic and acute back pain. Updated Cochrane reviews reach the same conclusion. [10,11] NSAIDs were statistically comparable to other widely used treatments, including physiotherapy, spinal manipulation, paracetamol, opioids, and muscle relaxants.[12,13] Thus, there is a lack of effective treatments for chronic pain, and new nonopioidergic treatments remain urgently needed. The pharmaceutical industry has spent billions of dollars searching for novel drugs for chronic pain unsuccessfully.

In this chapter, we present the latest evidence that a substantial component of placebo effects can be predicted by biological and behavioral parameters: genetic biomarkers, brain anatomy and function, personality characteristics, and language usage. Moreover, we briefly review the growing evidence that in well-controlled placebo studies (under neutral conditions, hidden conditions, or in properly explained and openly administered conditions) the evidence points to the possibility of large and sustained pain relief from placebo treatments. The combination of predictability and persistent analgesia imply that a placebo itself may be viewed as a viable treatment for chronic pain. Its basic psychological mechanisms—positive but appropriately calibrated expectation, hope, interpersonal care and connection, and learning processes shaped by selective attention to positive outcomes—overlap with psychological and behavioral treatments that can be delivered in a nondeceptive fashion.[14] Thus, we conclude the chapter by a call for a concerted effort to demonstrate the viability of treating chronic pain using optimized placebo protocols.

Placebos as a viable means for sustained relief from chronic pain

Overall placebo responses in clinical trials are large, but in part, are due to natural history (improvement that would have occurred without the placebo), regression to the mean, and other statistical artifacts related to selective attrition.[15] Estimating causal effects of a placebo requires comparing placebo groups with natural history controls, which tends to be rare in clinical trials but has been used in some studies.[16] The latter data show prevalence of placebo analgesia across multiple types of chronic pain. Placebo treatments can cause sustained effectiveness rivaling in magnitude to that of active drug treatments.[17] For example, meta-analyses of expectancy effects[18] and placebo effects in clinical samples[19] have found effect sizes in the Cohen's d = 0.5 range, and in more advantageous combinations of suggestion and psychosocial support, they can be quite large.[20-24] Note also that a recent meta-analysis of placebo effect sizes relative to no treatment in chronic back pain (CBP)[25] suggests smaller effects overall, but shows that most studies are limited in quality and duration.

Placebo treatments engage multiple brain circuits implicated in supraspinal sensitization, as well as in pain and nociception related circuitry,[26] descending modulation of the spinal cord,[27-29] and spinal cord activity.[30] Thus, placebo manipulations seem able to control spinal cord nociceptive inputs, their supraspinal projections, and the brain circuitry's ability to modulate the transformation of nociception to pain perception. Within the circuitry involved in placebo responses, the ventromedial prefrontal cortex (VMPFC) and dorsolateral prefrontal cortex (DLPFC) seem to play chief roles, including via their ability to modulate subcortical affective and motivational circuitry. The VMPFC projects to the hippocampus, nucleus accumbens, amygdala, hypothalamus, and brainstem (dorsal raphe, periaqueductal gray [PAG]) to provide contextual meaning-based control over affect and physiology.[31-33] It is consistently involved in placebo effects, including responding to placebos believed to be more expensive (a suggestion effect),[34] placebo-induced opioid release,[35] and placebo effects in social rejection.[36] Moreover, these circuits are further involved in depression,[37] posttraumatic stress disorder (PTSD),[38,39] drug craving and relapse,[40] social anxiety disorder,[41] chronic pain,[42,43] and others. A reason for this broad involvement in psychopathology may be its role in conceptualizing the self in a situational context, which is related to multiple forms of thought, including spontaneous and self-referential thought, future-oriented, prospective thought,[44,45] theory of mind,[46] and cognitive maps of conceptual relationships.[47]

Recent theoretical advances provide a framework for why context can exert such powerful effects,[36] and how learning-related signals affect prediction errors to shape learning,[46,48,49] resulting in placebo effects that do not diminish over time.[48] Predictive processing theories emphasize that the brain actively constructs a model of the underlying causes of sensory and interoceptive signals. Perceptions are viewed as *inferences* about the underlying state of the world and self, including pain. Predictive learning depends strongly on the underlying meaning of the cues as interpreted by the organism.[50] This provides an explanation for why verbal suggestions can be powerful in humans, even eliciting robust hormonal responses in some cases,[51] and provides a common pathway for conditioning, treatment history, suggestion, interpersonal (e.g., doctor-patient) interactions, and effects of physical context (e.g., the place in which one is treated; the look and feel of an injection) based on their *meaning* to the patient. This meaning is conceptual and constructed based on integration of multiple aspects of the external and internal (body state) context. The semantic category labels we apply to objects influence the nature of the emotional and brain responses they elicit.[52] For example, labeling an experience as belonging to one category or another influences how we generalize across pain-predictive cues, shaping pain and autonomic activity.[53–55] A key aspect of predictive processing is that it drives learning, providing an explanation for why placebo effects can persist and even grow over time. It is not simply the presence of a pain-predictive cue that drives learning, but awareness that the cue is linked to pain, and attribution of unique signal value to the cue.

Is a placebo predictable? And what are the clinical implications?

As reviewed above, placebo effects hinge on concrete brain circuitry and behavioral phenomena that can be experimentally studied and manipulated. Thus, a key question is whether we can take advantage of these biological and behavior properties to predict who is likely to respond to a placebo. Being able to predict placebo responders—who will respond strongly to a placebo and who will not—is highly desirable and has nontrivial implications for both clinical practice and clinical trial designs. First, knowing who is likely to benefit from a placebo minimizes ethical concerns related to prescribing placebos to the wrong patients. Recent encouraging findings on open-label placebos[56]— placebos given without deception, with the patients' full knowledge that they are receiving a placebo—suggests that this could be a viable pathway if the right individuals and conditions can be identified. Second, it could be used in replacement of other treatments, even if temporary, to reduce the burden of harmful side effects of many pharmacological treatments.[57] And third, the ability to predict placebo responses would provide a stronger, more controlled way to prescreen patients in the context of randomized controlled trials. We now turn to some promising new research that is paving the path forward in predicting placebo responders using genetic, brain, personality, and language features.

Genetic predictors of placebo responses

Determining whether genes influence the neurological pathways engaged during response to placebo treatment and, therefore, are predictive of placebo responders, is an area of active investigation. However, placebo genomics, like the related field of pharmacogenomics (i.e., the study of how genes influence response to active treatments), is stymied by the related challenges of low statistical power and lack of reproducibility. With tens of thousands of genes and even more possible polymorphisms, a large amount of data is necessary to begin to assess which genes might affect placebo responsiveness. Currently, for example, the LDhub repository in the field of genetics accepts a sample size of, at minimum, 5,000 for genome-wide association findings, and some studies now include over 1 million participants. One way to tackle the power problem is to use candidate gene analysis, a process of identifying individual genes that influence outcomes in the placebo arms of clinical trials. Still, candidate gene analyses often fail to replicate, because of the very small underlying effects of any single polymorphism and large numbers of tests.[58]

The search for placebo genes, or the placebome, is made more difficult because clinical trials are not often replicated, and the potential for gene-drug interactions can often mask important effects that influence placebo outcomes. This potential for placebo response pathways to be modified by drugs raises an interesting question that faces many clinicians, researchers, and drug manufacturers: do the effects of drugs and placebos interact or do they operate via independent mechanisms? The common "belief" is that drug and placebo effects may be additive in some cases.[59] But there is growing evidence that drugs like naloxone can abrogate response to placebo,[60] implying interdependence of placebo and opioid responses; gene-drug-placebo interactions have been demonstrated in other cases as well (Figure 2.1.1).[62–65] Hence, it is important to examine what happens if there are differential effects in the drug and placebo arms, and, further, if these effects vary by genotype. This topic is explored in further detail in Chapter 2.2.

It is difficult to disentangle the attributions of placebos in the context of genetic effects, but use of the pharmacogenomics approach to identify populations that might differentially respond to a placebo or drugs are warranted to add a deeper understanding to and more accurate interpretation of clinical trial results. Further, with the low cost and ease of genetic testing, identification of genes that might predict placebo responsiveness would aid in assembling appropriate sample sizes and ensuring appropriate treatment for individual patients in clinical care and, therefore, deserves serious further investigation.

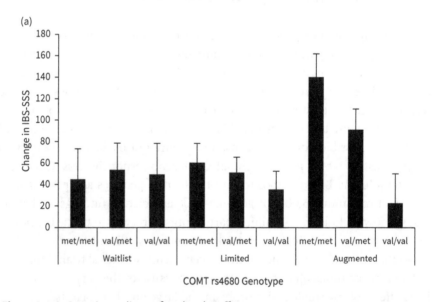

Figure 2.1.1 Genetic predictors for placebo effects.
(A) IBS outcomes (IBS-SSS) by COMT genotype and varying placebo treatments.[65]
(B) Major cardiovascular disease outcomes by COMT genotype in the WHS.[62] (C) Placebo and aspirin response in cardiovascular disease prevention by COMT genotype in the WHS. (D) Placebo and vitamin E response in cardiovascular disease prevention by COMT genotype in the WHS.[62]

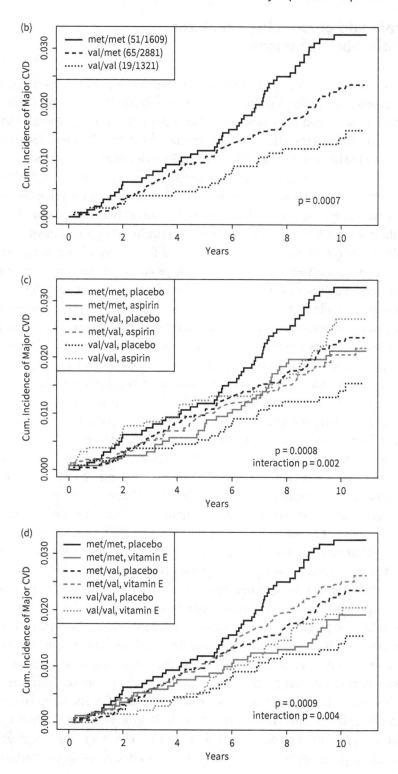

Figure 2.1.1 Continued

Brain and personality predictors of placebo responses

Only few studies have so far examined the neurobiology of placebo responses in chronic pain patients within the settings of RCTs. In a series of two RCTs, Apkarian lab tested the proposition that biological and psychological factors predetermine placebo effects in CBP patients.[23,24] A first RCT was designed to discover the brain regions and the personality traits involved in placebo effects, and a second one was designed to validate these discoveries. The study was implemented sequentially, meaning that CBP patients from the validation RCT were randomly assigned based on their expression of a placebo signature derived in the discovery RCT. Importantly, both RCTs included a no-treatment arm.

In the discovery RCT, the patients visited the lab on six occasions over 8 weeks and underwent identical scanning protocols on four of these visits. A battery of questionnaires was collected at each visit to capture patients' psychological profile and current emotional and pain states. The 43 patients in the placebo treatment group were exposed to multiple treatment periods and stratified into responders and nonresponders based on their pain ratings. The stratified patients were also compared to 20 patients randomly assigned to a no-treatment group that underwent the same protocol (Figure 2.1.2A). Brain networks constructed from resting state functional connectivity show that placebo responders, at baseline, displayed stronger functional connectivity between both ventral (VLPFC) and dorsolateral prefrontal cortex (DLPFC) and the sensorimotor cortex, as well as weaker connectivity between the dorsolateral prefrontal cortex and the PAG (frontal-PAG in Figure 2.1.2B). Personality questionnaires measuring emotion regulation and interoceptive awareness further dissociated placebo responders and nonresponders.[24] A logistic regression model was built based on data from the discovery RCT, combining the brain and questionnaire parameters,[23] and this model—a placebo biosignature—was used to predict placebo responders a priori in the validation RCT.[23]

In the validation RCT, a new group of 77 patients with CBP were classified as placebo responders or nonresponders based on the aforementioned.[23] The predicted placebo responders and nonresponders were identified prior to the randomization and were then allocated to placebo treatment, naproxen treatment, or no-treatment arms. The use of three treatment arms permitted researchers to disentangle the effect of pure placebo responses from the one embedded with the response to the drug (Figure 2.1.2C). The results demonstrate that placebo effects are is predictable at the group level, as within the placebo arm, patients a priori predicted as placebo responders show significant changes in pain—improvement of 21% from baseline pain—in contrast to no

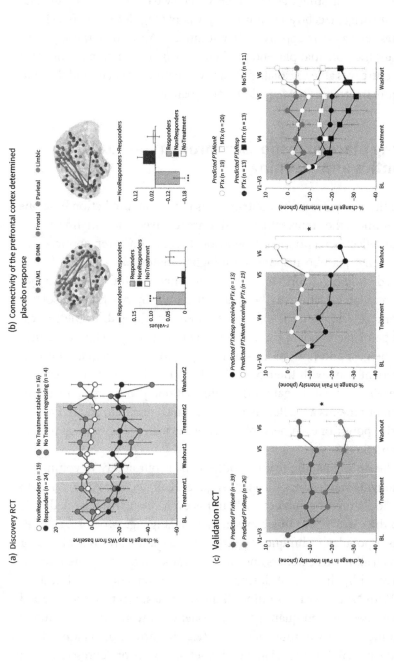

Figure 2.1.2 Neurobiological determinants that predict placebo effects in randomized controlled trials. (A) In the discovery RCT, significant changes in pain intensity were most frequent in CBP receiving placebo pills (56% response rate) than in CBP patients receiving no treatment (20% response rate). (B) Edges between the DLPFC/VLPFC and the sensorimotor cortex (positive weight) or the PAG (negative weight) determined placebo responses. (C) Predicted placebo responses were determined by applying the derived biosignature in a new group of CBP patients randomized in a validation RCT. Changes in pain intensity after the stratification between predicted placebo responders and nonresponders irrespectively of treatment (left), only in the placebo group (middle), and across both treatment arms with the no-treatment arm altogether (right).

minimal pain relief in those predicted as nonresponders.[23] Within the naproxen treatment arm, patients predicted as no-responders showed 15% pain
relief from baseline, but pain relief in those predicted as placebo responders
doubled to 32%, suggesting that pain relief could be partitioned into pure placebo and pure drug placebo analgesia of equivalent magnitudes (~10%–15%),
and that these effects were approximately additive.[23] Altogether, the approach
demonstrates the potential placebo predictability in a validation cohort, that
the biosignature was able to isolate pure active treatment effects, and that placebo and pure treatment showed additivity of pain relief.

Predicting placebo responses through the study of semantics and meaning

Genetic, brain, and personality contributions to placebo prediction have one
aspect in common: they represent traits that are relatively static in time, which
may in turn reflect perception and behavior. There is, however, an increased
appreciation that placebo responses are highly context-dependent,[66,67] and
perhaps predicting behavior from static traits only taps into one of the potential sources of variation in behavior: the built-in machinery isolated
from its context. The reality is, of course, more complicated. In the context
of chronic pain, each patient carries their own pain story—How were they
treated in the past and how successful were previous treatments? And how
does the patient cope with their pain? While qualitatively it makes sense to
simply interview patients to gather this information, quantifying it in an objective manner remains a challenge in psychological research, and to harness
the predictive power of each person's experiences with pain, we must turn to
novel methodologies.

One of the distinguishing features of humans is our ability to communicate our thoughts and feelings through language. Language provides a wealth
of information about the subjects' self and is even popularly regarded as "a
window to the soul."[68,69] In this context, natural language processing (NLP)
emerged as a popular technique to extract language features out of text or
speech, which allows researchers and clinicians alike to quantify latent topics
being addressed by the patient during a normal conversation or clinical interview.[70] With NLP, we can examine all the words a subject uses to respond
to any given question and quantify the prevalence of words that map into a
given semantic category or topic of interest (e.g., in chronic pain patients, are
the words the patient is using related to themes of anxiety or depression? And
what are common descriptors for their pain? Do patients use words more
related to emotion or physical descriptors?). This allows us to capture and

quantify important psychological constructs without addressing them explicitly, yet still in an objective and impartial way.

Berger et al.[70] tested whether this technique can be used to predict placebo responses in CBP patients. The premise here is that as patients speak about their life, in particular, how they cope with pain and their previous experiences in the medical system, we could gather enough information that could predict, in an ecological manner, who is likely to respond to an inert placebo pill versus who will not. If successful, it could also give us clearer insight into the psychological dimensions that subtend placebo responsiveness. In parallel to the brain and behavior study reported above, we looked at language use in the two separate studies described above. The first study was designed to identify and generate a placebo prediction model. The second was designed to validate the prior model in an independent dataset and establish generalizability (see Figure 2.1.3. for an overview of the methods and language features).

In Berger et al. study a set of language parameters collected at the end of the treatment phase did indeed identify placebo responders (i.e., patients who received significant analgesia from the placebo pill) with 79% accuracy.[70] Patients who responded to the placebo described their pain experiences using words semantically proximal to *afraid, fear, loss, awareness, identity, magnify, drives,* and *achievements.* Patients who did not respond to the placebo used words more proximal to *force* (i.e., physical forces), *stigma,* and *leisure.* Through these parameters, a predictive model was generated including four key orthogonal parameters: semantic similarity to *stigma, force,* and *magnify*; and number of words related to *achievement.* Representative examples of patients' speech as well as group differences for the semantic distance features are depicted in Figure 2.1.3. A second study was then conducted to validate and test the generalizability of the predictive language model. In this study, patients were instead interviewed before the treatment to assess the predictability of the model, and were randomized to either receive a placebo pill, or a naproxen pill. They were asked to describe themselves, to narrate a recent event, to describe their pain, and their past experiences in medical settings regarding their pain condition. Patients and researchers were blinded to which pill the patient received. By applying the predictive model from study 1 to study 2, the model predicted placebo responders with good accuracy (AUC = .71), but not drug responders (AUC = .52). This model could not predict spontaneous recovery in the no-treatment arms of study 1 and study 2 (AUC = .55), thus showing the model is predicting specific analgesic effects caused by a placebo and not attributable to, for example, regression to the mean effects. In fact, patients predicted to be placebo responders showed larger analgesic effects to the placebo compared to patients who were predicted to be nonresponders (30% vs. 3% change in pain, respectively).

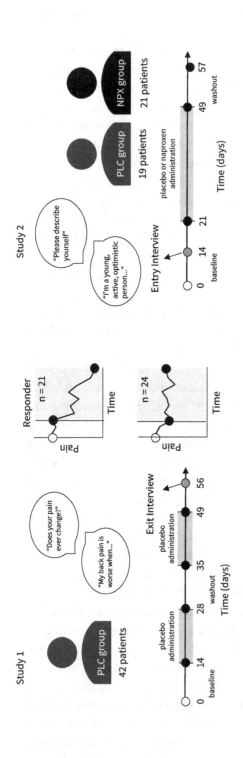

Figure 2.1.3 Language use predictive of placebo effects.

Methodology and natural language processing results are shown. In an interview participants are asked questions pertaining to their personality, mood, and pain. The answers are recorded, transcribed, and several language features are extracted, see. These parameters are then fed to a machine-learning algorithm that can predict who is a placebo responder and who is not, based on patterns of language use. In the first study (upper left), patients were divided into two arms: a set of patients with chronic back pain who received a placebo for two 2-week periods with a 1-week washout period in between, and a set of patients received no treatment (i.e., control condition). Patients rated their pain twice a day for the duration of the study and were determined to be placebo responders or not based on whether they had a significant pain reduction, compared to preintervention pain ratings. Study 2 (upper right) was conducted in an independent sample of patients with chronic back pain with similar characteristics to those in study 1, but the interview was performed before the start of the treatment and is, therefore, unbiased. Further, to test the specificity of prediction, the model was also tested in an arm of patients receiving Naproxen (NPX). Patients who do not respond to placebo (PTxNonR) used language more closely related to the terms *force* and *stigma*, whereas patients who respond to the placebo (PTxResp) used words more closely related to *magnify* (data from[69]). Below each topic is an example of patient speech related to each semantic topic, for each of the studies.

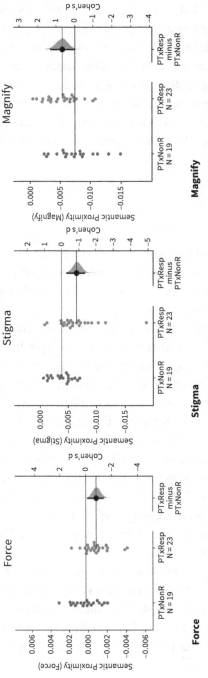

Force

"I was working for a moving company, and I really didn't know how to move, you know bend at the knees and lift with the knees, but I didn't really pay attention"

Study 1. PTxNonR

"What they explained to me when I first got hurt is that, okay so, I'm pulling in this motion, the body is not used to it, and the fibers spasm"

Study 2. PTxNonR

Stigma

"I have a very bad back for a guy. It's not straight and strong like it should be, it's kind of like curved. It upsets me'

Study 1. PTxNonR

"it's hard not to be discriminatory against fat people because that's the way society is set up. It's very hard, I understand, but at the same time we still need your help"

Study 2. PTxNonR

Magnify

"If I'm having a bad day, it's like I'm more focused on the pain"

Study 1. PTxResp

"What aggravates pain is walking long distances, even though I'm being told by physical therapy that's one thing I need to do, so…"

Study 2. PTxResp

Figure 2.1.3 Continued

In summary, how the subjects speak about themselves, their pain, and their medical expectations can provide important cues as to whether a patient will respond to a placebo or not. It is likely these language parameters reflect the subjects' state at the time, considering a multiplicity of psychological factors, which further enhances its predictive ability—even beyond that shown by a large set of psychological questionnaires which instead measure more stable traits.[71] This approach has strong ecological validity because it follows what would happen in a clinical context, where based on clinical interview, one must decide how to treat a patient. Although these studies remain mostly preliminary, advancing this technology can provide new opportunities for scientists and clinicians alike.

Concluding remarks

Historically, decades of research on predicting placebo responders has yielded a mixed picture, with findings of personality predictors in some studies failing to replicate or be consistent in others.[72] In addition, small changes in context—including the name of the placebo "drug"—have been found to substantially alter who responds to a placebo, resulting in low correlations in placebo responses across contexts[73] that interact with people's predispositions in some cases.[74] Similarly, placebo responses have been found to be uncorrelated across different outcomes. This variability fits within a pattern evidenced by personality research more broadly: Responses in a situation are driven by person x situation interactions.[75] For example, rather than "anxiety" being a trait characteristic that predicts responses across situations, a person may be high-anxiety in one situation (e.g., at a party) but low-anxiety in another (e.g., parachuting) or vice versa. Placebo responses may be similar: A "responder" to a cream may not be a "responder" to soothing verbal suggestions and vice versa. To the extent that these effects are large and vary across individuals, stable genetic, brain, and personality traits that are not influenced by these variables must have small predictive effects.

The current studies present a counterpoint to this picture, suggesting that placebo effects may be predictable based on genetics or pretreatment brain structure or activity. They build on earlier studies finding that larger placebo analgesia and similar context-based pain modulation is predicted by trait optimism;[76] low trait anxiety and fear of pain, for example,[77] and high trait engagement and behavioral activation.[78]

What does this mean for the ability to predict the magnitude of an individual's placebo responses, and how can these findings coexist?

Larger-scale, preregistered studies are needed to test the effects found in earlier smaller-scale studies, particularly in genetics and neuroimaging, where large numbers of variables and tests can lead to selection biases. Alternatively, stable characteristics may indeed predict placebo responses. Such responses may apply only to narrow contexts. For example, the COMT gene may predict placebo responses only with a particular outcome measure in a particular population, and it will work if other factors—the interpersonal setting, prior associations, and perceived characteristics of the placebo—are tightly controlled and uniform across patients. On the other hand, they may predict placebo responses more broadly, perhaps as part of a general disposition or ability to engage in positive expectations and attend to potential treatment gains. Further research is needed to adjudicate between these possibilities. A productive avenue would be replication of observed placebo prediction effects in prior studies with a "near-context" replication, controlling and reproducing the original context as tightly as possible, as well as other "far-transfer" tests. In sum, the results of recent studies are promising, but we have a lot of work to do.

References

1. Wager TD, Atlas LY. The neuroscience of placebo effects: Connecting context, learning and health. *Nature Reviews Neuroscience.* 2015;16(7):403–418. https://doi:10.1038/nrn3976
2. Tuttle AH, Tohyama S, Ramsay T, et al. Increasing placebo responses over time in U.S. clinical trials of neuropathic pain. *Pain.* 2015;156(12):2616–2626. https://doi:10.1097/j.pain.0000000000000333
3. Dahlhamer J, Lucas J, Zelaya, C, et al. Prevalence of chronic pain and high-impact chronic pain among adults—United States, 2016. *MMWR Morbidity and Mortality Weekly Report.* 2018;67(36):1001–1006. https://doi:10.15585/mmwr.mm6736a2
4. Manchikanti L, Giordano J, Boswell MV, Fellows B, Manchukonda SR, Pampati V. Psychological factors as predictors of opioid abuse and illicit drug use in chronic pain patients. *Journal of Opioid Management.* 2007;3(2):89–100. doi:10.5055/jom.2007.0045.
5. Geha P, deAraujo I, Green B, Small DM. Decreased food pleasure and disrupted satiety signals in chronic low back pain. *Pain.* 2014;155(4):712–722. https://doi:10.1016/j.pain.2013.12.027
6. Lin Y, De Araujo I, Stanley G, Small D, Geha P. Chronic pain precedes disrupted eating behavior in low-back pain patients. *PLoS ONE.* 2022;17(2):e0263527. https://doi:10.1371/journal.pone.0263527
7. Apkarian VA, Sosa Y, Krauss BR, et al. Chronic pain patients are impaired on an emotional decision-making task. *Pain.* 2004;108(1):129–136. https://doi:10.1016/j.pain.2003.12.015
8. Flor H, Turk DC, Berndt Scholz O. Impact of chronic pain on the spouse: Marital, emotional and physical consequences. *Journal of Psychosomatic Research.* 1987;31(1):63–71. https://doi:10.1016/0022-3999(87)90099-7
9. Jalal H, Buchanich JM, Roberts MS, Balmert LC, Zhang K, Burke DS. Changing dynamics of the drug overdose epidemic in the United States from 1979 through 2016. *Science.* 2018;361(6408):eaau1184. https://doi:10.1126/science.aau1184

10. Enthoven WT, Roelofs PD, Deyo RA, van Tulder MW, Koes BW. Non-steroidal anti-inflammatory drugs for chronic low back pain. Cochrane Back and Neck Group, ed. *Cochrane Database of Systematic Reviews.* 2016;2(2):CD012087. doi:10.1002/14651858. CD012087.

11. van der Gaag WH, Roelofs PD, Enthoven WT, van Tulder MW, Koes BW. In: Cochrane Back and Neck Group, eds. Non-steroidal anti-inflammatory drugs for acute low back pain. *Cochrane Database of Systematic Reviews.* Published online April 16, 2020. https:// doi:10.1002/14651858.CD013581

12. Chou R, Deyo R, Friedly J, et al. Systemic pharmacologic therapies for low back pain: A systematic review for an American College of Physicians clinical practice guideline. *Annals of Internal Medicine.* 2017;166(7):480. https://doi:10.7326/M16-2458

13. Ferreira ML, Ferreira PH, Latimer J, Herbert R, Maher CG. Does spinal manipulative therapy help people with chronic low back pain? *Australian Journal of Physiotherapy.* 2002;48(4):277–284. https://doi:10.1016/S0004-9514(14)60167-7

14. Ashar YK, Chang LJ, Wager TD. Brain mechanisms of the placebo effect: An affective appraisal account. *Annual Review of Clinical Psychology.* 2017;13:73–98. https://doi:10.1146/ annurev-clinpsy-021815-093015

15. Kienle GS, Kiene H. The powerful placebo effect: Fact or fiction? *Journal of Clinical Epidemiology.* 1997;50(12):1311–1318. https://doi:10.1016/s0895-4356(97)00203-5

16. Hróbjartsson A, Gøtzsche PC. Placebo interventions for all clinical conditions. *Cochrane Database of Systematic Reviews.* 2010;(1):CD003974. doi:10.1002/14651858.CD003974. pub3.

17. Chappell AS, Desaiah D, Liu-Seifert H, et al. A double-blind, randomized, placebo-controlled study of the efficacy and safety of duloxetine for the treatment of chronic pain due to osteoarthritis of the knee: Duloxetine and chronic pain due to osteoarthritis of the knee. *Pain Practice.* 2011;11(1):33–41. https://doi:10.1111/j.1533-2500.2010.00401.x

18. Peerdeman KJ, van Laarhoven AI, Peters ML, Evers AW. An integrative review of the influence of expectancies on pain. *Frontiers in Psychology.* 2016 Aug 23;7:1270. doi:10.3389/ fpsyg.2016.01270.

19. Lennep J, Han PA, Trossèl F, Perez RSGM, et al. Placebo effects in low back pain: A systematic review and meta-analysis of the literature. *European Journal of Pain.* 2021;25(9):1876– 1897. https://doi:10.1002/ejp.1811

20. Haake M. German acupuncture trials (Gerac) for chronic low back pain: Randomized, multicenter, blinded, parallel-group trial with 3 groups. *Archives of Internal Medicine.* 2007;167(17):1892. https://doi:10.1001/Archinte.167.17.1892

21. Kaptchuk TJ, Kelley JM, Conboy LA, et al. Components of placebo effect: Randomised controlled trial in patients with irritable bowel syndrome. *British Medical Journal.* 2008;336(7651):999–1003. https://doi:10.1136/bmj.39524.439618.25

22. Tétreault P, Mansour A, Vachon-Presseau E, Schnitzer TJ, Apkarian AV, Baliki MN. Brain connectivity predicts placebo response across chronic pain clinical trials. *PLOS Biology.* 2016;14(10):e1002570. https://doi:10.1371/journal.pbio.1002570

23. Vachon-Presseau E, Abdullah TB, Berger SE, Huang L, Griffith JW, Schnitzer TJ, Apkarian AV. Validating a biosignature-predicting placebo pill response in chronic pain in the settings of a randomized controlled trial. *Pain.* 2022 May 1;163(5):910–922. doi:10.1097/ j.pain.0000000000002450.

24. Vachon-Presseau E, Berger SE, Abdullah TB, et al. Brain and psychological determinants of placebo pill response in chronic pain patients. *Nature Communications.* 2018;9(1):3397. https://doi:10.1038/s41467-018-05859-1

25. Strijkers RHW, Schreijenberg M, Gerger H, Koes BW, Chiarotto A. Effectiveness of placebo interventions for patients with nonspecific low back pain: A systematic review and meta-analysis. *Pain.* 2021;162(12):2792–2804. https://doi:10.1097/j.pain.0000000000002272

26. Zunhammer M, Bingel U, Wager TD; for the Placebo Imaging Consortium. Placebo effects on the neurologic pain signature: A meta-analysis of individual participant functional magnetic resonance imaging data. *JAMA Neurology*. 2018;75(11):1321. http://doi:10.1001/jamaneurol.2018.2017

27. Grahl A, Onat S, Büchel C. The periaqueductal gray and Bayesian integration in placebo analgesia. *eLife*. 2018;7:e32930. https://doi:10.7554/eLife.32930

28. Wager TD, Rilling JK, Smith EE, et al. Placebo-induced changes in fMRI in the anticipation and experience of pain. *Science*. 2004;303(5661):1162–1167. https://doi:10.1126/science.1093065

29. Zubieta JK. Placebo effects mediated by endogenous opioid activity on opioid receptors. *Journal of Neuroscience*. 2005;25(34):7754–7762. https://doi:10.1523/JNEUROSCI.0439-05.2005

30. Eippert F, Finsterbusch J, Bingel U, Büchel C. Direct evidence for spinal cord involvement in placebo analgesia. *Science*. 2009;326(5951):404–404. https://doi:10.1126/science.1180142

31. Price JL, Drevets WC. Neurocircuitry of mood disorders. *Neuropsychopharmacol*. 2010;35(1):192–216. https://doi:10.1038/npp.2009.104

32. Roy M, Shohamy D, Wager TD. Ventromedial prefrontal-subcortical systems and the generation of affective meaning. *Trends in Cognitive Sciences*. 2012;16(3):147–156. https://doi:10.1016/j.tics.2012.01.005

33. Zhang L, Losin EAR, Ashar YK, Koban L, Wager TD. Gender biases in estimation of others' pain. *Journal of Pain*. 2021;22(9):1048–1059. https://doi:10.1016/j.jpain.2021.03.001

34. Geuter S, Eippert F, Hindi Attar C, Büchel C. Cortical and subcortical responses to high and low effective placebo treatments. *NeuroImage*. 2013;67:227–236. https://doi:10.1016/j.neuroimage.2012.11.029

35. Wager TD, Scott DJ, Zubieta JK. Placebo effects on human μ-opioid activity during pain. *Proceedings of the National Academy of Sciences USA*. 2007;104(26):11056–11061. https://doi:10.1073/pnas.0702413104

36. Koban L, Kross E, Woo CW, Ruzic L, Wager TD. Frontal-brainstem pathways mediating placebo effects on social rejection. *Journal of Neuroscience*. 2017;37(13):3621–3631. https://doi:10.1523/JNEUROSCI.2658-16.2017

37. Schmaal L, Yücel M, Ellis R, et al. Brain structural signatures of adolescent depressive symptom trajectories: A longitudinal magnetic resonance imaging study. *Journal of the American Academy of Child & Adolescent Psychiatry*. 2017;56(7):593–601.e9. https://doi:10.1016/j.jaac.2017.05.008

38. Etkin A, Wager TD. Functional neuroimaging of anxiety: A meta-analysis of emotional processing in PTSD, social anxiety disorder, and specific phobia. *Artificial Juridical Person*. 2007;164(10):1476–1488. https://doi:10.1176/appi.ajp.2007.07030504

39. Weaver SS, Kroska EB, Ross MC, et al. Sacrificing reward to avoid threat: Characterizing PTSD in the context of a trauma-related approach–avoidance conflict task. *Journal of Abnormal Psychology*. 2020;129(5):457–468. https://doi:10.1037/abn0000528

40. Goldstein RZ, Volkow ND. Dysfunction of the prefrontal cortex in addiction: Neuroimaging findings and clinical implications. *Nature Reviews Neuroscience*. 2011;12(11):652–669. https://doi:10.1038/nrn3119

41. Hahn A, Stein P, Windischberger C, et al. Reduced resting-state functional connectivity between amygdala and orbitofrontal cortex in social anxiety disorder. *NeuroImage*. 2011;56(3):881–889. https://doi:10.1016/j.neuroimage.2011.02.064

42. Nieminen LK, Pyysalo LM, Kankaanpää MJ. Prognostic factors for pain chronicity in low back pain: a systematic review. *PR9*. 2021;6(1):e919. https://doi:10.1097/PR9.0000000000000919

43. Smallwood RF, Laird AR, Ramage AE, et al. Structural brain anomalies and chronic pain: A quantitative meta-analysis of gray matter volume. *Journal of Pain*. 2013;14(7):663–675. https://doi:10.1016/j.jpain.2013.03.001

44. Bąbel P. Classical conditioning as a distinct mechanism of placebo effects. *Frontiers in Psychiatry*. 2019;10:449. https://doi:10.3389/fpsyt.2019.00449

45. Satterthwaite TD, Green L, Myerson J, Parker J, Ramaratnam M, Buckner RL. Dissociable but inter-related systems of cognitive control and reward during decision making: Evidence from pupillometry and event-related fMRI. *NeuroImage*. 2007;37(3):1017–1031. https://doi:10.1016/j.neuroimage.2007.04.066

46. Benedetti F, Carlino E, Pollo A. How placebos change the patient's brain. *Neuropsychopharmacology*. 2011;36(1):339–354. https://doi:10.1038/npp.2010.81

47. Constantinescu AO, O'Reilly JX, Behrens TEJ. Organizing conceptual knowledge in humans with a gridlike code. *Science*. 2016;352(6292):1464–1468. https://doi:10.1126/science.aaf0941

48. Jepma M, Koban L, van Doorn J, Jones M, Wager TD. Behavioural and neural evidence for self-reinforcing expectancy effects on pain. *Nature Human Behaviour*. 2018;2(11):838–855. https://doi:10.1038/s41562-018-0455-8

49. Jepma M, Wager TD. Multiple potential mechanisms for context effects on pain. *Pain*. 2013;154(5):629–631. https://doi:10.1016/j.pain.2013.02.011

50. Ploghaus A, Tracey I, Clare S, Gati JS, Rawlins JNP, Matthews PM. Learning about pain: The neural substrate of the prediction error for aversive events. *Proceedings of the National Academy of Sciences USA*. 2000;97(16):9281–9286. https://doi:10.1073/pnas.160266497

51. Benedetti F. Placebo analgesia. *Neurological Sciences*. 2006;27(S2):s100–s102. https://doi:10.1007/s10072-006-0580-4

52. Satpute AB, Lindquist KA. The default mode network's role in discrete emotion. *Trends in Cognitive Sciences*. 2019;23(10):851–864. https://doi:10.1016/j.tics.2019.07.003

53. Koban L, Jepma M, Geuter S, Wager TD. What's in a word? How instructions, suggestions, and social information change pain and emotion. *Neuroscience & Biobehavioral Reviews*. 2017;81:29–42. https://doi:10.1016/j.neubiorev.2017.02.014

54. Lebois LAM, Hertzog C, Slavich GM, Barrett LF, Barsalou LW. Establishing the situated features associated with perceived stress. *Acta Psychologica (Amst)*. 2016;169:119–132. https://doi:10.1016/j.actpsy.2016.05.012

55. Lieberman MD, Eisenberger NI, Crockett MJ, Tom SM, Pfeifer JH, Way BM. Putting feelings into words: affect labeling disrupts amygdala activity in response to affective stimuli. *Psychological Science*. 2007;18(5):421–428. https://doi:10.1111/j.1467-9280.2007.01916.x

56. Kaptchuk TJ, Friedlander E, Kelley JM, et al. Placebos without deception: A randomized controlled trial in irritable bowel syndrome. *PLoS ONE*. 2010;5(12):e15591. https://doi:10.1371/journal.pone.0015591

57. Schedlowski M, Enck P, Rief W, Bingel U. Neuro-bio-behavioral mechanisms of placebo and nocebo responses: implications for clinical trials and clinical practice. *Pharmacological Reviews*. 2015;67(3):697–730. https://doi:10.1124/pr.114.009423

58. Duncan LE, Pollastri AR, Smoller JW. Why many geneticists and psychological scientists have discrepant views about gene–environment interaction (G×E) research. *American Psychologist*. 2014;69(3):249–268. https://doi:10.1037/a0036320

59. Atlas LY, Whittington RA, Lindquist MA, Wielgosz J, Sonty N, Wager TD. Dissociable influences of opiates and expectations on pain. *Journal of Neuroscience*. 2012;32(23):8053–8064. https://doi:10.1523/JNEUROSCI.0383-12.2012

60. Amanzio M, Benedetti F. Neuropharmacological dissection of placebo analgesia: Expectation-activated opioid systems versus conditioning-activated specific subsystems. *Journal of Neuroscience*. 1999;19(1):484–494.

61. Schenk LA, Sprenger C, Geuter S, Büchel C. Expectation requires treatment to boost pain relief: An fMRI study. *Pain*. 2014;155(1):150–157. https://doi:10.1016/j.pain.2013.09.024

62. Hall KT, Nelson CP, Davis RB, et al. Polymorphisms in catechol-O-methyltransferase modify treatment effects of aspirin on risk of cardiovascular disease. *Arteriosclerosis, Thrombosis, and Vascular Biology (ATVB)*. 2014;34(9):2160–2167. https://doi:10.1161/ATVBAHA.114.303845

63. Hall KT, Buring JE, Mukamal KJ, et al. COMT and alpha-tocopherol effects in cancer prevention: Gene-supplement interactions in two randomized clinical trials. *Journal of the National Cancer Institute*. 2019;111(7):684–694. https://doi:10.1093/jnci/djy204

64. Hall KT, Kossowsky J, Oberlander TF, et al. Genetic variation in catechol-O-methyltransferase modifies effects of clonidine treatment in chronic fatigue syndrome. *Pharmacogenomics Journal*. 2016;16(5):454–460. https://doi:10.1038/tpj.2016.53

65. Hall KT, Lembo AJ, Kirsch I, et al. Catechol-O-methyltransferase val158met polymorphism predicts placebo effect in irritable bowel syndrome. *PLoS ONE*. 2012;7(10):e48135. https://doi:10.1371/journal.pone.0048135

66. Atlas LY. A social affective neuroscience lens on placebo analgesia. *Trends in Cognitive Sciences*. 2021;25(11):992–1005. https://doi:10.1016/j.tics.2021.07.016

67. Horing B, Weimer K, Muth ER, Enck P. Prediction of placebo responses: A systematic review of the literature. *Frontiers in Psychiatry*. 2014 Oct 1;5:1079. doi:10.3389/fpsyg.2014.01079.

68. Pennebaker JW, Mehl MR, Niederhoffer KG. Psychological aspects of natural language use: Our words, our selves. *Annual Review of Psychology*. 2003;54:547–577. https://doi:10.1146/annurev.psych.54.101601.145041

69. Tausczik YR, Pennebaker JW. The psychological meaning of words: LIWC and computerized text analysis methods. *Journal of Language and Social Psychology*. 2010;29(1):24–54. https://doi:10.1177/0261927X09351676

70. Berger SE, Branco P, Vachon-Presseau E, Abdullah TB, Cecchi G, Apkarian AV. Quantitative language features identify placebo responders in chronic back pain. *Pain*. 2021;162(6):1692–1704. https://doi:10.1097/j.pain.0000000000002175

71. Vachon-Presseau E, Berger SE, Abdullah TB, Griffith JW, Schnitzer TJ, Apkarian AV. Identification of traits and functional connectivity-based neurotraits of chronic pain. *PLoS Biology*. 2019;17(8):e3000349. https://doi:10.1371/journal.pbio.3000349

72. Kern A, Kramm C, Witt CM, Barth J. The influence of personality traits on the placebo/nocebo response: A systematic review. *Journal of Psychosomatic Research*. 2020;128:109866. https://doi:10.1016/j.jpsychores.2019.109866

73. Whalley B, Hyland ME, Kirsch I. Consistency of the placebo effect. *Journal of Psychosomatic Research*. 2008;64(5):537–541. https://doi:10.1016/j.jpsychores.2007.11.007

74. Hyland ME. Motivation and placebos: do different mechanisms occur in different contexts? *Philosophical Transactions of the Royal Society B: Biological Sciences*. 2011;366(1572):1828–1837. https://doi:10.1098/rstb.2010.0391

75. Lyby PS, Aslaksen PM, Flaten MA. Is fear of pain related to placebo analgesia? *Journal of Psychosomatic Research*. 2010;68(4):369–377. https://doi:10.1016/j.jpsychores.2009.10.009

76. Geers AL, Wellman JA, Fowler SL, Rasinski HM, Helfer SG. Placebo expectations and the detection of somatic information. *Journal of Behavioral Medicine*. 2011;34(3):208–217. https://doi:10.1007/s10865-010-9301-9

77. Koban L, Wager TD. Beyond conformity: Social influences on pain reports and physiology. *Emotion*. 2016;16(1):24–32. https://doi:10.1037/emo0000087

78. Schweinhardt P, Seminowicz DA, Jaeger E, Duncan GH, Bushnell MC. The anatomy of the mesolimbic reward system: A link between personality and the placebo analgesic response. *Journal of Neuroscience*. 2009;29(15):4882–4887. https://doi:10.1523/JNEUROSCI.5634-08.2009

2.2

Molecular mechanisms of placebo responses

From genes to pathways

Hailey Yetman, Marta Peciña, Arun Tiwari, Jan Vollert, and Kathryn Hall

Introduction

The molecular drivers of placebo effects in experimental placebo analgesia are difficult to study without access to real-time physical sampling. For some conditions, (e.g., immunosuppression), researchers are able to utilize animal models to investigate conditioning and associative learning processes that can induce placebo effects. However, human studies are limited to blood-based analyses and surrogate biomarkers of the molecular response to placebo treatments. Using *omics* technologies and pharmacological interventions, placebo researchers are now able to examine biochemical, genetic, and gene expression effects that can be utilized to model and predict placebo responsiveness.

Signaling in the brain is dependent on synaptic activity. Synaptic activity involves the release and uptake of neurotransmitters. Depending on the duration of signals, changes in dendritic branching, synapse maturation, or the pruning of synapses can occur. While little is known about the molecular changes induced in response to placebo treatment, even less is known about how they might induce longer term effects on altered synaptic connectivity over time.[1] In addition to neurological changes, there is growing evidence of molecular endocrine and immunologic modulation as a result of placebo treatment.[1,2] Studying neurological, cellular, and molecular processes and how they interact to influence placebo effects could provide levers to modify and control placebo effects and, thus, represent a new frontier in placebo science.

Genome-wide association studies and retrospective analyses

Genome-wide association studies (GWAS) investigating the influence of genetic variation on response to placebo controls in secondary analyses of placebo-controlled randomized clinical trials have identified several genetic loci that may be associated with response to placebo treatment.[3] Many of these genetic loci, collectively termed the *placebome*, (Table 2.2.1)[4-7] are now reported in the GWAS catalog under the trait "response to placebo."[8]

Irritable bowel syndrome: prospective clinical trials of placebo effects

Irritable bowel syndrome (IBS) is a functional gastrointestinal disorder. Symptoms vary and clinical presentation is heterogenous, but the core

Table 2.2.1 GWAS reveal genes that are associated with outcomes in the placebo treatment arm of some clinical trials

Condition	Outcome	Genes	P	Source
IBS	IBS-SSS	NAV2	4.93E-06	12
		ANTXRL	4.93E-06	
		LINC02006	1.87E-06	
Major depression	MADRS	STAC1	1.25E-08	30
Asthma	QOL	CAMTA1	2.53E-06	33
Asthma	Wheezing	BBS9	1.11E-07	5
		NAV2	7.21E-06	
Rheumatoid arthritis	QOL	Intergenic	1.46E-06	33
COVID-19	Day of last COVID-19 symptom	NPR3	1.17E-06	6
		DEC1	3.95E-08	
Cardiovascular disease	Major coronary event	FHIT	2.87E-08	7
		ACOT6	2.45E-08	
Hypertension	White-coat effect	CACNA2D3	6.08E-07	35
		LOC101927108	4.50E-07	
		SORBS1	2.17E-07	
		ADAM12	7.88E-05	

symptoms include ongoing or bowel-movement related abdominal pain, bloating, as well as frequent constipation, diarrhea, or both.[9] Quality of life can be severely affected for patients, and effects on social and professional life can be detrimental.[10] In most cases, causes are unknown and long-term cures are not available. Symptom management can be difficult, especially for pain; the widely used nonsteroidal anti-inflammatory drugs (NSAIDS) like ibuprofen are not an option, as they are known to have significant side effects negatively affecting the gut. Similarly, opioids are not a viable option for long-term treatment because their leading side effect is constipation, ignoring their addictive potential. At the same time, IBS has been reported to have high rates of placebo responsiveness,[10] making it an interesting case study for placebo research.

Based on previous findings,[11] a prospective study of IBS patients randomized to different types of placebos was designed and a GWAS to examine the effects of placebos on IBS Symptom Severity Score (IBS-SSS) was conducted.[12] A gene transcription network created from the genes associated with treatment response at the genome-wide suggestive level revealed that one of the top hits was *EGR1*. *EGR1*, or early growth response gene, is major mediator of synaptic plasticity and neuronal activity in both physiological and pathological conditions. *EGR1* is known to be activated by stress, early life experiences, and cognitive learning tasks, and it affects synaptic plasticity.[13] In the study by Wang et al., *EGR1* was found to be downregulated in whole blood samples during placebo treatment, suggesting that *EGR1* might be influential to this placebo response inducing pathway. The androgen receptor was another strongly networked hit. The androgen receptor is involved in testosterone signaling, which has been shown to modulate visceral hypersensitivity in IBS. Examination of hormone levels in this study revealed that testosterone was associated with levels of pain intensity.[14] Subsequent subanalyses of this dataset found that variants of rs4680 of catechol-O-methyltransferase (*COMT*), an enzyme that metabolizes catecholamines including dopamine, epinephrine, and norepinephrine, were associated with placebo responses, consistent with previous findings about IBS and placebo analgesia.[11,15] Specifically, participants that were homozygous for a version of the gene that contained a transversion corresponding to a substitution of valine (val) to methionine (met) tended to show greater improvement with placebo treatment in terms of overall IBS-SSS.[12]

The special case of pain as outcome

Pain is of special interest in placebo research for two reasons. First, placebo effects and placebo responses are higher in pain-related outcomes than most other outcomes, according to the literature.[16] Second, as pain can be safely, ethically, and reversibly induced in healthy participants, it has become the classic model to study placebo. Since treatment options for chronic pain are limited, the use of placebos and open-label placebos for pain has been discussed.[17] Pain in IBS is hard to classify and has historically been labeled as "nociceptive pain," which is defined as pain resulting from inflammation of body tissue or other activation of an otherwise healthy nervous system. However, clinically it has long been acknowledged that pain and gut and bowel symptoms in IBS form a negative, reinforcing feedback loop. This nuance indicates that IBS pain is related to chronic alterations in the nervous system, which can be solely a consequence of neuroplasticity in reaction to long-lasting symptoms, but also be fostered by genetic predisposition. Therefore, IBS pain has recently been reclassified as "nociplastic pain" (i.e., pain resulting from functional changes in pain processing nervous pathways).[18]

With these aspects in mind, a pain-focused reanalysis of previously published data of placebo effects in IBS was conducted.[19] Placebo-mediated pain relief in severity and frequency subscales within the IBS-SSS in 212 patients.[20] Using a gene dosage model, increasing number of met alleles in *COMT* single nucleotide polymorphisms (SNP) rs4680 was associated with a significantly greater reduction in IBS pain severity from baseline to week 6 ($p = 0.03$), but not frequency ($p = 0.20$). Participants homozygous for the low activity met allele (met/met) had the greatest reduction in pain severity. This result remained when stratifying for treatment arms or including women only. In an additional exploratory GWAS of change in pain severity, 24 SNPs in close proximity on chromosome 7 reached genome-wide suggestive significance ($p < 5 * 10{-6}$). This genomic region is near gene *SNX13*, which is associated with intracellular trafficking and has been previously associated with chronic widespread pain and a reduced biodiversity of the gut microbiome.[21] When analyzing improvement of pain frequency during the trial, five SNPs within close proximity on chromosome 18 reached genome-wide significance. These SNPs mapped closely to the *L3MBTL4* gene that encodes the histone methyl-lysine binding protein and was previously linked to pain severity in dysmenorrhea (pain with menses).[22] While these are clearly exploratory results, they open interesting routes of research to investigate the genetic and neurophysiological basis of pain in functional disorders like IBS.

With these molecular-based studies, placebo researchers are beginning to uncover how placebo effects might be mediated at a molecular level. As molecular techniques evolve, collaboration between researchers and translational studies to incorporate behavioral, neural, and blood-based data are essential to isolate the underlying molecular mechanism of placebo effects.

Genetics of placebo responses in major depressive disorder

The genetic studies of placebo responses are relatively sparse as compared to studies on antidepressant response. Similar to antidepressant responses, placebo responses are a complex trait and show considerable interindividual variability with 35%–40% responding to placebo treatments in clinical trials.[23] More importantly, up to 67.6% of the variability in antidepressant responses can be attributed to placebo.[24] Several sociodemographic and clinical factors have been explored for possible association with placebo responses with largely inconsistent findings. These include female sex, non-Caucasian ancestry, fewer years of education, lower neuroticism scores, lower severity of depression at baseline, no/successful prior use of antidepressants, length of the trial, and the number of study centers, among others.[23,25]

The genetic studies of placebo responses in depression have largely focused on hypothesis-based candidate gene studies and more recently on hypothesis-free GWAS. One of the earliest candidate gene studies on placebo response analyzed functional genetic variations in COMT (Val158met, rs4680) and monoamine oxidase inhibitor (MAO)-A (rs6323) identified the G or G/G coding for higher activity of MAO to be associated with reduced placebo responses.[26] We conducted a larger study focused on the 34 genes (532 SNPs) from the monoaminergic and hypothalamic-pituitary-adrenal axis pathways for association with placebo responses ($n = 257$). Individuals for this study were derived from the placebo arm of multicenter, double-blind, randomized, placebo-controlled trials for bupropion (Wellbutrin XL). SNPs in the serotonin receptor 2A (HTR2A, rs2296972) and serotonin transporter (5-HTT or SLC6A4, rs4251417) were marginally associated with placebo remission and SNP rs6609257 in monoamine oxidase A (MAOA) with placebo responses.[27] Overall, these associations with genes from the monoaminergic system suggest that both placebo and antidepressant drugs may act via similar disease-related pathways.[28] This is further supported by the observation of the nominal association of a SNP in the inflammatory cytokine, interleukin-6 (IL-6, rs2066992), with both placebo and duloxetine responses.[29]

Currently, large-scale GWAS of placebo response in individuals with depression is lacking. The only GWAS study for placebo responses, conducted in 205 individuals, identified rs76767803 (C > T) present upstream of the STAC1 gene to be associated at the genome-wide significance level.[30] Individuals with the T/T genotype showed the least mean decrease in symptoms and lack of symptom improvement over time. In terms of symptom dimensions, this variant showed association with questions measuring negative thought, lack of energy, and sadness. Further, the T/T genotype was reported to be associated with decreased expression of the STAC1 gene in the medulla and frontal cortex regions. STAC1 gene is highly expressed in substantia innominate (SI) and locus ceruleus (LC). SI is the main source of cholinergic innervations to the cortical regions and has been shown to be involved in cognitive processes, including attention, learning, and memory. LC sends noradrenergic projections to several brain regions including the prefrontal cortex, and its dysfunction has been associated with many neurological and neuropsychiatric diseases including depression and anxiety.[31] Thus, the STAC1 gene may influence placebo responses by modulating cognitive processes.[30]

Overall, both candidate genes, as well as the GWAS, suggest that the placebo responses utilize a mechanism similar to that used by active medications. However, the studies of the genetics of placebo responses are still in a nascent stage and face limitations, such as lack of replication, much like the initial genetic studies of depression and anxiety. The current sample sizes are relatively small, derived from clinical trials, and are potentially heterogeneous because of different ascertainment criteria. The recent GWAS of antidepressant responses suggest that sample sizes of more than 10,000 may be required to detect significant genome-wide associations.[32] Therefore, similar sample sizes may be required for placebo response studies. In the absence of such large samples, methods such as polygenic risk score analyses that aggregate SNP effect across the genome can help us to understand the genetic architecture and overlap of placebo responses with other traits (e.g., neuroticism, openness) and neuropsychiatric disorders.

Inflammatory diseases and placebos: asthma and arthritis

In a GWAS of the placebo arms of a clinical trials of patients with asthma, the top hit was CAMTA1, a calmodulin binding activator.[33] The protein encoded by this gene is also involved in calcium signaling. The white-coat effect, or the change in systolic blood pressure from before to during a clinical visit, is an established phenomenon associated with placebo responses.[34] A GWAS of the white-coat effect showed an association with CACNA2D3, a gene also associated with calcium signaling, also suggesting a role for calcium signaling in placebo responses.[35]

In some clinical trials, it can be challenging to assess what portion of an effect is attributed to the placebo because patients often take medication simultaneously. The US Food and Drug Administration mandates that patients with rheumatoid arthritis participating in a clinical trial should not be taken off ongoing treatments (i.e., methotrexate) and that they must be switched from a placebo to an active drug within a short period of time if they are randomly assigned to a placebo. In a GWAS of patients from multiple studies of rheumatoid arthritis, almost every trial had patients who were maintained on methotrexate.[33] In context of placebo, previous studies have shown that certain drugs can perturb placebo responsiveness. In this study, the effect of dexamethasone could not be separated from that of placebo.

COVID-19 symptoms and placebo

While placebos are no match for treating conditions of cellular (cancer), bacterial (pneumonia), or viral (COVID-19) proliferation, they can influence symptoms and the side effects of treatment.[36] Further differential effects by genotype in drug and placebo treatment arms can mask both the drug and potential placebo effects in a clinical trial.[37] In a recent randomized trial of colchicine for remission of COVID symptoms, a genomic locus that maps to the pappalysin 1 gene (PAPPA) with links to venous abnormalities was found to be associated with remission in the placebo but not the colchicine treatment arm. Another locus that mapped proximal to the gene encoding NPR3 was associated with remission in both the placebo and colchicine treatment arms. NPR3 is a natriuretic peptide receptor that is involved in the renin-angiotensin system. While these observations are not likely to be linked to placebo effects proper, they suggest there is a potential for differences in response to a placebo and a drug by genotype, or gene-drug/placebo interactions to mask subpopulations that might benefit or be harmed by some drug therapies. These observations underscore the importance of accounting for genetic variation in placebo treatment response in randomized clinical trials.

There are significant limitations to use of GWAS at the genome-wide level. Reproducibility of findings is a major limitation of genetic studies in general. This is particularly difficult with placebo studies, which have, to date, focused on retrospective studies because of the high cost of clinical trials and challenges inherent in funding and recruiting for large placebo focused studies. However, the heterogeneity across clinical trials in disease area, patient population, trial duration, drug treatment regimens, and outcomes pose significant challenges to reproducibility.[38] Generally, many patient factors cannot be excluded or controlled for retrospectively, so retrospective trials provide limited insight into genetic effects on placebo responses. Thus, prospective trials examining the genetic underpinnings of placebos are necessary to investigate how genetics can influence response to placebo treatments.

Other approaches: in vivo molecular imaging and pharmacological studies

In addition to the evidence provided by the field of genomics, in vivo molecular imaging and pharmacological studies have contributed significantly to our understanding of the molecular mechanisms implicated in placebo effects. Among the many different peptides and neurotransmitter systems, the opioid system has been consistently involved in placebo analgesia and antidepressant placebo effects.[39-42] The opioid systems consist of opioid peptides (β-endorphin, endomorphins, enkephalins, and dynorphins) and their opioid receptor sites (μ, β-endorphin, the endomorphins, enkephalins and δ enkephalins, and κ dynorphins). In particular, the μ-opioid receptors (MORs) are critically involved in analgesia, reward, stress responses, and the regulation of emotions. The original study that demonstrated the biological bases of placebo effects used the MOR antagonist naloxone, or placebo, in patients who underwent wisdom tooth extraction.[43] This study showed that patients who received naloxone reported higher pain scores than those who received placebo, suggesting placebo effects reduced pain by engaging endogenous MORs. These findings were followed up by a number of molecular imaging studies using the μ-opioid receptor radioligand [^{11}C]carfentanil in the context of a placebo analgesia manipulation. In a first attempt to use this approach, Zubieta et al. demonstrated that the administration of a placebo with expectations of analgesia was associated with the activation of the endogenous opioid system and μ-opioid receptors in vivo in the rostral and subgenual, the dorsolateral prefrontal cortex, anterior insular cortex, and the nucleus accumbens.[42] Beyond the field of placebo analgesia, the opioid system has also been implicated in antidepressant placebo effects, both using in vivo molecular imaging and pharmacological approaches.[39,44] Here, the authors demonstrated that the administration of antidepressant placebos is associated with increased opioid release, which can be blocked by the μ-opioid antagonist naltrexone. These studies confirmed that the role of the opioid system in placebo effects expands beyond pain processing to modulate mood responses.

Apart from the opioidergic system, several studies have linked the mesolimbic system to placebo analgesia. This hypothesis was first investigated in patients with Parkinson's disease using the D2/3 radioligand [^{11}C]raclopride.[45] This study revealed that the expectation of motor improvement in responses to a placebo treatment was associated with dopamine release in the ventral striatum. Interestingly, no relationship was found between placebo-induced dopamine release and the placebo effects on motor function. The study investigated the role of dopamine neurotransmission in placebo analgesia. This study showed that placebo administration was associated with the activation of dopamine D2/D3 neurotransmission localized in the striatum.[46] Dopamine activation was positively correlated with the individual expectations of analgesia, the update of those expectations during the study period, and the magnitude of analgesia. This hypothesis was also tested in patients with depression using the D2/3 radioligand [^{11}C]raclopride.[47] In this case, the administration of a placebo was also associated with dopamine activation in the ventral striatum; however, placebo-induced dopamine release was not associated with the patient's expectations of antidepressant effects or their actual improvement of depressive symptoms.

Another neurotransmitter system implicated in placebo analgesia is the endocannabinoid system. This system, comprised of cannabinoid CB1 and CB2 receptors and their endogenous ligands, including N-arachidonoyl ethanolamine (anandamide, AEA) and 2-arachidonoyl glycerol (2-AG), is thought to be involved in pain and reward processing, both of which are engaged during the development of placebo effects. Using a conditioning paradigm, investigators demonstrated that the cannabinoid receptor 1 (CBR1) antagonist SR 141716A (Rimonabant) blocked nonopioid, ketorolac-conditioned placebo analgesia, but not opioid placebo responses after morphine conditioning.[48] A different study used a combined candidate gene and in vivo molecular imaging approach to demonstrate an interaction between the cannabinoid and the opioid system during placebo analgesia.[49] This study combined genotyping information from the functional missense variant Pro129Thr of the gene coding fatty acid amide hydrolase (FAAH), the major degrading enzyme of endocannabinoids, and a placebo analgesia experiment using [^{11}C]carfentanil and [^{11}C]raclopride molecular imaging. FAAH Pro129/Pro129 homozygotes had greater endogenous opioid system activation, but not dopamine, in widespread regions cortically and subcortically. The effects of FAAH on placebo-induced regional activation of µ-opioid neurotransmission were significantly correlated with placebo analgesia.

This evidence demonstrates the role of opioid and nonopioid mechanisms in placebo effects across different clinical conditions. These processes are important to understanding the interindividual variability that leads to recovery from any illness. Opioid, dopamine, and endocannabinoid neurotransmission seem to modulate various elements of placebo effects, including value representation, expectancy update, and changes in sensory and emotional ratings over time. Further, the circuitry involved in placebo analgesia also has the potential to modulate several functions beyond pain, such as stress regulation, neuroendocrine and autonomic functions, mood, reward, and contextual processing.

Conclusions

As biological research techniques become more precise, researchers and physicians have the opportunity to move toward personalized medicine by utilizing an individual's genetic profile to make treatment decisions. Understanding the molecular drivers of placebo effects and responses in randomized clinical trials is critical to identifying who responds to placebos, and importantly, who responds to drug treatment. Genomics, neuroimaging, and pharmacology have all proven to be useful in identifying molecular factors that influence outcomes in clinical trials. While these approaches are still in their early stages, it appears there are a variety of genes involved in drug response; some overlap, and some differ from those that affect outcomes in the placebo treatment arms. Further, these studies have elucidated the potential for gene-drug interactions that can potentially mask the subpopulations of patients that respond to placebos or particular drugs.

We are a long way from elucidating all the pathways involved in placebo responses (and effects) and understanding how they overlap and potentially interact with disease pathophysiological networks. What is clear is that broad collaborations across disease and treatment paradigms that collect biological samples for OMICS and deep-learning analyses are needed to accelerate our understanding of the molecular mechanisms of placebos.

References

1. Wager TD, Atlas LY. The neuroscience of placebo effects: Connecting context, learning and health. *Nature Reviews Neuroscience.* 2015;16(7):403–418. http://doi:10.1038/nrn3976
2. Prossin A, Koch A, Campbell P, Laumet G, Stohler CS, Dantzer R, Zubieta JK. Effects of placebo administration on immune mechanisms and relationships with central endogenous opioid neurotransmission. *Molecular Psychiatry.* 2022;27(2):831–839. doi:10.1038/s41380-021-01365-x.
3. Ozdemir V, Endrenyi L. Rethinking clinical trials and personalized medicine with placebogenomics and placebo dose. *OMICS.* 2021;25(1):1–12. http://doi:10.1089/omi.2020.0208
4. Hall KT, Loscalzo J, Kaptchuk T. Pharmacogenomics and the placebo response. *ACS Chemical Neuroscience.* 2018;9(4):633–635. http://doi:10.1021/acschemneuro.8b00078

5. Wang RS, Croteau-Chonka DC, Silverman EK, Loscalzo J, Weiss ST, Hall KT. Pharmacogenomics and placebo response in a randomized clinical trial in asthma. *Clinical Pharmacology and Therapeutics.* 2019;106(6):1261–1267. http://doi:10.1002/cpt.1646

6. Dube MP, Lemacon A, Barhdadi A, et al. Genetics of symptom remission in outpatients with COVID-19. *Scientific Reports.* 2021;11(1):10847. http://doi:10.1038/s41598-021-90365-6

7. Yeo A, Li L, Warren L, et al. Pharmacogenetic meta-analysis of baseline risk factors, pharmacodynamic, efficacy and tolerability endpoints from two large global cardiovascular outcomes trials for darapladib. *PLoS ONE.* 2017;12(7):e0182115. http://doi:10.1371/journal.pone.0182115

8. Buniello A, MacArthur JAL, Cerezo M, et al. The NHGRI-EBI GWAS catalog of published genome-wide association studies, targeted arrays and summary statistics 2019. *Nucleic Acids Research.* 2019;47(D1):D1005–D1012. http://doi:10.1093/nar/gky1120

9. Ford AC, Sperber AD, Corsetti M, Camilleri M. Irritable bowel syndrome. *Lancet.* 2020;396(10263):1675–1688. http://doi:10.1016/S0140-6736(20)31548-8

10. Buono JL, Carson RT, Flores NM. Health-related quality of life, work productivity, and indirect costs among patients with irritable bowel syndrome with diarrhea. *Health and Quality of Life Outcomes.* 2017;15(1):35. http://doi:10.1186/s12955-017-0611-2

11. Hall KT, Lembo AJ, Kirsch I, et al. Catechol-O-methyltransferase val158met polymorphism predicts placebo effect in irritable bowel syndrome. *PLoS ONE.* 2012;7(10):e48135. http://doi:10.1371/journal.pone.0048135

12. Wang R-S, Lembo AJ, Kaptchuk TJ, et al. Genomic effects associated with response to placebo treatment in a randomized trial of irritable bowel syndrome: Original research. *Frontiers in Pain Research (Lausanne).* 2022;2:775386. http://doi:10.3389/fpain.2021.775386.

13. Duclot F, Kabbaj M. The role of early growth response 1 (EGR1) in brain plasticity and neuropsychiatric disorders. *Frontiers in Behavioral Neuroscience.* 2017;11:35. http://doi:10.3389/fnbeh.2017.00035

14. Rastelli D, Robinson A, Lagomarsino VN, Matthews LT, Hassan R, Perez K, Dan W, Yim PD, Mixer M, Prochera A, Shepherd A, Sun L, Hall K, Ballou S, Lembo A, Nee J, Rao M. Diminished androgen levels are linked to irritable bowel syndrome and cause bowel dysfunction in mice. *Journal of Clinical Investigation.* 2022;132(2):e150789. http://doi:10.1172/JCI150789.

15. Yu R, Gollub RL, Vangel M, Kaptchuk T, Smoller JW, Kong J. Placebo analgesia and reward processing: integrating genetics, personality, and intrinsic brain activity. *Human Brain Mapping.* 2014;35(9):4583–4593. http://doi:10.1002/hbm.22496

16. Shaibani A, Frisaldi E, Benedetti F. Placebo response in pain, fatigue, and performance: Possible implications for neuromuscular disorders. *Muscle Nerve.* 2017;56(3):358–367. http://doi:10.1002/mus.25635

17. Kaptchuk TJ, Hemond CC, Miller FG. Placebos in chronic pain: Evidence, theory, ethics, and use in clinical practice. *British Medical Journal.* 2020;370:m1668. http://doi:10.1136/bmj.m1668

18. Kosek E, Cohen M, Baron R, et al. Do we need a third mechanistic descriptor for chronic pain states? *Pain.* 2016;157(7):1382–1386. http://doi:10.1097/j.pain.0000000000000507

19. Lembo A, Kelley JM, Nee J, et al. Open-label placebo vs double-blind placebo for irritable bowel syndrome: A randomized clinical trial. *Pain.* 2021;162(9):2428–2435. http://doi:10.1097/j.pain.0000000000002234

20. Vollert J, Wang R, Regis S, Yetman H, Lembo AJ, Kaptchuk TJ, Cheng V, Nee J, Iturrino J, Loscalzo J, Hall KT, Silvester JA. Genotypes of pain and analgesia in a randomized trial of irritable bowel syndrome. *Frontiers in Psychiatry.* 2022 Mar 23;13:842030. doi:10.3389/fpsyt.2022.842030.

21. Freidin MB, Stalteri MA, Wells PM, et al. An association between chronic widespread pain and the gut microbiome. *Rheumatology (Oxford)*. 2021;60(8):3727–3737. http://doi:10.1093/rheumatology/keaa847

22. Hirata T, Koga K, Johnson TA, et al. Japanese GWAS identifies variants for bust-size, dysmenorrhea, and menstrual fever that are eQTLs for relevant protein-coding or long noncoding RNAs. *Scientific Reports*. 2018;8(1):8502. http://doi:10.1038/s41598-018-25065-9

23. Furukawa TA, Cipriani A, Atkinson LZ, et al. Placebo response rates in antidepressant trials: a systematic review of published and unpublished double-blind randomised controlled studies. *Lancet Psychiatry*. 2016;3(11):1059–1066. http://doi:10.1016/S2215-0366(16)30307-8

24. Rief W, Nestoriuc Y, Weiss S, Welzel E, Barsky AJ, Hofmann SG. Meta-analysis of the placebo response in antidepressant trials. *Journal of Affective Disorders*. 2009;118(1–3):1–8. http://doi:10.1016/j.jad.2009.01.029

25. Holmes RD, Tiwari AK, Kennedy JL. Mechanisms of the placebo effect in pain and psychiatric disorders. *Pharmacogenomics Journal*. 2016;16(6):491–500. http://doi:10.1038/tpj.2016.15

26. Leuchter AF, McCracken JT, Hunter AM, Cook IA, Alpert JE. Monoamine oxidase A and catechol-o-methyltransferase functional polymorphisms and the placebo response in major depressive disorder. *Journal of Clinical Psychopharmacology*. 2009;29(4):372–377. http://doi:10.1097/JCP.0b013e3181ac4aaf

27. Tiwari AK, Zai CC, Sajeev G, Arenovich T, Muller DJ, Kennedy JL. Analysis of 34 candidate genes in bupropion and placebo remission. *International Journal of Neuropsychopharmacology*. 2013;16(4):771–781. http://doi:10.1017/S1461145712000843

28. Benedetti F, Carlino E, Pollo A. How placebos change the patient's brain. *Neuropsychopharmacology*. 2011;36(1):339–354. doi:10.1038/npp.2010.81

29. Maciukiewicz M, Marshe VS, Tiwari AK, et al. Genetic variation in IL-1beta, IL-2, IL-6, TSPO and BDNF and response to duloxetine or placebo treatment in major depressive disorder. *Pharmacogenomics*. 2015;16(17):1919–1929. http://doi:10.2217/pgs.15.136

30. Maciukiewicz M, Marshe VS, Tiwari AK, et al. Genome-wide association studies of placebo and duloxetine response in major depressive disorder. *Pharmacogenomics Journal*. 2018;18(3):406–412. http://doi:10.1038/tpj.2017.29

31. Poe GR, Foote S, Eschenko O, et al. Locus coeruleus: A new look at the blue spot. *Nature Reviews Neuroscience* 2020;21(11):644–659. http://doi:10.1038/s41583-020-0360-9

32. Pain O, Hodgson K, Trubetskoy V, Ripke S, Marshe VS, Adams MJ, Byrne EM, Campos AI, Carrillo-Roa T, Cattaneo A, Als TD, Souery D, Dernovsek MZ, Fabbri C, Hayward C, Henigsberg N, Hauser J, Kennedy JL, Lenze EJ, Lewis G, Müller DJ, Martin NG, Mulsant BH, Mors O, Perroud N, Porteous DJ, Rentería ME, Reynolds CF 3rd, Rietschel M, Uher R, Wigmore EM, Maier W, Wray NR, Aitchison KJ, Arolt V, Baune BT, Biernacka JM, Bondolfi G, Domschke K, Kato M, Li QS, Liu YL, Serretti A, Tsai SJ, Turecki G, Weinshilboum R; GSRD Consortium; Major Depressive Disorder Working Group of the Psychiatric Genomics Consortium; McIntosh AM, Lewis CM. Identifying the common genetic basis of antidepressant response. *Biological Psychiatry Global Open Science*. 2022; (2):115–126. doi:10.1016/j.bpsgos.2021.07.008.

33. Haug-Baltzell A, Bhangale TR, Chang D, et al. Previously reported placebo-response-associated variants do not predict patient outcomes in inflammatory disease phase III trial placebo arms. *Genes & Immunity*. 2019;20(2):172–179. http://doi:10.1038/s41435-018-0018-z

34. Suonsyrja T, Hannila-Handelberg T, Fodstad H, Donner K, Kontula K, Hiltunen TP. Renin-angiotensin system and alpha-adducin gene polymorphisms and their relation to responses to antihypertensive drugs: Results from the GENRES study. *American Journal of Hypertension*. 2009;22(2):169–175. http://doi:10.1038/ajh.2008.343

35. Ogata S, Kamide K, Asayama K, et al. Genome-wide association study for white coat effect in Japanese middle-aged to elderly people: The HOMED-BP study. *Clinical and Experimental Hypertension*. 2018;40(4):363–369. http://doi:10.1080/10641963.2017.1384481

36. Amanzio M, Mitsikostas DD, Giovannelli F, Bartoli M, Cipriani GE, Brown WA. Adverse events of active and placebo groups in SARS-CoV-2 vaccine randomized trials: A systematic review. *Lancet Regional Health Europe*. 2022;12:100253. http://doi:10.1016/j.lanepe.2021.100253

37. Hall KT, Loscalzo J, Kaptchuk TJ. Systems pharmacogenomics: Gene, disease, drug and placebo interactions—A case study in COMT. *Pharmacogenomics*. 2019;20(7):529–551. http://doi:10.2217/pgs-2019-0001

38. Hall KT, Vase L, Tobias DK, et al. Historical controls in randomized clinical trials: Opportunities and challenges. *Clinical Pharmacology and Therapeutics*. 2021;109(2):343–351. http://doi:10.1002/cpt.1970

39. Pecina M, Bohnert AS, Sikora M, et al. Association between placebo-activated neural systems and antidepressant responses: Neurochemistry of placebo effects in major depression. *JAMA Psychiatry*. 2015;72(11):1087–1094. http://doi:10.1001/jamapsychiatry.2015.1335

40. Petrovic P, Kalso E, Petersson KM, Ingvar M. Placebo and opioid analgesia: Imaging a shared neuronal network. *Science*. 2002;295(5560):1737–1740. http://doi:10.1126/science.1067176

41. Eippert F, Bingel U, Schoell ED, et al. Activation of the opioidergic descending pain control system underlies placebo analgesia. *Neuron*. 2009;63(4):533–543. http://doi:10.1016/j.neuron.2009.07.014

42. Zubieta JK, Bueller JA, Jackson LR, et al. Placebo effects mediated by endogenous opioid activity on mu-opioid receptors. *Journal of Neuroscience*. 2005;25(34):7754–7762. http://doi:10.1523/JNEUROSCI.0439-05.2005

43. Levine JD, Gordon NC, Fields HL. The mechanism of placebo analgesia. *Lancet*. 1978;2(8091):654–657. http://doi:10.1016/s0140-6736(78)92762-9

44. Pecina M, Chen J, Lyew T, Karp JF, Dombrovski AY. Mu opioid antagonist naltrexone partially abolishes the antidepressant placebo effect and reduces orbitofrontal cortex encoding of reinforcement. *Biological Psychiatry: Cognitive Neuroscience and Neuroimaging*. 2021;6(10):1002–1012. http://doi:10.1016/j.bpsc.2021.02.009

45. de la Fuente-Fernandez R, Stoessl AJ. The placebo effect in Parkinson's disease. *Trends in Neurosciences*. 2002;25(6):302–306. http://doi:10.1016/s0166-2236(02)02181-1

46. Scott DJ, Stohler CS, Egnatuk CM, Wang H, Koeppe RA, Zubieta JK. Individual differences in reward responding explain placebo-induced expectations and effects. *Neuron*. 2007;55(2):325–336. http://doi:10.1016/j.neuron.2007.06.028

47. Pecina M, Sikora M, Avery ET, et al. Striatal dopamine D2/3 receptor-mediated neurotransmission in major depression: Implications for anhedonia, anxiety and treatment response. *European Neuropsychopharmacology*. 2017;27(10):977–986. http://doi:10.1016/j.euroneuro.2017.08.427

48. Benedetti F, Amanzio M, Rosato R, Blanchard C. Nonopioid placebo analgesia is mediated by CB1 cannabinoid receptors. *Nature Medicine*. 2011;17(10):1228–1230. http://doi:10.1038/nm.2435

49. Pecina M, Martinez-Jauand M, Hodgkinson C, Stohler CS, Goldman D, Zubieta JK. FAAH selectively influences placebo effects. *Molecular Psychiatry*. 2014;19(3):385–391. http://doi:10.1038/mp.2013.124

2.3

Dynamic regulation of genes in placebo responsiveness in alcohol use disorder and co-occurring pain

Chamindi Seneviratne, Susan G. Dorsey, and Luana Colloca

Introduction

Alcohol misuse is attributed to development of more than 200 diseases, including alcohol use disorder (AUD), and 2%–10% of all deaths reported worldwide each year.[1] The percentage of those who progress on to developing AUD has remained around 10% of the U.S. population in the past decade.[2] More importantly, a significant proportion of those who misuse alcohol also experience moderate-to-severe pain. Pain and AUD are complex and common conditions that contribute significantly to the global disease burden.[3,4] Chronic pain (CP) affects 20% of the world's adult population,[5] while a quarter of the adult population in the United States and in many countries around the world consume alcohol in harmful quantitates (i.e., alcohol misuse).[6,7] In fact, CP is one of the most common comorbid conditions observed with AUD, and some studies have indicated that the prevalence of comorbidity can be well over 50% in those who seek treatment for AUD.[8,9]

Response to placebos and in general to pharmacologic treatments is highly variable among individuals and the genetic makeup of a person (i.e., the variations in DNA sequence) among individuals may contribute to the response heterogeneity (see also Chapter 2.2). However, the conversion of DNA sequence into functional products (i.e., gene expression) is not a linear or static process.[10] It is a process governed by constant interplay between DNA sequence variation that does not change during a person's lifetime under normal or healthy conditions, and environmental exposures. This fundamental concept is particularly important in the understanding of molecular dysregulation in AUD (and CP), as attributes such as the type, frequency, and quantity often vary considerably. The purpose of this chapter is to highlight these mechanisms and studies conducted to identify specific dynamically regulated genes that are associated with placebo responsiveness in individuals with AUD. We begin with a discussion on neurobiological dysregulation highlighting the dynamic nature of pathophysiology. Moreover, we discuss research conducted to identify specific genes whose expression alterations drive molecular changes underlying placebo responses in AUD and CP both separately and comorbidly, and finally discuss future directions addressing gaps in current knowledge.

Neurobiology of alcohol use disorder and pain

A mechanistic understanding of the relationship between AUD and pain disorders is important for effective treatment and prevention of both conditions. Laboratory human studies and animal models have demonstrated bidirectional associations between CP syndromes and alcohol misuse and AUD.[11-13] One line of evidence suggests that the analgesic properties of acute alcohol consumption contribute to higher prevalence of alcohol misuse and AUD among those with CP syndromes, while other evidence argues that the aberrant neurobiological mechanisms underlying CP may in fact promote the journey from alcohol use to misuse to AUD.[14]

Repeated exposure to alcohol over time offsets the homeostatic threshold between reward and stress, leading to emotional distress or negative affect, termed as *hyperkatifeia*, resulting in a motivational shift in drinking behaviors from positive to negative reinforcement in those who are vulnerable to developing AUD.[15,16] The dysregulated homeostasis manifests as the pathological state of addiction[17] characterized by three stages that are repeated cyclically: compulsive alcohol seeking, uncontrollable alcohol consumption, and increased "emotional pain" and distress when alcohol is inaccessible.[18] The process of transition from acute to CP in CP disorders (i.e., pain chronification) shares common features with the neurobiological processes underlying AUD.[19] Similar to the dysregulation caused by repeated alcohol exposures, repeated acute pain episodes dysregulate the homeostasis between reward and stress.[20] Further, recurrent acute pain episodes hypersensitize the aversion/stress system and hyposensitize the reward system, consequently offsetting pain threshold within endogenous pain relief pathways.[21] This offset will require stronger subsequent stimuli to activate the reward systems to alleviate pain. In this light, both AUD and CP conditions overlap with each other in terms of neurobiology and can be considered as dysregulated states of homeostasis between stress and reward systems.

The reward and stress stimuli are processed in the brain through dynamic and complex interplay between phasic and tonic release of neurotransmitters and neuronal firing.[22-24] Under physiological states, most neurotransmitters such as dopamine, endorphins, and glutamine, are in fact maintained at steady levels in the extracellular space via feedback mechanisms. Repeated exposures over time alter the neurochemical balance leading to development of alcohol tolerance or aversion to pain. These dynamic processes are not uniform across individuals in either condition, neither do they uniformly occur within an individual when exposed to differing conditions or over time. Research has shown significant variation in neurobiological regulation in alcohol use/misuse and AUD as well as pain syndromes influenced by both environmental and biological factors such as a person's genetic background. These differences affect how individuals respond to treatment with pharmacological or behavioral therapies. Moreover, the neurobiological processes underlying AUD comorbid with pain syndromes constitute a state that differs from either condition alone, requiring focused research for the development of neurobiology-based treatment strategies including a better understanding of the placebo responses in populations with comorbid AUD and pain. An important question would be whether this overlap in neural mechanisms alter placebo responses.

The placebo component underlying drinking and treatment for AUD in clinical trials

Responses to treatment of alcohol misuse arise from highly complex interactions between responses to treatment itself (process-A in Figure 2.3.1) and pharmacological effects underlying continued drinking during or around treatment (process-B in Figure 2.3.1) that may feedback to moderate treatment responses. Genetic variations can influence each of these mechanisms, along with other environmental and biological factors. While larger phase 2 trials have been employed to study placebo effects involving process-A, studies exploring placebo effects underlying process-B are mostly limited to smaller "laboratory-based" mechanistic studies.

Randomized placebo-controlled trials have a long history in the alcohol and drug addiction field,[25] but most trials have utilized placebos purely as a comparator group. A landmark study by Litten et al. revealed that the placebo responses in improving percentage of abstinent days across 51 AUD treatment trials that tested acamprosate, naltrexone or a combination ranged from 20.8% to 93.5%.[26] A variability of this magnitude in placebo responses

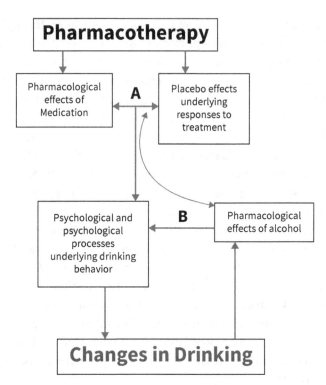

Figure 2.3.1 Processes underlying response to treatment of alcohol misuse. Simplified schematic presentation of (A) interactive effects between an active pharmacologic agent (i.e., medication) and placebo effects associated with responses to pharmacologic treatment. The cumulative interactive effects of these two components are referred to as "process-A" in the text. (B) feedback effects of pharmacologic properties of altered drinking amounts, which is referred to as "process-B" in the text. Processes A and B interact with each other to elicit overall effects of medication treatments to alter drinking patterns.

makes it difficult to discern a quantifiable treatment effect for modestly effective investigational medications. Therefore, identifying factors that influence placebo responses in AUD trials, including genomic factors, is crucial for the development of efficacious medications. A few studies have looked at the effects of variation of DNA sequence among individuals, at specific locations within genes hypothesized to moderate treatment responses (i.e., candidate genetic associations) including placebo responses in AUD trials (Table 2.3.1). As stated above, the information encoded in DNA sequence of a gene is used in the synthesis of end products (i.e., protein or noncoding RNA) through *gene expression*. None of the above-mentioned studies have explored whether the candidate genetic associations (i.e., associations with DNA

Table 2.3.1 Genetic associations within placebo arms of AUD pharmacotherapy trials

Gene	Outcome Measure	Genetic Association with Placebo Responses (N)	Treatment Duration	Tested Active Pharmacologic Agent (Dose)	Adjunctive treatments*	Source
GABBR1	(1) Percentage of days abstinent (2) Average DPD	Improved in rs29220-GG/GC genotype carriers compared to CC carriers (N = 21)	12 weeks	Baclofen (30–75 mg/day)	Brief compliance therapy	43
SLC6A4	Nighttime drinking intensity	Placebo treatment was associated with lower nighttime drinking intensity in individuals with early-onset alcoholism carrying 5-HTTLPR+rs25531-L$_A$L$_A$ genotypes (N = 7) who were experiencing higher levels of daily anxiety	12 weeks	Sertraline (50–200 mg/day)	Structured coping skills training sessions	44
OPRM1	Daily desire to drink	Greater desire to drink resulted in higher drinking in placebo treated rs1799971-AG/GG compared to AA (N = 77) genotype carriers	12 weeks	Naltrexone (50 mg/day)	Structured coping skills training sessions	45
OPRM1	DPD	DPD correlated positively with cue-elicited activation of mPFC and VS in rs1799971-AG/GG compared to AA carriers	7 days	Naltrexone (50 mg/day)	None	46

(continued)

Table 2.3.1 Continued

Gene	Outcome Measure	Genetic Association with Placebo Responses (N)	Treatment Duration	Tested Active Pharmacologic Agent (Dose)	Adjunctive treatments*	Source
OPRM1 and SLC6A3 combination	(1) Average DPD (2) Percent heavy drinking days	Improved in carriers of: 1) SLC6A3:rs28363170-9R,9R/9R,10R and OPRM1:rs1799971-GG, compared to AA/AG carriers (N = 17) 2) SLC6A3:rs28363170-10R,10R and OPRM1:rs1799971-AA/AG, compared to GG carriers (N = 28)	5 days	Naltrexone (25–50 mg/day)	None	47
SLC6A3 COMT DRD2 DRD4	Drinking in a bar lab	(1) Greater alcohol cue-elicited VS activation and (2) higher number of standard drinks** consumed by carriers of greater number of alleles in the following dopamine-related genetic composite: SLC6A3:rs28363170l-9R, COMT: rs4680-A, DRD2:rs1076560-T, and/or DRD4 long allele (N = 24)	8 days	Aripiprazole (titrated to 15 mg)	none	48

CBI, cognitive behavioral intervention; DPD, drinks per day; **represent adjunctive treatments common to both placebo and active medication arms; *standard drink, an alcoholic beverage that contains 14 grams of pure alcohol in the United States.; mPFC, medial frontal cortex; VS, ventral striatum.

sequence variation) with placebo responses resulted through altered expression of relevant genes. Further, the findings have not been widely replicated by independent research, and the placebo groups often consisted of adjunctive behavioral therapies that varied widely across studies. Nevertheless, it is intriguing that the genetic variants that were associated with lower placebo responses showed greater response to the active pharmacologic agent, and suggested mechanisms underlying these opposing effects within individuals based on their genetic variation require further scrutiny.

Treatment of AUD or alcohol misuse is further complicated by continued drinking exerting pharmacological and other psychological processes such as craving or expectancies of reinforcing effects of alcohol associated with drinking behavior, in addition to pharmacologic effects of medications and placebo effects associated with undergoing treatment as discussed above. To explore pharmacological and placebo responses underlying drinking behavior (process-B in Figure 2.3.1), researchers have utilized experimental paradigms involving controlled bar-like settings where participants are served alcohol and monitored or observed by research staff for various outcome measures. These studies commonly involve *placebo alcohol beverages* such as fruit juice laced with small volumes of about 1% alcohol that are too low to elicit any pharmacological effects of alcohol or floated on top to provide the odor of alcohol, and in some studies, commercially available nonalcoholic beverages such as nonalcoholic beer or wine that are similar in texture and appearance to the regular alcohol beverages of the same type or brand. Another masking strategy is to present participants with false breath alcohol concentration readings following placebo alcohol consumption. Interestingly, several studies have reported responses to placebo alcohol similar to consuming regular alcohol in genetically specified subgroups (Table 2.3.2). Of note, the studies listed in Table 2.3.2 have utilized a candidate genetic analysis approach of known functional polymorphisms within genes hypothesized to underlie placebo responses. For example, the 7-repeat elements in DRD4 gene have been shown to blunt the intracellular response to dopamine,[27] which may translate to increased drug seeking, or the 5-HTTLPR-LL genotype that were shown to be associated with greater transcription rates resulting in increased copies of serotonin transporters and clearance of serotonin at the synapses. Further, the 5-HTTLPR-LL genotype has also been reported to be associated with treatment response to several pharmacologic agents for the treatment of AUD.[28,29]

As with studies on treatment responses, it is unknown whether gene expression alterations played an intermediary role in genetic associations observed with responses to placebo alcohol consumption. As expression of genes is

Table 2.3.2 Genetic associations with placebo responses underlying drinking

Gene	Genetic Association with Placebo Responses (N)	Source
DRD4	Noncarriers of exon-3 VNTR 7-repeat elements perceived themselves to be more sociable compared to carriers, when they consumed placebo alcohol beverages that were both concealed as regular alcohol or unmasked mimicking open-label placebo administration	49
GABRG1	3-UTR rs6447493-TT genotype carriers had strong stimulatory response to placebo as measured on the Biphasic Alcohol Effects Scale, while there were no genotype-based differences observed in response to high doses of alcohol	50
GABRA2	Carriers of rs279871-AA genotype exposed to aromas of their preferred alcoholic drink while infused with saline (placebo) than did AG subjects; during the alcohol session, there were no group differences	51
GABRA2	Carriers of the minor alleles for a haplotype that spanned across GABRA2 reported lower mean "negative" alcohol effects scores than individuals homozygous for the common allele in response to placebo alcohol	52
OXTR	rs1488467-GG carriers demonstrated greater aggression compared to rs1488467-CG as measured by the Response Choice Aggression Paradigm scale; alcohol group showed opposite effects	53

sensitive to environmental and biological factors, meticulous study design is crucial for identifying specific genes responsive to placebos. Findings from a recent study by our group demonstrated that the sequence of alcohol administration may in fact influence gene expression alterations associated with placebo responses in cross-over trials.[30] In this study, the mRNA expression levels of SLC6A4 gene were significantly higher when placebo alcohol was administered in the first sequence compared to later sequences in the absence of measurable amounts of alcohol in blood during placebo alcohol administration days. Whether and how these alterations occurred during placebo administration remain to be explored in future studies.

Gene expression profiling of placebo responsiveness to AUD comorbid with pain

Gene expression profiling can be used to identify molecular mechanisms of CP conditions and pain states, patients who are likely to respond favorably to pharmacologic or placebo interventions from nonresponders, and novel therapeutic targets to reduce pain through intracellular signaling pathways that are engaged or repressed during placebo interventions. Two recent hypothesis-generating transcriptome-wide analyses have aided in identifying gene expression biomarkers beyond the capacity of smaller candidate approaches with strong mechanistic bases (Table 2.3.3). A transcriptome-wide study by Theken et al. reported that 39 of 47 genes enriched in inflammatory pathways differentially expressed in both complete responders to ibuprofen treatment and the placebo group.[31] Although the pain tolerance scores were significantly lower in the placebo group compared to ibuprofen responders, the overlap of the differentially expressed genes between the two groups is promising and suggestive of molecular mechanisms that can potentially be harnessed to improve treatment outcomes. Two other studies have also reported expression alterations in inflammatory genes in response to treatment with a placebo in those with irritable bowel syndrome[32] and knee osteoarthritis,[33] further highlighting the role of inflammatory pathways underlying placebo responses.

Table 2.3.3 Genes and pathways with altered expression in responses to placebo interventions

Condition	Genes/ Pathways	Effect	P-Value	Study Design	Source
Surgical extraction of bony impacted third molars	Phagosome formation	Differentially expressed 3.17 ± 0.42 hours after placebo administration from baseline	1.41×10^{-8}	PBMC transcriptomics	31
	iCOS-iCOSL signaling in T helper cells		3.01×10^{-8}		
	CD28 signaling in T helper cells		5.98×10^{-8}		
	Role of macrophages, fibroblasts and endothelial cell in RA		6.31×10^{-8}		
	Role of NFAT in regulation of immune response		1.40×10^{-7}		
Irritable bowel syndrome	EGR1	Reduced after 6 weeks of placebo	2.00×10^{-2}	Whole blood transcriptomics	32
Knee osteoarthritis	Col1A and Col6	Elevated after 10 days of placebo	$< 5.00 \times 10^{-2}$	Candidate gene analysis in synovial MSC	33

RA, rheumatoid arthritis; MSC, mesenchymal stem cells; NFAT, nuclear factor of activated T cell gene.

Both AUD and CP are heterogeneous, vary widely among individuals, and share many pathophysiological commonalities. Both conditions have large and genetically moderated placebo effects on disease progression and response to treatments.[26,34] Despite these facts and the high prevalence of AUD and CP co-occurrence, influence of genetic variation on placebo responsiveness, or the underlying gene expression alterations, remains an unexplored area of research at present. Nevertheless, there is convincing indirect evidence of genetic mechanisms common to CP and AUD that may drive the differential expression of genes.

The OPRM1 gene is the most widely studied candidate gene in AUD mechanistic and treatment trials as it encodes the mu-opioid receptors that are the primary target molecule of naltrexone, one of the three US Food and Drug Administration–approved medications to treat AUD. Mu-opioid receptors constitute the primary site of action of endogenous opioid peptides[35] and, therefore, are widely implicated in pathophysiology and treatment responses to CP conditions. In humans, molecular studies have revealed a functional difference of mu-opioid receptors (i.e., differences in expression levels and/or function of the protein molecule/the receptor) based on which of the alleles of single-nucleotide polymorphism (rs1799971; also known as A118G or Asn440Asp) present in the exon 1 of OPRM1 gene. The rs1799971-G allelic variant compared to AA variant, was associated with lower expression of mu-opioid receptors at the surface in smokers and those with AUD,[36,37] and decreased agonist binding and forskolin-induced cAMP activation.[38] By using mu-opioid selective agonist radiotracer [^{11}C] carfentanil and positron emission tomography, Pecina et al. demonstrated a reduction of baseline mu-opioid receptor availability in regions implicated in pain and affective regulation in healthy volunteers carrying rs1799971-G allele.[39] Lower endogenous opioid and dopamine system activation in G-allele carriers to a placebo during expectation of analgesia in several brain regions, including anterior insula, amygdala, thalamus, and brainstem, and higher neuroticism scores may increase vulnerability to stress and depression. Colloca et al. expanded upon these findings to explore epistasis of variations in OPRM1 with two other genes including catechol-O-methyltransferase (COMT) and fatty acid amide hydrolase (FAAH) that have been reported to be associated with placebo hypoalgesia.[40] The carriers of rs1799971-AA (genotype that showed greater response in Pecina et al) combined with FAAH rs324420-CC (Pro/Pro) and COMT gene rs4680-AA (met/met) polymorphisms together showed significant placebo effects. Placebo responsiveness underlying both treatment of AUD and drinking varied in carriers of these genotypes, suggesting potential common genetic mechanisms underlying AUD comorbid with CP (see Tables 2.3.1 and 2.3.2).

Gaps in transcriptomic research on placebo responses

Studying expression profiles of genes provides the opportunity to decipher the function of genes under varying conditions. Such changes in gene expression patterns are possibly governed by varying patterns of drinking, such as type, frequency, and quantity. Likewise, pain disorders also vary on a continuum influenced by a multitude of factors that potentially and bidirectionally affect placebo effects and responses. While gene expression analyses, especially at a transcriptome-wide level, are only beginning to emerge, it is crucial to consider several factors that could propagate and accelerate such analyses. These may include: (1) systematic and standardized assessment of alcohol and other substance use, (2) inclusion of comorbid AUD and CP populations in CP and AUD clinical trials respectively, (3) improvement of access to clinical large data for exploratory analyses of moderating effects, (4) improvement of methodological aspects in reporting findings (i.e., assessment of changes from baseline in the placebo arms of RCTs rather than reporting results of the active agent "relative to placebo"), and (5) longitudinal biological studies to capture dynamic changes in gene expression driving molecular responses to treatment and disease progression. It should also be noted that the gene expression profiles of different postmortem brain regions from diseased individuals were estimated to correlate only 74%–79% with that of peripheral blood from living individuals.[41,42] This is another area of research that requires more innovative approaches to accurately capture molecular changes in response to psychosomatic phenomena such as placebo effects and responses.

There are only a few evidence-based treatments available for the treatment of substance co-use, and even fewer to address CP among individuals with comorbid opioid use disorder and/or AUD.[9] As gene expression is the intermediary between genotype and phenotype that is sensitive to environmental changes and closest to genotype, gene expression findings can have enormous translational potential for developing novel approaches to treatment and diagnosis.

References

1. World Health Organization. Alcohol [Internet]. World Health Organization; 2022 [cited 2023 Jul 6]. Available from: https://www.who.int/news-room/fact-sheets/detail/alcohol
2. National Institute on Alcohol Abuse and Alcoholism. *Alcohol use disorder (AUD) in the United States: Age groups and demographic characteristics.* [Internet]. National Institute on

Alcohol Abuse and Alcoholism; 2023 [cited 2023 Jul 6]. Available from: https://www. niaaa.nih.gov/alcohols-effects-health/alcohol-topics/alcohol-facts-and-statistics/ alcohol-use-disorder-aud-united-states-age-groups-and-demographic-characteristics

3. Mills SEE, Nicolson KP, Smith BH. Chronic pain: A review of its epidemiology and associated factors in population-based studies. *British Journal of Anaesthesia.* 2019;123(2):e273–e283.

4. Maleki N, Oscar-Berman M. Chronic pain in relation to depressive disorders and alcohol abuse. *Brain Sciences.* 2020;10(11):826. doi:10.3390/brainsci10110826.

5. Goldberg DS, McGee SJ. Pain as a global public health priority. *BMC Public Health.* 2011;11:770.

6. Hingson RW, Zha W, White AM. Drinking beyond the binge threshold: Predictors, consequences, and changes in the U.S. *American Journal of Preventive Medicine.* 2017;52(6):717–727.

7. Creswell KG, Chung T, Skrzynski CJ, et al. Drinking beyond the binge threshold in a clinical sample of adolescents. *Addiction.* 2020;115(8):1472–1481.

8. Abdin E, Subramaniam M, Vaingankar JA, Chong SA. The role of sociodemographic factors in the risk of transition from alcohol use to disorders and remission in Singapore. *Alcohol and Alcoholism.* 2014;49(1):103–108.

9. Witkiewitz K, Vowles KE. Alcohol and opioid use, co-use, and chronic pain in the context of the opioid epidemic: A critical review. *Alcoholism: Clinical and Experimental Research.* 2018;42(3):478–488.

10. Alvarez M, Schrey AW, Richards CL. Ten years of transcriptomics in wild populations: What have we learned about their ecology and evolution? *Molecular Ecology.* 2015;24(4):710–725.

11. Zale EL, Maisto SA, Ditre JW. Interrelations between pain and alcohol: An integrative review. *Clinical Psychology Review.* 2015;37:57–71.

12. Alford DP, German JS, Samet JH, Cheng DM, Lloyd-Travaglini CA, Saitz R. Primary care patients with drug use report chronic pain and self-medicate with alcohol and other drugs. *Journal of General Internal Medicine.* 2016;31(5):486–491.

13. Paulus DJ, Bakhshaie J, Ditre JW, et al. Emotion dysregulation in the context of pain and alcohol use among Latinos in primary care. *Journal of Studies on Alcohol and Drugs.* 2017;78(6):938–944.

14. Cucinello-Ragland JA, Edwards S. Neurobiological aspects of pain in the context of alcohol use disorder. *International Review of Neurobiology.* 2021;157:1–29.

15. Koob GF. Alcoholism: allostasis and beyond. *Alcohol Clin Exp Res.* 2003;27(2):232–243. doi:10.1097/01.ALC.0000057122.36127.C2

16. Koob GF. Anhedonia, Hyperkatifeia, and Negative Reinforcement in Substance Use Disorders. *Curr Top Behav Neurosci.* 2022;58:147–165. doi:10.1007/7854_2021_288

17. Koob GF, Buck CL, Cohen A, et al. Addiction as a stress surfeit disorder. *Neuropharmacology.* 2014;76 Pt B(0 0):370–382. doi:10.1016/j.neuropharm.2013.05.024

18. Koob GF, Le Moal M. Drug abuse: hedonic homeostatic dysregulation. *Science.* 1997;278(5335):52–58. doi:10.1126/science.278.5335.52

19. Yeung EW, Craggs JG, Gizer IR. Comorbidity of alcohol use disorder and chronic pain: genetic influences on brain reward and stress systems. *Alcoholism: Clinical and Experimental Research.* 2017;41(11):1831–1848.

20. Borsook D, Linnman C, Faria V, Strassman AM, Becerra L, Elman I. Reward deficiency and anti-reward in pain chronification. *Neurosci Biobehav Rev.* 2016;68:282–297. doi:10.1016/j. neubiorev.2016.05.033.

21. Zhang Q, Manders T, Tong AP, et al. Chronic pain induces generalized enhancement of aversion. *Elife.* 2017;6:e25302. doi:10.7554/eLife.25302.

22. Wanat MJ, Willuhn I, Clark JJ, Phillips PE. Phasic dopamine release in appetitive behaviors and drug addiction. *Current Drug Abuse Reviews.* 2009;2(2):195–213.

23. Grace AA. The tonic/phasic model of dopamine system regulation and its implications for understanding alcohol and psychostimulant craving. *Addiction*. 2000;95(8s2):119–128.

24. Gee TA, Weintraub NC, Lu D, et al. A pain-induced tonic hypodopaminergic state augments phasic dopamine release in the nucleus accumbens. *Pain*. 2020;161(10):2376.

25. Testa M, Fillmore MT, Norris J, et al. Understanding alcohol expectancy effects: Revisiting the placebo condition. *Alcoholism: Clinical and Experimental Research*. 2006;30(2):339–348.

26. Litten RZ, Castle IJ, Falk D, et al. The placebo effect in clinical trials for alcohol dependence: An exploratory analysis of 51 naltrexone and acamprosate studies. *Alcoholism: Clinical and Experimental Research*. 2013;37(12):2128–2137.

27. Asghari V, Sanyal S, Buchwaldt S, Paterson A, Jovanovic V, Van Tol HH. Modulation of intracellular cyclic AMP levels by different human dopamine D4 receptor variants. *Journal of Neurochemistry*. 1995;65(3):1157–1165.

28. Seneviratne C, Johnson BA. Serotonin transporter genomic biomarker for quantitative assessment of ondansetron treatment response in alcoholics. *Frontiers in Psychiatry*. 2012;3:23.

29. Muhonen LH, Lahti J, Alho H, Lonnqvist J, Haukka J, Saarikoski ST. Serotonin transporter polymorphism as a predictor for escitalopram treatment of major depressive disorder comorbid with alcohol dependence. *Psychiatry Research*. 2011;186(1):53–57.

30. Cornell J, Conchas A, Wang XQ, et al. Validation of serotonin transporter mRNA as a quantitative biomarker of heavy drinking and its comparison to ethyl glucuronide/ethyl sulfate: A randomized, double-blind, crossover trial. *Alcoholism: Clinical and Experimental Research*. 2022;46(10):1888–1899. doi: 10.1111/acer.14931.

31. Theken KN, Hersh EV, Lahens NF, et al. Variability in the analgesic response to ibuprofen is associated with cyclooxygenase activation in inflammatory pain. *Clinical Pharmacology and Therapeutics*. 2019;106(3):632–641.

32. Wang RS, Lembo AJ, Kaptchuk TJ, et al. Genomic effects associated with response to placebo treatment in a randomized trial of irritable bowel syndrome. *Frontiers in Pain Research (Lausanne)*. 2021;2:775386.

33. Tucker JD, Goetz LL, Duncan MB, et al. Randomized, placebo-controlled analysis of the knee synovial environment following platelet-rich plasma treatment for knee osteoarthritis. *Physical Medicine and Rehabilitation (PMR)*. 2021;13(7):707–719.

34. Hall KT, Loscalzo J, Kaptchuk TJ. Genetics and the placebo effect: the placebome. *Trends in Molecular Medicine*. 2015;21(5):285–294.

35. Dumitrascuta M, Bermudez M, Ballet S, Wolber G, Spetea M. Mechanistic understanding of peptide analogues, DALDA, [Dmt(1)]DALDA, and KGOP01, binding to the mu opioid receptor. *Molecules*. 2020;25(9):2087. doi:10.3390/molecules25092087.

36. Ray R, Ruparel K, Newberg A, et al. Human mu opioid receptor (OPRM1 A118G) polymorphism is associated with brain mu-opioid receptor binding potential in smokers. *Proceedings of the National Academy of Sciences USA*. 2011;108(22):9268–9273.

37. Weerts EM, McCaul ME, Kuwabara H, et al. Influence of OPRM1 Asn40Asp variant (A118G) on [11C]carfentanil binding potential: preliminary findings in human subjects. *International Journal of Neuropsychopharmacology*. 2013;16(1):47–53.

38. Kroslak T, Laforge KS, Gianotti RJ, Ho A, Nielsen DA, Kreek MJ. The single nucleotide polymorphism A118G alters functional properties of the human mu opioid receptor. *Journal of Neurochemistry*. 2007;103(1):77–87.

39. Pecina M, Love T, Stohler CS, Goldman D, Zubieta JK. Effects of the mu opioid receptor polymorphism (OPRM1 A118G) on pain regulation, placebo effects and associated personality trait measures. *Neuropsychopharmacology*. 2015;40(4):957–965.

40. Colloca L, Wang Y, Martinez PE, et al. OPRM1 rs1799971, COMT rs4680, and FAAH rs324420 genes interact with placebo procedures to induce hypoalgesia. *Pain*. 2019;160(8):1824–1834.

41. Liu X, Finucane HK, Gusev A, et al. Functional architectures of local and distal regulation of gene expression in multiple human tissues. *American Journal of Human Genetics*. 2017;100(4):605–616.

42. Qi T, Wu Y, Zeng J, et al. Identifying gene targets for brain-related traits using transcriptomic and methylomic data from blood. *Nature Communications*. 2018;9(1):2282.

43. Morley KC, Luquin N, Baillie A, et al. Moderation of baclofen response by a GABAB receptor polymorphism: Rresults from the BacALD randomized controlled trial. *Addiction*. 2018;113(12):2205–2213.

44. Kranzler HR, Armeli S, Tennen H, Covault J. 5-HTTLPR genotype and daily negative mood moderate the effects of sertraline on drinking intensity. *Addiction Biology*. 2013;18(6):1024–1031.

45. Kranzler HR, Armeli S, Covault J, Tennen H. Variation in OPRM1 moderates the effect of desire to drink on subsequent drinking and its attenuation by naltrexone treatment. *Addiction Biology*. 2013;18(1):193–201.

46. Schacht JP, Anton RF, Voronin KE, et al. Interacting effects of naltrexone and OPRM1 and DAT1 variation on the neural response to alcohol cues. *Neuropsychopharmacology*. 2013;38(3):414–422.

47. Anton RF, Voronin KK, Randall PK, Myrick H, Tiffany A. Naltrexone modification of drinking effects in a subacute treatment and bar-lab paradigm: Influence of OPRM1 and dopamine transporter (SLC6A3) genes. *Alcoholism: Clinical and Experimental Research*. 2012;36(11):2000–2007.

48. Schacht JP, Voronin KE, Randall PK, Anton RF. Dopaminergic genetic variation influences aripiprazole effects on alcohol self-administration and the neural response to alcohol cues in a randomized trial. *Neuropsychopharmacology*. 2018;43(6):1247–1256.

49. Creswell KG, Sayette MA, Manuck SB, Ferrell RE, Hill SY, Dimoff JD. DRD4 polymorphism moderates the effect of alcohol consumption on social bonding. *PLoS ONE*. 2012;7(2):e28914.

50. Arias AJ, Covault J, Feinn R, et al. A GABRA2 variant is associated with increased stimulation and "high" following alcohol administration. *Alcohol*. 2014;49(1):1–9.

51. Karekin DA, Liang T, Wetherill L, et al. A polymorphism in GABRA2 is associated with the medial frontal response to alcohol cues in an fMRI study. *Alcoholism: Clinical and Experimental Research*. 2010;34(12):2169–2178.

52. Hart M, Weerts EM, McCaul ME, et al. GABRA2 markers moderate the subjective effects of alcohol. *Addiction Biology*. 2013;18(2):357–369.

53. Johansson A, Bergman H, Corander J, et al. Alcohol and aggressive behavior in men: Moderating effects of oxytocin receptor gene (OXTR) polymorphisms. *Genes, Brain and Behavior*. 2012;11(2):214–221.

2.4

Placebos meet proteomics

Predicting and monitoring placebo effects by plasma proteins

Karin Meissner, Christine von Toerne, Dominik Lutter,
Stefanie M. Hauck, and Matthias Tschoep

Introduction

Placebo responses and effects play a central role in interpretation of clinical trials. The gold standard for evaluating the efficacy of new interventions is still the placebo-controlled randomized clinical trial (RCT) design, which compares experimental treatment with a placebo intervention. The specific effect of the active treatment is defined as the difference between improvement in the active group compared to the placebo group. The effect in the placebo group depends on the size of placebo effects and other effects (e.g., regression to the mean) that are generally called placebo responses. The ability to isolate and, therefore, predict placebo effect sizes in clinical trials is of greatest interest for clinical researchers, as it would allow the exclusion of participants with expectedly high placebo effects and thus increase the specific treatment effects. In addition, more knowledge of the molecular fingerprint of placebo effects may permit estimation of placebo effect sizes without the inclusion of a placebo control group. Plasma proteomics is a promising approach to identify novel biomarkers that allow researchers to predict and track the placebo effects from circulating proteins in an unbiased fashion.

Proteomics

The technique of proteomics belongs to a group of approaches that analyze global information in so-called -ome layers such as the genome, the transcriptome, or the proteome. Proteomics technology has significantly driven the discovery of novel protein biomarkers in health and disease, and an increasing number of clinical trials is currently validating these new biomarkers in clinical settings. A systematic review on the use of protein/peptide biomarkers and proteomics in clinical trials, for example, revealed several hundred registered studies aiming to discover and evaluate protein biomarkers for patient stratification, diagnosis, and prognosis.[1] First examples show that proteomic biomarkers can be successfully applied in clinical settings.[2] CKD273, for example, is a proteomic classifier based on 273 urinary peptides that has been validated for the early detection of chronic kidney disease and for prognosis of its progression. In addition, initial attempts have been made to track individual responses to treatment through proteomic profiling.[3]

The use of proteomics techniques dates back to the 1990s, when the first articles on mass spectrometry (MS) in combination with capillary electrophoresis were published.[4] Since then, mass spectrometry has greatly improved in terms of sensitivity and accuracy, making it possible to identify a large number of proteins in a single mass spectrometric run.[5] Today's proteomics platforms allow the evaluation of thousands of proteins from various biological matrixes (e.g., plasma, saliva, urine, and tissues).[6] A typical workflow starts with proteolysis of intact proteins extracted from the respective biological sample by a protease (mostly trypsin) with sequence-specific activity. This generates a complex mixture of peptides in appropriate size, which are then further separated using liquid chromatography (LC), before elution and electrospray ionization transfer into the mass spectrometer. Peptide masses (MS1) and their derived fragments (MS2) are analyzed in high accuracy and allow identification of peptides/proteins, while recorded intensities allow their relative quantification.[7] Absolute quantification is possible by the use of isotope labeled peptides, but frequently relative quantification of protein or peptide abundance is sufficient.[1] Meanwhile, LC-MS is used in virtually all areas of biomedical analysis.[8]

Placebo effects and their molecular background in nausea

We recently performed the first randomized controlled placebo study that used a comprehensive proteomics approach to learn more about the molecular basis of placebo effects.[9] The goal of our proteomic approach was twofold: first, we aimed to characterize the molecular correlates of placebo effects at the time of its greatest intensity; second, we wondered whether we could identify protein signatures at baseline, which would distinguish between placebo responders and non-responders. To this end, we performed a proof-of-principle study in healthy volunteers. Importantly, we included a no-treatment (NT) group to disentangle genuine placebo effects from other influences, such as regression to the mean, spontaneous changes, and habituation effects.

The study design comprised two experimental days on which nausea was induced by a virtual vection drum for 20 minutes.[9] On the second day, participants were randomly allocated to one of two placebo interventions ($n = 30$ each) or NT ($n = 30$). The two placebo interventions were implemented by mock transcutaneous electrical nerve stimulation (TENS) at a dummy acupuncture point and differed in terms of somatosensory stimulation (yes or no). All groups were stratified by gender. An additional 10 participants were randomly allocated to active TENS at the acupuncture point PC6 to allow for blinded administration of the placebo interventions. Results confirmed significant placebo effects on our three nausea indices, namely mean intensity of nausea, motion sickness severity, and the ratio of normogastric to tachygastric activity (normo-to-tachy ratio; NTT) in the electrogastrogram (the latter only in women). Because somatosensory stimulation did not modulate placebo effects,[10] the two placebo groups were combined ($n = 60$) for proteomic analyses.[9]

Plasma proteomics approach

For each of our 90 participants, we performed proteomic analyses of plasma samples collected at baseline and after 20 minutes of nausea stimulation on both experimental days. We used a MS-based discovery proteomics approach for a maximum of unbiased identifications and quantifications of plasma proteins (Figure 2.4.1). Working with undepleted plasma (i.e., without exclusion of high-abundance proteins) was a compromise between analytical depth and reproducibility on the quantification level.[11] In contrast to data-dependent approaches (DDA-MS) in previous shotgun proteomic approaches, we pursued the newer data-independent approach (DIA-MS). One big difference between the approaches is that in DDA-MS (referred to as MS/MS), the fragmentation of the peptide (also referred to as fragment ion) that is needed for peptide identification is triggered by the presence of a number of high- intense peptides (also referred to as precursor ion and Top N method), whereas in DIA-MS the fragmentation is triggered systematically regardless of precursor ion intensities. As a result, DIA does not suffer from the data-dependent ion selection problem leading to under-sampling.[12] The resulting, more complete, data matrix is better suited to be compared over

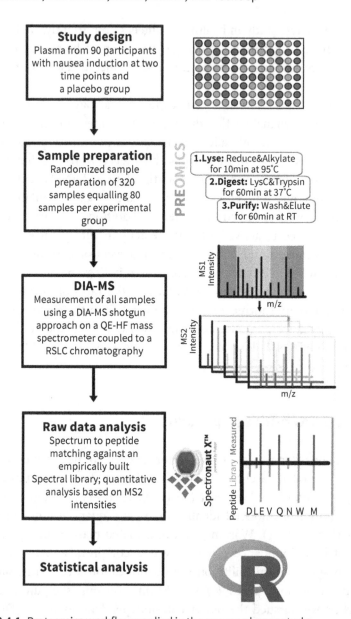

Figure 2.4.1 Proteomics workflow applied in the nausea plasma study.

Abbreviations: DIA-MS, data-independent acquisition mass spectrometry; QE-HF, QExactive high field mass spectrometer from Thermo Fisher Scientific; RSLC, (short for) Ultimate 3000 rapid separation liquid chromatography system using nano flow from Thermo Fisher Scientific; MS2, fragment spectrum as spectrum from spectrum (also named MS/MS).

hundreds of samples from a study cohort. This approach was possible due to faster MS technologies with a higher resolution, needed for a later deconvolution of mixed spectra. In the first years of DIA-MS analysis, when our study was performed, matching of the complex mixed spectra was only achievable by comparing them to empirically built libraries, in contrast to in-silico built spectral libraries used in DDA-MS. Meanwhile, direct DIA (i.e., without the need of spectral libraries) is possible.[13] We thus searched our DIA files against an in-house library generated from selected MS data encompassing 57 files of plasma and serum preparations. These tailored libraries allow for an increase in analytical depth by combining results from different sample preparation approaches such as fractionated plasma or depleted plasma samples without unnecessarily increasing the search space.[14] The final spectral library generated in Spectronaut software (Biognosys, Schlieren, Switzerland) contained 1,811 protein groups, 10,445 proteotypic peptides, and 26,805 peptide-precursors. The MS-based proteomics approach on peripheral plasma identified 711 proteins represented by 3.224 peptides and 14.588 peptide-precursors.[9]

Prediction of protein fold changes by experimental factors

To predict protein changes on Day 2 by experimental factors (sex, group, and day-adjusted scores (DAS) of nausea, motion sickness, and the gastric NTT-ratio) we performed a linear regression approach.[9] Each of the protein and nausea measurements were modeled independently, including predictive interaction terms. Proteins 89, 84, and 95 could be predicted by at least one experimental factor for the three nausea measures, respectively. To further translate this primary level of information into meaningful biological knowledge, gene ontology (GO) enrichment analyses was performed on the three protein sets. This bioinformatics approach compares the frequency of proteins in the study set with the frequency of proteins in the provided population set for each GO term. A hypergeometric distribution test is then used to check for over-representation ("enrichment"). One of the most significantly enriched GO terms in our regression models including NTT was "regulation of grooming behavior," with the key proteins "neurexin-1" (NRXN1) and "contactin-associated protein-like 4" (CNTNAP4) involved in empathic behavior.[15] Most strikingly, social grooming has been linked by several authors to the evolutionary antecedents of the doctor-patient-relationship and placebo effects.[16,17] One further key protein in models including NTT was reelin (RELN), which is known to functionally interact with the trust-enhancing neuropeptide oxytocin.[18] Taken together by following an unbiased proteomics approach, we were able to identify biological processes that support the assumption that bonding and social attachment mechanisms play a central role for the generation of placebo effects.[9]

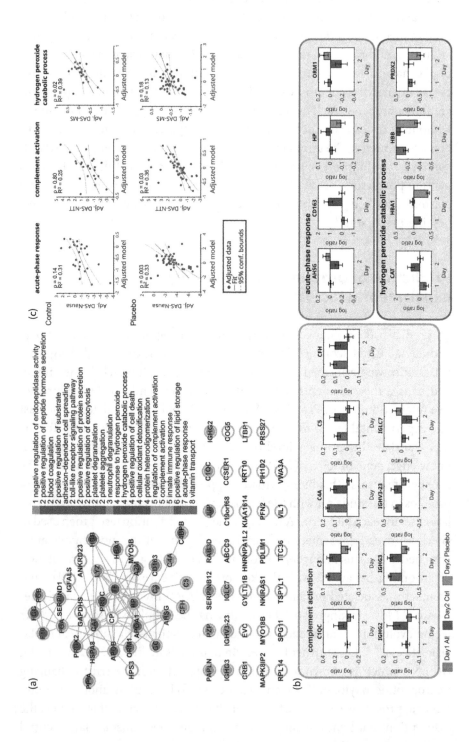

Figure 2.4.2 Placebo-related proteins.

StringDB network and Gene Ontology (GO) enrichment analysis of placebo-related proteins. (A) StringDB network of placebo-related proteins. Nodes are colored according to Gene Ontology (GO) term group association. Numbers refer to functional clusters. GO functional clusters were created based on shared members (proteins). Edges refer to StringDB interactions. (B) Expression patterns for selected GO term proteins. Barplots depict average log expression (nausea vs. baseline measurement) of all protein-associated peptides. Barplot colors refer to day and group. Error bars denote standard error of the mean. Boxes around barplots indicate GO term membership, and the color of the boxes refer to GO functional cluster associated in panel A. (C) The fitted GO term–based linear multiple regression models to predict day-adjusted scores (DAS) of nausea measures. Acute-phase response proteins predict DAS-Nausea in control (top) and placebo group (bottom); complement activation proteins predict DAS-normo-to-tachy-ratio in control and placebo groups; hydrogen peroxide catabolic process proteins predict DAS-motion sickness (MS) in control and placebo groups; Model p-values (FDR-corrected) and model R-squared are specified in the plots. Blue dots are model outputs for each data point. The linear fit and 95% confident bands are denoted by solid and dashed red lines, respectively.

Figure from Meissner K, Lutter D, von Toerne C, et al. Molecular classification of the placebo effect in nausea. *PLoS ONE.* 2020;15(9):e0238533, Fig. 5, via Creative Commons Attribution (CC BY) license.

To identify proteins that were significantly affected by the placebo intervention independent of changes in nausea measures, we performed an analysis of covariance (ANCOVA) for each vection-drum induced protein fold change on Day 2 with "group" and "sex" as categorical predictive variables and fold changes on Day 2 as covariate.[9] To further increase statistical power, ANCOVA was performed on the peptides instead of protein data, thereby increasing the sample size for large individual proteins up to 1,000-fold. The ANCOVAs revealed 74 proteins that were regulated differently on Day 2 in the placebo group as compared to the NT control group. A GO enrichment analyses for these 74 placebo-related proteins identified 21 nonredundant enriched GO terms related to eight functional protein clusters (Figure 2.4.2). Among those, the GO term 'complement activation' showed a striking protein pattern for 8 out of 9 proteins, each decreased in the placebo group compared to control (Figure 2.4.2). We next performed a multiple linear regression approach for each enriched GO term to predict DAS-scores based on protein fold changes. We found significant associations in the placebo group for DAS-Nausea and "acute phase-response" as well as DAS-NTT and "blood coagulation" and "complement activation." In the control group, DAS-motion sickness was predicted by three different GO terms (Figure 2.4.2).[9]

The close relationship between placebo effects and proteins involved in the acute phase response and complement activation suggests that placebo treatment may attenuate microinflammatory responses to the stress of nausea induction. This hypothesis fits well with results from experimental and clinical studies indicating attenuation of proinflammatory cytokines by expectancy-based placebo interventions.[19-21] By using a classical placebo pain paradigm, for example, placebo-induced expectation of pain relief reduced the proinflammatory cytokine IL-18 quantified from plasma samples.[20] Strikingly, the amount of IL-18 reduction in the placebo condition correlated with both placebo analgesia and the associated release of endogenous opioids in the brain's reward system. Results suggest a close link between placebo effects, central changes, and stress-responsive innate immune responses. Further, a clinical trial in cardiac patients found a reduction of the proinflammatory cytokine IL-6 in the experimental group that had received a psychotherapeutic intervention to optimize treatment expectations before undergoing cardiac surgery.[21] Taken together, our results are in line with empirical evidence from other studies that interventions that induce positive treatment expectations can down-regulate peripheral inflammatory processes. Like Prossin et al.,[20] we found a close link between these peripheral changes and placebo-induced symptom improvement. Results thus support the notion that biomarkers of placebo effects are quantifiable from circulating blood.

Prediction of placebo responders by plasma proteins at baseline

As mentioned above, the a priori identification of placebo responders would be of greatest interest for clinical research, because the exclusion of placebo responders would enhance the specific treatment effect, defined as the verum-placebo difference. There are plenty of studies that aimed to identify personality traits of placebo responders;[22] however, this line of research was not as successful as initially thought. Meanwhile, several studies have identified gene variants that can explain a significant amount of variance in placebo effects (see Chapter 2.2). For example, the catechol-O-methyltransferase (COMT) genotype was shown to predict placebo effects in pain, irritable bowel syndrome, and fatigue in cancer survivors.[23–27] The predictive value of individual gene variants for the size of placebo effects is limited, but can be increased by considering multiple variables, such as more than one genetic variant, brain imaging outcomes, personality traits, and/or experimental factors.[24,26] This is not surprising, as it is well known that the

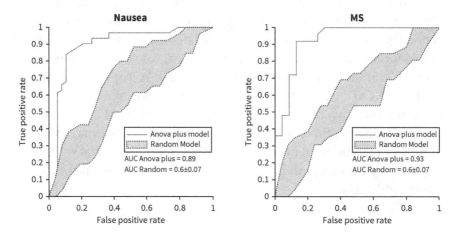

Figure 2.4.3 Receiver operating characteristic curves.
Prediction of placebo responders by Day 2 baseline proteins. *Placebo responders* were defined as participants showing a reduction of at least 50% in day-adjusted scores for nausea (DAS-Nausea) and motion sickness (DAS-MS), respectively. The blue line refers to the "ANOVA plus model." The yellow area refers to the range of all 10 "RANDOM model" permutations, area under the curve values in mean, and standard deviation given.

Figure adapted from Meissner K, Lutter D, von Toerne C, et al. Molecular classification of placebo effects in nausea. *PLoS ONE*. 2020;15(9):e0238533, Fig. 6b, via Creative Commons Attribution (CC BY) license.

magnitude of placebo effects depends on a variety of contextual factors.[28] The use of proteomics to identify protein biomarkers that predict placebo effects in specific treatment contexts appears to be a promising complement to placebo genomics.

To evaluate the potential of proteomics to identify placebo responders, we tested whether placebo responders could be predicted by protein abundances at baseline of our second experimental day, on which the placebo intervention took place.[9] *Placebo responders* were defined as participants in the placebo groups who showed at least a 50% reduction of nausea or motion sickness from Day 1 to Day 2. We then performed a three-step predictive approach. We first identified a number of predictive candidate proteins using ANOVA to select those with differential abundances between responders and non-responders. Additional predictive proteins were selected performing sequential feature selection with the ANOVA proteins as starting set. Subsequently, we used this protein list to train a support vector machine to predict responders from nonresponders on the three nausea scores. This "ANOVA plus model" was then compared to a control reference model based on a random selection of proteins ("RANDOM model"). Models were compared based on receiver operating characteristics curves following a 10-fold cross validation with 10 independent permutations. This approach revealed area under curve estimates of 0.86 for nausea and 0.93 for motion sickness, respectively, compared to 0.6 ± 0.07 for the "RANDOM model" (Figure 2.4.3). The proteins selected for the ANCOVA plus model contained immunoglobulins and serum proteases, both involved in the regulation of complement activation.[9] We can conclude from this that proteomic signatures from plasma are eligible to predict placebo responders with surprisingly high accuracy. The next step is to replicate and validate the results in larger samples and under different conditions.

Proteomics for future placebo research

In a seminal paper, Hall et al.[29] introduced the term *placebome* for a "hypothesized group of genome-related or derived molecules (i.e., genes, proteins, or miRNAs) that affect an individual's response to placebo treatment" (p. 286). With our study on the molecular background of placebo effects in nausea, we have provided the first empirical evidence that plasma proteomics is a promising tool to predict placebo responders in clinical trials.[9] Identifying placebo responders could also be of relevance for clinical practice, as treatment approaches including the patient-provider-interaction could be modified in order to enhance the individual placebo component, and hence the treatment's benefit for the patient.[29] Thus, the identification of specific plasma biomarkers to predict placebo effects would be an important step toward personalized medicine.

At the same time, we went one-step further by showing that the technique of plasma proteomics also has potential to identify biomarkers to monitor placebo responses in clinical trials. Tracking placebo effects using circulating proteins would also be an important methodological advance, paving the way for replacing expensive placebo control groups in the future with simple blood samples. This is even more important as expectations underlying placebo effects are not constant but seem to vary over time[30,31] as well as with contextual factors, such as the type and characteristics of a specific treatment.[32,33]

Pros and cons of using plasma proteomics for placebo research

A major advantage of proteomics is its unbiased approach, as data are analyzed largely independent of a priori hypotheses. This facilitates the discovery of proteins as novel biomarker candidates.[6] Plasma proteomics appears promising in this regard, as plasma samples are routinely used in clinics and sample handling is standardized. In addition, proteomics in urine and saliva may also prove to be a useful source for detecting biomarkers of placebo effects. Further, the elucidation of patterns in protein expression changes by plasma proteomics may shed light on key mechanisms underlying placebo effects that could be further investigated in mechanistic experiments, longitudinal studies, and clinical trials. Through increased sensitivity and speed, modern MS approaches allow a higher throughput and a comprehensive analysis of hundreds of proteins in one run.[11] Multiomics approaches, integrating genetic, proteomic, metabolomic and other "omic" data,[34] offer even more potential to understand the molecular basis of placebo effects, paving the way from personalized medicine to the development of new drugs and behavioral interventions that maximize placebo effects.

There are certainly also disadvantages of using plasma proteomics in placebo research. First of all, sample analysis is associated with high costs and only specialized centers can provide this type of analysis. Second, further limitations exist through the necessity of successive measurements during the DIA-MS approach, which reduces reproducibility. Third, in plasma and other body fluids, protein concentrations have an extreme difference in dynamic range, leading to limited sensitivity and identification of low abundant proteins. This limitation can at least partially be overcome by alternative approaches such as the proximity extension assays utilizing antibodies for detection and enabling signal amplification and quantification by nucleotide-based methods.[35,36] Fourth, large validation studies are necessary to follow-up and validate initial discoveries of potential biomarkers related to placebo effects that are hampered by high costs and low scientific merit.[37] Once established, however, selected biomarkers can be monitored by ELISA or other routine clinical lab procedures.

Conclusions

The application of plasma proteomics and other "omic" technologies holds great translational potential for placebo research and clinical trial methodology and should be pursued further. However, much remains to be done until protein biomarkers are identified that reliably predict placebo responders and allow the magnitude of placebo effects to be estimated in the absence of a placebo.

References

1. He T. Implementation of proteomics in clinical trials. *Proteomics Clinical Applications.* 2019;13(2):e1800198. http://doi:10.1002/prca.201800198
2. Latosinska A, Frantzi M, Vlahou A, Merseburger AS, Mischak H. Clinical proteomics for precision medicine: The bladder cancer case. *Proteomics Clinical Applications.* 2018;12(2). doi:10.1002/prca.201700074.
3. Li QR, Chen WJ, Shen JW, et al. Personalized evaluation based on quantitative proteomics for drug-treated patients with chronic kidney disease. *Journal of Cellular and Molecular Medicine.* 2016;8(3):184–194. http://doi:10.1093/jmcb/mjw015
4. Aebersold R. A mass spectrometric journey into protein and proteome research. *Journal of the American Society for Mass Spectrometry.* 2003;14(7):685–695.
5. Beretta L. Proteomics from the clinical perspective: Many hopes and much debate. *Nature Methods.* 2007;4(10):785–786. http://doi:10.1038/nmeth1007-785
6. Moaddel R, Ubaida-Mohien C, Tanaka T, et al. Proteomics in aging research: A roadmap to clinical, translational research. *Aging Cell.* 2021;20(4):e13325. http://doi:10.1111/acel.13325
7. Sinha A, Mann M. A beginner's guide to mass spectrometry–based proteomics. *Biochemistry.* 2020;42(5):64–69.
8. Brandtzaeg OK, Johnsen E, Roberg-Larsen H, et al. Proteomics tools reveal startlingly high amounts of oxytocin in plasma and serum. *Scientific Reports.* 2016;6:31693. http://doi:10.1038/srep31693

9. Meissner K, Lutter D, von Toerne C, et al. Molecular classification of the placebo effect in nausea. *PloS ONE.* 2020;15(9):e0238533.
10. Aichner S, Haile A, Hoffmann V, Olliges E, Tschöp MH, Meissner K. The role of tactile stimulation for expectation, perceived treatment assignment and the placebo effect in an experimental nausea paradigm. *Frontiers in Neuroscience.* 2019;13:1212. doi:10.3389/fnins.2019.01212.
11. Geyer PE, Kulak NA, Pichler G, Holdt LM, Teupser D, Mann M. Plasma proteome profiling to assess human health and disease. *Cell Systems.* 2016; 2(3):185–195.
12. Pino LK, Just SC, MacCoss MJ, Searle BC. Acquiring and analyzing data independent acquisition proteomics experiments without spectrum libraries. *Molecular & Cellular Proteomics.* 2020;19(7):1088–1103.
13. Bekker-Jensen DB, Bernhardt OM, Hogrebe A, et al. Rapid and site-specific deep phosphoproteome profiling by data-independent acquisition without the need for spectral libraries. *Nature Communications.* 2020;11(1):1–12.
14. Pacharra S, Marcus K, May C. Sample fractionation techniques for CSF peptide spectral library generation. *Methods in Molecular Biology.* 2019;2044:69–77. http://doi.10.1007/978-1-4939-9706-0_5
15. Misra V. The social brain network and autism. *Annals of Neurosciences.* 2014;21(2):69.
16. Benedetti F. Placebo and the new physiology of the doctor-patient relationship. *Physiological Reviews.* 2013;93(3):1207–1246.
17. Colloca L, Miller FG. How placebo responses are formed: A learning perspective. *Philosophical Transactions of the Royal Society B: Biological Sciences.* 2011;366(1572):1859–1869.
18. Peñagarikano O. Oxytocin in animal models of autism spectrum disorder. *Developmental Neurobiology.* 2017;77(2):202–213.
19. Hashish I, Harvey W, Harris M. Anti-inflammatory effects of ultrasound therapy: Evidence for a major placebo effect. *British Journal of Rheumatology.* 1986;25(1):77–81. http://doi:10.1093/rheumatology/25.1.77
20. Prossin A, Koch A, Campbell P, Laumet G, Stohler CS, Dantzer R, Zubieta JK. Effects of placebo administration on immune mechanisms and relationships with central endogenous opioid neurotransmission. Molecular Psychiatry. 2022;27(2):831–839. doi:10.1038/s41380-021-01365-x.
21. Rief W, Shedden-Mora MC, Laferton JA, et al. Preoperative optimization of patient expectations improves long-term outcome in heart surgery patients: Results of the randomized controlled PSY-HEART trial. *Bone Marrow Concentrate in Medicine.* 2017;15(1):4. http://doi:10.1186/s12916-016-0767-3
22. Kern A, Kramm C, Witt CM, Barth J. The influence of personality traits on the placebo/nocebo response: A systematic review. *Journal of Psychosomatic Research.* 2020;128:109866.
23. Aslaksen PM, Forsberg JT, Gjerstad J. The opioid receptor mu 1 (OPRM1) rs1799971 and catechol-O-methyltransferase (COMT) rs4680 as genetic markers for placebo analgesia. *Pain.* 2018;159(12):2585–2592.
24. Colloca L, Wang Y, Martinez PE, et al. OPRM1 rs1799971-COMT rs4680-FAAH rs324420 genes interact with placebo procedures to induce hypoalgesia. *Pain.* 2019;160(8):1824.
25. Hall KT, Lembo AJ, Kirsch I, Ziogas DC, Douaiher J, Jensen KB, Conboy LA, Kelley JM, Kokkotou E, Kaptchuk TJ. Catechol-O-methyltransferase val158met polymorphism predicts placebo effect in irritable bowel syndrome. *PLoS One.* 2012;7(10):e48135. doi:10.1371/journal.pone.0048135.
26. Yu R, Gollub RL, Vangel M, Kaptchuk T, Smoller JW, Kong J. Placebo analgesia and reward processing: Integrating genetics, personality, and intrinsic brain activity. *Human Brain Mapping.* 2014;35(9):4583–4593.

27. Zhou ES, Hall KT, Michaud AL, Blackmon JE, Partridge AH, Recklitis CJ. Open-label placebo reduces fatigue in cancer survivors: A randomized trial. *Supportive Care in Cancer.* 2019;27(6):2179–2187.
28. Di Blasi Z, Harkness E, Ernst E, Georgiou A, Kleijnen J. Influence of context effects on health outcomes: A systematic review. *Lancet.* 2001;357(9258):757–762.
29. Hall KT, Loscalzo J, Kaptchuk TJ. Genetics and the placebo effect: The placebome. *Trends in Molecular Medicine.* 2015;21(5):285–294.
30. Laferton JAC, Vijapura S, Baer L, et al. Mechanisms of perceived treatment assignment and subsequent expectancy effects in a double-blind placebo controlled RCT of major depression. *Frontiers in Psychiatry.* 2018;9:424. http://doi:10.3389/fpsyt.2018.00424
31. Stone DA, Kerr CE, Jacobson E, Conboy ScD LA, Kaptchuk TJ. Patient expectations in placebo-controlled randomized clinical trials. *Journal of Evaluation in Clinical Practice.* 2005;11(1):77–84.
32. Meissner K, Fässler M, Rücker G, et al. Differential effectiveness of placebo treatments: A systematic review of migraine prophylaxis. *JAMA Internal Medicine.* 2013;173(21):1941–1951.
33. Meissner K, Linde K. Are blue pills better than green? How treatment features modulate placebo effects. *International Review of Neurobiology.* 2018;139:357–378.
34. Hasin Y, Seldin M, Lusis A. Multi-omics approaches to disease. *Genome Biology.* 2017;18(1):83. http://doi:10.1186/s13059-017-1215-1
35. Darmanis S, Nong RY, Vanelid J, et al. ProteinSeq: High-performance proteomic analyses by proximity ligation and next generation sequencing. *PLoS ONE.* 2011;6(9):e25583. http://doi:10.1371/journal.pone.0025583
36. Petrera A, von Toerne C, Behler J, et al. Multiplatform approach for plasma proteomics: Complementarity of Olink proximity extension assay technology to mass spectrometry-based protein profiling. *Journal of Proteome Research.* 2021;20(1):751–762. http://doi:10.1021/acs.jproteome.0c00641
37. Mischak H. How to get proteomics to the clinic? Issues in clinical proteomics, exemplified by CE-MS. *Proteomics Clinical Applications.* 2012;6(9–10):437–442. http://doi:10.1002/prca.201200027

3

PLACEBOS AND NOCEBOS ACROSS CONDITIONS

Within this Section, an in-depth exploration awaits, unravels intriguing realms in sleep, chronic pain, cough, immunopharmacology, sports and exercise, migraine clinical trials, and the COVID-19, shedding light on the placebo and nocebo effects and their potential to shape the future of healthcare and well-being.

The profound connection between sleep and chronic pain unfolds, where sleep disturbances reveal tangible consequences on pain perception and management is explored in Chapter one. Over-the-counter cough medicines, with their viscous sweet syrups and a multitude of excipients, tap into the power of placebos to provide relief for cough, where the influence of placebo effects is significant. This is the topic of Chapter two.

In the field of immunopharmacology as detailed in Chapter three, strategies to behaviorally condition placebo responses unfold. By pairing novel tastes with immunomodulatory drugs, an opportunity arises to minimize drug dosages while modifying immune functions.

Sports and exercise present their own enigmas when it comes to placebo effects. Psychological factors that enhance performance in sports, alongside affective responses to exercise, become focal points of exploration in Chapter four.

The often overlooked nocebo responses take center stage in migraine clinical trials. Chapter five indicates as examining their impact on treatment profiles, adverse events, and treatment adherence, sheds light on their vital role in optimizing patient adherence and outcomes.

Finally, the challenges posed by the COVID-19 era are confronted in Chapter six. From the clinical expression of the illness to the efficacy and acceptance of treatments and vaccines, placebo and nocebo effects permeate every aspect.

3.1

The role of sleep disturbance in endogenous pain modulation through opioidergic, placebo, and positive affective mechanisms

Patrick H. Finan, Luana Colloca, Stella Iacovides, and Gilles J. Lavigne

Introduction

As pain disorders have increased in prevalence over the past decade,[1,2] chronic pain has emerged as the world's leading cause of disability.[3,4] At the same time, surgeries have also increased in volume, creating new opportunities to ensnare patients from the recursive loops of inflammation and tissue healing. For example, elective lumbar fusion surgeries increased by 62% between 2004 and 2015,[5] despite variable success rates and substantial risk for prolonged pain.[6] Despite the rise in pain and disability, pharmaceutical drug development has offered few safe and effective long-term solutions for chronic pain. As such, there remains an intense focus on the identification of modifiable clinical correlates and mechanisms of pain that may unlock novel targets for intervention to improve pain-related outcomes. Out of this clinical research need, sleep has emerged as an important clinical and physiological correlate that is strongly and bidirectionally associated with pain.[7-9] This chapter will focus on how sleep improves pain through endogenous pain modulation, a neurobiological process that operates via opioidergic, placebo, and positive affective mechanisms.

Effects of sleep disturbance on pain, opioids and opioid analgesia

Numerous cross-sectional, microlongitudinal, macrolongitudinal, and experimental studies over the past 2 decades have supported the association between sleep and pain, with a preponderance of studies demonstrating that the temporal effect of sleep on future pain is stronger and more reliable than the effect of pain on future sleep.[8,10,11] This observation underscores the importance of identifying mechanisms—likely at multiple biological, psychological, and social levels—that explain how pain-related processes are altered when sleep is disturbed.

Mu-opioid receptors (MORs) are prevalent in all of the spinal and supraspinal brain regions comprising the classic descending pain modulatory pathway. Engaging MORs through administration of exogenous opioids or opioid antagonists produces profound analgesia or hyperalgesia, respectively, across species (for a comprehensive review, see Fields[12]). Evidence in rodents and humans suggests that opioid analgesia is diminished in the context of sleep disturbance. Total sleep deprivation downregulates rats' μ and δ opioid receptors,[13] the principal receptors involved in opioid analgesia, and diminishes the antinociceptive effects of morphine in the periaqueductal gray (PAG) and the rostral ventral medulla (RVM).[14,15] Additionally, accumulated sleep debt from daily moderate sleep restriction in mice both increases sensitivity to noxious stimuli and attenuates the effects of the opioid agonist morphine.[16] Animal studies provide further evidence that the analgesic effect of systemically administered opioids is decreased by REM-sleep deprivation.[17,18] In humans, healthy, pain-free participants who reported greater subjective sleepiness demonstrated reduced analgesia from codeine.[19] Short-sleeping healthy participants also demonstrated altered cerebral MOR binding potential in the anterior cingulate and dorsolateral prefrontal cortices during a laboratory pain induction.[20] In a controlled experimental setting, sleep disruption via forced awakenings reduced the analgesic effect of morphine on cold pressor withdrawal latency threefold.[21] Clinically, poor sleep is associated with increased opioid dose requirements following burn injury.[22] These findings represent important aspects of the sleep-related endogenous modulation, although caution is needed because it is likely that not a single effect of sleep deprivation affects endogenous opioid modulation; rather it is the consequence of a complex sequence or parallel series of adjustments that body processes put in place for survival.

The proposed mechanisms by which sleep deprivation reduces the efficacy of the opioid analgesic pathway include: (1) inhibiting the synthesis of endogenous opioids, (2) downregulating central opioid receptors, (3) and reducing the affinity of μ- and δ-opioid receptors.[8,23,24] Selective REM-sleep fragmentation for a 5-day period increases the spontaneous firing rate and greater firing regularity in the cholinergic output neurons in the medial habenula of mice.[25] Also, REM-sleep deprivation in rats decreases the antinociceptive effect induced by the administration of morphine into the PAG.[14] Given that activation of the μ-opioid receptors at the PAG by endogenous or exogenous opioids leads to the activation of the descending inhibitory pain pathways and inhibition of the descending facilitatory pain pathways,[12] one mechanism by which REM-sleep deprivation decreases morphine analgesia may involve the modulation of the descending pain modulatory system.[14]

Finally, it is important to note that the effect of sleep disturbance on opioid analgesia is more complex in patients with obstructive sleep apnea (OSA). OSA appears to complicate opioid-based pain management by increasing both pain sensitivity[26] and opioid sensitivity.[27] In children with OSA, recurrent hypoxemia is associated with increased sensitivity to opioids[28] and reduced opioid requirement for analgesia.[29] Similar findings are observed in male volunteers with high risk for OSA: nocturnal hypoxemia enhances the analgesic effect of a μ-opioid agonist, hypoxia decreases pain sensitivity and enhances potency for opioid analgesia.[30] Collectively, these findings suggest the clinical context of sleep disturbance (e.g., sleep disordered breathing vs. insomnia) must be taken into account when assessing the effect of sleep disturbance on opioid analgesia. Moreover, other physiological homeostatic process such as cardiovascular[31] and endothelial function,[32] can be disrupted by persistent sleep disturbance, creating a multisystem spectrum of dysfunction that not only aggravates physical health, but also create vulnerabilities in mental health and affective functioning.

Effects of sleep on positive affective analgesia

Positive affective analgesia refers to the process by which pleasant feeling states inhibit the experience of pain. Experimentally, this phenomenon is observed when a constant noxious stimulus results in lower pain ratings when it is paired with positively valence, emotionally evocative stimuli (e.g., erotic images or music) versus neutral (e.g., a chair) or negative (e.g., mutilation) stimuli.[33-37] The analgesic effect of positive affect is also observed in intensive experience sampling studies of pain and affect dynamics among patients with chronic pain.[38-42] Positive affective analgesia is engendered by the activation of descending pain modulatory circuits that respond to rewarding and pleasurable affective input in the cortex (e.g., insula; anterior cingulate cortex)[36] and inhibit activity in core pain processing regions (e.g., PAG).[43,44] Compared with controls, patients with major depressive disorder[45] and patients with chronic musculoskeletal pain[33,46] show deficient positive affective analgesia.

Sleep is a major homeostatic regulator of emotional health,[47,48] and studies generally reveal a stronger association between sleep and positive affective states than negative affective states.[49,50] Disruption of sleep continuity, a common experience among patients with chronic pain,[51,52] is particularly detrimental to next-day positive affect relative to other forms of sleep loss.[38] A recent daily diary study in patients with temporomandibular disorder—a chronic orofacial pain condition—showed that minutes spent awake after sleep onset prospectively predicted lower next-morning positive affect, which in turn predicted greater pain over the course of that day.[53]

These findings appear to extend and generalize to the effects of various sleep disturbances (both self-reported and experimentally induced) on positive affective analgesia, which have been directly assessed in four studies of which we are aware. Clinically significant insomnia symptoms are associated with an attenuation of the analgesic benefit of positive, relative to neutral and negative visual stimuli.[54] In contrast, retrospective reports of poor sleep quality over the previous month are associated with an attenuation of the positive affective inhibition of the nociceptive flexion response, but not pain perception.[55] A single night of experimental sleep continuity disruption significantly attenuates positive affective analgesia in response to visual emotional stimuli (assessed via ratings of pain perception).[49] A smaller sleep continuity disruption study in healthy participants failed to show sleep-related differences in self-reported pain ratings between rewarding and neutral music.[37] That study revealed, however, that sleep disruption attenuated activation within the nucleus accumbens—a neural hub of the valuation of rewarding and aversive stimuli—during pain onset and increased the functional connectivity of the nucleus accumbens and the anterior midcingulate cortex, a brain region associated with cognitive control.[37] Other recent work in healthy participants has similarly shown attenuated pain-related nucleus accumbens function following total sleep deprivation.[56] An important caveat here is that both the DelVentura et al.[54] and Finan et al.[49] studies showed that sleep disturbance also attenuated negative affective hyperalgesia, consistent with a general abolishment of affective pain modulation rather than a selective effect on positive affective analgesia. Together, these findings suggest that sleep disturbance may alter the brain's ability to effectively discriminate between affective and pain stimuli, thereby diminishing the ability of affective stimuli to modulate pain. This may occur via a devaluing of affective stimuli, as evidenced by diminished nucleus accumbens function, and/or via a degradation of attentional resources,[57,58] consistent with earlier findings from Tiede et al.[59] that showed a significant reduction in distraction analgesia following experimental sleep restriction.

Nocturnal considerations in evaluating mechanisms of sleep and pain

Sleep is neither coma nor anesthesia. Nociception remains potent during sleep and can evoke a brain protective response that can be variable across sleep stages.[60] Indeed, experimental pain stimulation during sleep can induce transient nocturnal brain, heart and muscle activities, all of which may be categorized as arousal. These effects persist for 3–15 seconds and contribute to a preparatory awake fight or fight reaction, expressed as a full return of consciousness with a potential emotional reaction. Sleep arousal is a marker of sleep disruption when it reoccurs more than 7–14 times per hour of sleep and is correlated with diurnal fatigue, loss of attention or cognitive alteration, and sleepiness.[61-64] The pain-related arousal response rate to experimental pain stimulation is higher in light Stage N2 sleep, lower in deep Stage N3 (i.e., slow wave sleep), and intermediate in REM sleep. The magnitude of experimental stimulation during N3 sleep (characterized by slow wave activity associated with a subjective sense of feeling "refreshed" upon awakening) and during REM sleep (characterized by low muscle tone, high brain activity, and more vivid dreams) need to be higher to trigger arousal and awakening.[65-69]

The effect of sleep on endogenous pain modulation and placebo analgesia

Endogenous pain modulation describes the process by which nociceptive neurons originating in the spinal cord are functionally altered by neuronal activity within an interconnected network of subcortical (e.g., PAG and RVM) and cortical (e.g., anterior cingulate cortex (ACC), ventromedial prefrontal cortex (vmPFC), and anterior insula) brain regions.[70-72] It is now clear that several of these descending modulatory pathways regulate the excitation and facilitation,[73,74] as well as the inhibition [75] of nociceptive signaling, and that sleep disturbance potentiates these descending effects.[76]

Several studies of sleep and conditioned pain modulation—a quantitative sensory pain inhibition task that is at least partly regulated by endogenous opioidergic circuits[77-79]—highlight the broader effects of sleep on endogenous pain modulation. Smith and colleagues[24] reported that experimental sleep disruption, via forced awakenings throughout the night, impaired conditioned pain modulation in healthy female participants. Such findings have been replicated,[80,81] and support several observational studies linking insomnia and general sleep disruption with impairments in conditioned pain modulation.[82-84] Placebo analgesia remains active during sleep, despite the fact that pain is not perceived at a conscious level.[85] Memories associated with a persuasive placebo analgesia conditioning paradigm applied immediately before sleep are consolidated during sleep and influence expectations for pain relief the next morning, and these effects are augmented when REM sleep is shorter than normal.[86] Laverdure-Dupont and colleagues explored in healthy participants occurrence of placebo effects to acute heat painful stimulations following a conditioning procedure conducted before sleep. The paradigm included 3-night procedures—habituation, placebo analgesia and control nights—delivered in a counterbalanced manner. Presleep conditioning created reinforced expectations of analgesia before the night when placebo effects were tested. Participants reported a decrease in pain, anxiety, and associated sleep disturbance during the placebo night, along with a 10% reduction in brain arousals evoked by the painful stimulation during REM sleep. REM sleep may contribute to reinforce expectations of analgesia. Expectations created before sleep likely induced a reduction of nocturnal pain and subjective sleep disturbances. Moreover, REM sleep predicted placebo-induced expectations of pain relief.

Use of clonidine, an alpha 2 adrenergic agonist that blunts REM sleep, further modulates expectation-mediated placebo effects.[87] Chouchou and colleagues pharmacologically manipulated REM and sleep deprivation. After a habituation night in a sleep laboratory, participants underwent a conditioning procedure in the evening. Following conditioning, participants were randomly assigned to either clonidine—a selective alpha-2 agonist that interferes with the REM/NREM sleep cycle—or inert control pills. Participants and staff were blinded to the randomization. Results showed that REM-sleep deprivation was associated with an increase in placebo analgesia.

A decade of studies on healthy participants has contributed to the advance of mechanistic knowledge of placebo effects in physiological conditions.[88] However, there is a need to translate this knowledge into patient-oriented research conducted directly with patients in clinical settings. Some evidence is beginning to support this approach. For example, Mun et al.[53] recently showed that sleep modulates pain expectancies, which are a key component of placebo analgesic effects. In that study, which gathered naturalistic data from patients with temporomandibular disorder, daily expectancies for pain set in the morning mediated the prospective effect of the previous night's total sleep time on next-day pain severity.[53] Thus, a night of shorter total sleep time was associated with higher next-morning pain expectancies, which was sequentially associated with higher next-evening pain reports.

Colloca et al. has recently conducted a study in patients with chronic pain associated with temporomandibular disorders (TMD) matched with healthy controls (HC). The goal of this study was to understand how sleep quality and insomnia severity, assessed using the Pittsburgh Sleep Quality Index and the Insomnia Severity Index could affect placebo analgesia.

Participants suffering from chronic (orofacial) pain displayed either good or poor sleep quality as compared to HC. Controlling for sex, age, and pain sensitivity, TMD and HC participants underwent a well-established classical conditioning placebo manipulation to determine occurrence and magnitude of placebo effects in a laboratory setting. They found that the magnitudes of placebo effects were comparable. However, we found a main effect of sleep quality on placebo analgesia. Namely, the TMD cohort was characterized by those with good sleep quality and those with poor quality. Those who had no sleep disturbance showed greater placebo effects than those with poor sleep quality. They also found that participants with less than 6-hour sleep had smaller placebo analgesic effects compared to those with 6 to 9 hours of sleep. Moreover, those with increased pain interference had reduced placebo analgesia and sleep disturbance led to an impairment in conditioning learning.[89]

Poor sleep quality has been found to interfere with the mechanisms of descending pain inhibition.[20] Also, those with poor sleep quality and shorter sleep hours over night are likely to have altered endogenous opioid binding.[20] Also, good sleep quality has recently been linked to the OPRM1 rs1799971 single nucleotide polymorphism that has been strongly associated with placebo analgesia and endogenous opioid system function.[90,91]

Together, these findings highlight the pivotal role of sleep and sleep physiology in the endogenous modulation of pain via placebo induction and pain expectations. However, since not all are placebo "responders,"[92] it is important to consider the potential for other factors to synergize with sleep in driving variation in placebo analgesia. Future studies should determine whether the association of sleep and endogenous pain modulation systems varies as a function of sex/gender, race, and sociocultural context. Indeed, there is ample evidence that these sources of individual difference profoundly influence the incidence of sleep and pain disorders,[93,94] as well as the perception of pain[95] and endogenous pain modulation.[96] Beyond these fundamental individual difference variables, it is also important to consider the propensity for sleep-related memory consolidation, individual differences in prior pain-related experiences, sensitivity to suggestion and/or deception, and presence of comorbidities that modulate the so-called pain and sleep circular interaction.[97-100]

Conclusions

The circular aspects of the working model related to decrypting the influence of chronic pain on sleep should be updated, as it may be influenced by many more variables other than pain and sleep (see Figure 3.1.1).[101,102] Further, the basic notion that there is a bidirectional relationship between sleep and pain is complicated by the observation that the directional effect of sleep on pain is more consistently reported than the directional effect of pain on sleep[8,10] (though a meta-analysis of this observation has yet to be conducted). Further, whereas clinical trials of insomnia interventions in patients with chronic pain have reliably demonstrated strong improvements in sleep, clinical changes in pain have been weaker and less consistently observed.[103-107] Thus, it is likely that a host of mediators and moderators account for meaningful portions of variance in the association of sleep and pain, and these should be considered in study designs seeking to advance our understanding of this complex relationship. In redesigning our conceptualization of the sleep-pain interaction—and its mechanistic underpinnings in endogenous pain modulation—models should, for example, take into consideration the influence of sex and race, learning behavior, pain-relief expectation relative to prior experience, and the presence of sleep or pain comorbidities such as insomnia, sleep apnea, fibromyalgia, and temporomandibular disorders.[101,102,108-115] In assessing analgesia and the putative effect of substances such as cannabis or opioids on sleep quality, the influence of expectation and beliefs, the function of the corticostriatal reward and valuation circuits, and possible breathing risks all require special attention.[116-119] Of course, assessing the specificity of action and safety are not negotiable in study design. Finally, future investigations of the interaction of pain, sleep, and endogenous pain modulation will be enhanced by the identification of psychophysiological phenotypes in individuals who are responders and nonresponders to opioids, placebos, and positive affective stimuli, and such targeted approaches will contribute to innovation in the management of pain.[117,120,121]

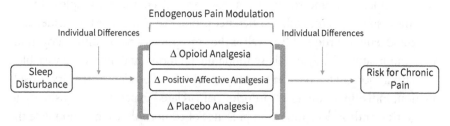

Figure 3.1.1 Proposed model for putative endogenous pain modulatory mechanisms accounting for the effect of sleep disturbance on chronic pain.

References

1. Zimmer Z, Zajacova A, Grol-Prokopczyk H. Trends in pain prevalence among adults aged 50 and older across Europe, 2004 to 2015. *Journal of Aging and Health.* 2020;32(10):1419–1432.
2. Zajacova A, Grol-Prokopczyk H, Zimmer Z. Pain trends among American adults, 2002–2018: Patterns, disparities, and correlates. *Demography.* 2021;58(2):711–738.
3. Blyth FM, Briggs AM, Schneider CH, Hoy DG, March LM. The global burden of musculoskeletal pain—Where to from here? *American Journal of Public Health.* 2019;109(1):35–40.
4. Wu A, March L, Zheng X, Huang J, Wang X, Zhao J, Blyth FM, Smith E, Buchbinder R, Hoy D. Global low back pain prevalence and years lived with disability from 1990 to 2017: Estimates from the Global Burden of Disease Study 2017. *Annals of Translational Medicine.* 2020;8(6):299. doi:10.21037/atm.2020.02.175.
5. Martin BI, Mirza SK, Spina N, Spiker WR, Lawrence B, Brodke DS. Trends in lumbar fusion procedure rates and associated hospital costs for degenerative spinal diseases in the United States, 2004 to 2015. *Spine (Phila Pa 1976).* 2019;44(5):369–376.
6. Buchbinder R, van Tulder M, Öberg B, et al. Low back pain: A call for action. *Lancet* 2018;391(10137):2384–2388.
7. Alexandre C, Latremoliere A, Finan PH. Effect of sleep loss on pain. In: Wood JN, ed. *The Oxford Handbook of the Neurobiology of Pain.* Oxford University Press; 2020:557–608.
8. Finan PH, Goodin BR, Smith MT. The association of sleep and pain: An update and a path forward. *Journal of Pain.* 2013;14(12):1539–1552.
9. Smith MT, Haythornthwaite JA. How do sleep disturbance and chronic pain inter-relate? Insights from the longitudinal and cognitive-behavioral clinical trials literature. *Sleep Medicine Reviews.* 2004;8(2):119–132.
10. Afolalu EF, Ramlee F, Tang NK. Effects of sleep changes on pain-related health outcomes in the general population: A systematic review of longitudinal studies with exploratory meta-analysis. *Sleep Medicine Reviews.* 2018;39:82–97.
11. Andersen ML, Araujo P, Frange C, Tufik S. Sleep disturbance and pain: A tale of two common problems. *Chest.* 2018;154(5):1249–1259.
12. Fields H. State-dependent opioid control of pain. *Nature Reviews Neuroscience.* 2004;5(7):565–575.
13. Fadda P, Tortorella A, Fratta W. Sleep deprivation decreases μ and δ opioid receptor binding in the rat limbic system. *Neuroscience Letters.* 1991;129(2):315–317.
14. Tomim DH, Pontarolla FM, Bertolini JF, et al. The pronociceptive effect of paradoxical sleep deprivation in rats: Evidence for a role of descending pain modulation mechanisms. *Molecular Neurobiology.* 2016;53(3):1706–1717.
15. Longordo F, Kopp C, Lüthi A. Consequences of sleep deprivation on neurotransmitter receptor expression and function. *European Journal of Neuroscience.* 2009;29(9):1810–1819.
16. Alexandre C, Latremoliere A, Ferreira A, et al. Decreased alertness due to sleep loss increases pain sensitivity in mice. *Nature Medicine.* 2017;23(6):768.
17. Skinner GO, Damasceno F, Gomes A, de Almeida OM. Increased pain perception and attenuated opioid antinociception in paradoxical sleep-deprived rats are associated with reduced tyrosine hydroxylase staining in the periaqueductal gray matter and are reversed by L-dopa. *Pharmacology Biochemistry and Behavior.* 2011;99(1):94–99.
18. Nascimento DC, Andersen ML, Hipólide DC, Nobrega JN, Tufik S. Pain hypersensitivity induced by paradoxical sleep deprivation is not due to altered binding to brain μ-opioid receptors. *Behavioural Brain Research.* 2007;178(2):216–220.
19. Steinmiller CL, Roehrs TA, Harris E, Hyde M, Greenwald MK, Roth T. Differential effect of codeine on thermal nociceptive sensitivity in sleepy versus nonsleepy healthy subjects. *Experimental and Clinical Psychopharmacology.* 2010;18(3):277.

20. Campbell CM, Bounds SC, Kuwabara H, et al. Individual variation in sleep quality and duration is related to cerebral mu opioid receptor binding potential during tonic laboratory pain in healthy subjects. *Pain Medications*. 2013;14(12):1882–1892.
21. Smith MT, Mun CJ, Remeniuk B, et al. Experimental sleep disruption attenuates morphine analgesia: findings from a randomized trial and implications for the opioid abuse epidemic. *Scientific Reports*. 2020;10(1):1–12.
22. Raymond I, Ancoli-Israel S, Choinière M. Sleep disturbances, pain and analgesia in adults hospitalized for burn injuries. *Sleep Medicine*. 2004;5(6):551–559.
23. Lautenbacher S, Kundermann B, Krieg J-C. Sleep deprivation and pain perception. *Sleep Medicine Reviews*. 2006;10(5):357–369.
24. Smith MT, Edwards RR, McCann UD, Haythornthwaite JA. The effects of sleep deprivation on pain inhibition and spontaneous pain in women. *Sleep*. 2007;30(4):494–505.
25. Ge F, Mu P, Guo R, et al. Chronic sleep fragmentation enhances habenula cholinergic neural activity. *Molecular Psychiatry*. 2021;26(3):941–954.
26. Khalid I, Roehrs TA, Hudgel DW, Roth T. Continuous positive airway pressure in severe obstructive sleep apnea reduces pain sensitivity. *Sleep*. 2011;34(12):1687–1691.
27. Lam KK, Kunder S, Wong J, Doufas AG, Chung F. Obstructive sleep apnea, pain, and opioids: Is the riddle solved? *Current Opinion in Anaesthesiology*. 2016;29(1):134.
28. Brown KA, Laferriere A, Lakheeram I, Moss IR. Recurrent hypoxemia in children is associated with increased analgesic sensitivity to opiates. *Journal of the American Society of Anesthesiologists*. 2006;105(4):665–669.
29. Brown KA, Laferrière A, Moss IR. Recurrent hypoxemia in young children with obstructive sleep apnea is associated with reduced opioid requirement for analgesia. *Journal of the American Society of Anesthesiologists*. 2004;100(4):806–810.
30. Doufas AG, Tian L, Padrez KA, et al. Experimental pain and opioid analgesia in volunteers at high risk for obstructive sleep apnea. *PLoS ONE*. 2013;8(1):e54807.
31. Patrick L, Renaud T, Claire A, et al. Sleep deprivation, sleep apnea and cardiovascular diseases. *Frontiers in Bioscience-Elite*. 2012;4(6):2007–2021.
32. Holmer BJ, Lapierre SS, Jake-Schoffman DE, Christou DD. Effects of sleep deprivation on endothelial function in adult humans: A systematic review. *Geroscience*. 2021;43(1):137–158.
33. Rhudy JL, DelVentura JL, Terry EL, et al. Emotional modulation of pain and spinal nociception in fibromyalgia. *Pain*. 2013;154(7):1045–1056.
34. Rhudy JL, Williams AE, McCabe KM, Rambo P. Affective modulation of nociception at spinal and supraspinal levels. *Psychophysiology*. 2005;42(5):579–587.
35. Roy M, Peretz I, Rainville P. Emotional valence contributes to music-induced analgesia. *Pain*. 2008;134(1):140–147.
36. Roy M, Piché M, Chen J-I, Peretz I, Rainville P. Cerebral and spinal modulation of pain by emotions. *Proceedings of the National Academy of Sciences*. 2009;106(49):20900–20905.
37. Seminowicz DA, Remeniuk B, Krimmel SR, Smith MT, Barrett FS, Wulff AB, Furman AJ, Geuter S, Lindquist MA, Irwin MR, Finan PH. Pain-related nucleus accumbens function: Modulation by reward and sleep disruption. *Pain*. 2019;160(5):1196–1207. doi:10.1097/j.pain.0000000000001498.
38. Finan PH, Garland EL. The role of positive affect in pain and its treatment. *Clinical Journal of Pain*. 2015;31(2):177–187.
39. Finan PH, Quartana PJ, Smith MT. Positive and negative affect dimensions in chronic knee osteoarthritis: Effects on clinical and laboratory pain. *Psychosomatic Medicine*. 2013;75(5):463–470.
40. Ong AD, Thoemmes F, Ratner K, Ghezzi-Kopel K, Reid MC. Positive affect and chronic pain: a preregistered systematic review and meta-analysis. *Pain*. 2020;161(6):1140.

41. Zautra AJ, Affleck GG, Tennen H, Reich JW, Davis MC. Dynamic approaches to emotions and stress in everyday life: Bolger and Zuckerman reloaded with positive as well as negative affects. *Journal of Personalized Medicine*. 2005;73(6):1511–1538.
42. Zautra AJ, Fasman R, Reich JW, et al. Fibromyalgia: Evidence for deficits in positive affect regulation. *Psychosomatic Medicine*. 2005;67(1):147–155.
43. Bushnell MC, Čeko M, Low LA. Cognitive and emotional control of pain and its disruption in chronic pain. *Nature Reviews Neuroscience*. 2013;14(7):502–511.
44. Villemure C, Bushnell MC. Mood influences supraspinal pain processing separately from attention. *Journal of Neuroscience*. 2009;29(3):705–715.
45. Terry EL, DelVentura JL, Bartley EJ, Vincent AL, Rhudy JL. Emotional modulation of pain and spinal nociception in persons with major depressive disorder (MDD). *Pain*. 2013;154(12):2759–2768.
46. Kamping S, Bomba IC, Kanske P, Diesch E, Flor H. Deficient modulation of pain by a positive emotional context in fibromyalgia patients. *Pain*. 2013;154(9):1846–1855.
47. Goldstein AN, Walker MP. The role of sleep in emotional brain function. *Annual Review of Clinical Psychology*. 2014;10:679.
48. Simon EB, Vallat R, Barnes CM, Walker MP. Sleep loss and the socio-emotional brain. *Trends in Cognitive Sciences*. 2020;24(6):435–450.
49. Finan PH, Quartana PJ, Remeniuk B, et al. Partial sleep deprivation attenuates the positive affective system: Effects across multiple measurement modalities. *Sleep*. 2017; 40(1):zsw017.
50. Palmer CA, Alfano CA. Sleep and emotion regulation: An organizing, integrative review. *Sleep Medicine Reviews*. 2017;31:6–16. doi:10.1016/j.smrv.2015.12.006.
51. Drewes AM, Svendsen L, Taagholt SJ, Bjerregård K, Nielsen KD, Hansen B. Sleep in rheumatoid arthritis: A comparison with healthy subjects and studies of sleep/wake interactions. *British Journal of Rheumatology*. 1998;37(1):71–81.
52. Mahowald MW, Mahowald ML, Bundlie SR, Ytterberg SR. Sleep fragmentation in rheumatoid arthritis. *Arthritis & Rheumatism*. 1989;32(8):974–983.
53. Mun CJ, Finan P, Weaver K, et al. The intra-day link between sleep disturbance and pain severity among individuals with temporomandibular joint disorder: Pain expectancy as a potential mechanism. *Journal of Pain*. 2021;22(5):611.
54. DelVentura JL, Terry EL, Bartley EJ, Rhudy JL. Emotional modulation of pain and spinal nociception in persons with severe insomnia symptoms. *Annals of Behavioral Medicine*. 2014; 47(3):303–315.
55. Huber FA, Toledo TA, Newsom G, Rhudy JL. The relationship between sleep quality and emotional modulation of spinal, supraspinal, and perceptual measures of pain. *Biological Psychology*. 2022;171:108352. doi:10.1016/j.biopsycho.2022.108352.
56. Krause AJ, Prather AA, Wager TD, Lindquist MA, Walker MP. The pain of sleep loss: A brain characterization in humans. *Journal of Neuroscience*. 2019;39(12):2291–2300.
57. Goel N, Rao H, Durmer JS, Dinges DF. Neurocognitive consequences of sleep deprivation. *Seminars in Neurology*. 2009;29(4):320–339. doi:10.1055/s-0029-1237117.
58. Whitney P, Hinson JM, Satterfield BC, Grant DA, Honn KA, Van Dongen H. Sleep deprivation diminishes attentional control effectiveness and impairs flexible adaptation to changing conditions. *Scientific Reports*. 2017;7(1):1–9.
59. Tiede W, Magerl W, Baumgärtner U, Durrer B, Ehlert U, Treede R-D. Sleep restriction attenuates amplitudes and attentional modulation of pain-related evoked potentials, but augments pain ratings in healthy volunteers. *Pain*. 2010;148(1):36–42.
60. Lavigne GJ, Sessle BJ. The neurobiology of orofacial pain and sleep and their interactions. *Journal of Dental Research*. 2016: 95(10):1109–1116. doi:10.1177/0022034516648264.

61. Halász P, Terzano M, Parrino L, Bódizs R. The nature of arousal in sleep. *Journal of Sleep Research*. 2004;13(1):1–23.

62. Gilmartin GS, Thomas RJ. Mechanisms of arousal from sleep and their consequences. *Current Opinion in Pulmonary Medicine*. 2004;10(6):468–474.

63. Yue HJ, Bardwell W, Ancoli-Israel S, Loredo JS, Dimsdale JE. Arousal frequency is associated with increased fatigue in obstructive sleep apnea. *Sleep and Breathing*. 2009; 13(4):331–339.

64. Janackova S, Sforza E. Neurobiology of sleep fragmentation: Cortical and autonomic markers of sleep disorders. *Current Pharmaceutical Design*. 2008;14(32):3474–3480.

65. Lavigne G, Zucconi M, Castronovo C, Manzini C, Marchettini P, Smirne S. Sleep arousal response to experimental thermal stimulation during sleep in human subjects free of pain and sleep problems. *Pain*. 2000;84(2–3):283–290.

66. Bentley AJ. Pain Perception during sleep and circadian influences: The experimental evidence. In: Lavigne G, Sessle BJ, ChoiniŠre M, Soja PJ, eds. *Sleep and Pain*. IASP Press; 2007:123–136.

67. Bentley AJ, Newton S, Zio CD. Sensitivity of sleep stages to painful thermal stimuli. *Journal of Sleep Research*. 2003;12:143–147.

68. Daya VG, Bentley AJ. Perception of experimental pain is reduced after provoked waking from rapid eye movement sleep. *Journal of Sleep Research*. 2010;19(2):317–322.

69. Lavigne G, Brousseau M, Kato T, et al. Experimental pain perception remains equally active over all sleep stages. *Pain*. 2004;110(3):646–655.

70. Melzack R. From the gate to the neuromatrix. *Pain*. 1999;82:S121–S126.

71. Price DD. *Psychological Mechanisms of Pain and Analgesia*. IASP press; 1999.

72. Wall P. The laminar organization of dorsal horn and effects of descending impulses. *Journal of Physiology*. 1967;188(3):403–423.

73. Porreca F, Ossipov MH, Gebhart GF. Chronic pain and medullary descending facilitation. *Trends in Neurosciences*. 2002;25(6):319–325.

74. Urban M, Gebhart G. Supraspinal contributions to hyperalgesia. *Proceedings of the National Academy of Sciences*. 1999;96(14):7687–7692.

75. Harrison R, Gandhi W, Van Reekum CM, Salomons TV. Conditioned pain modulation is associated with heightened connectivity between the periaqueductal grey and cortical regions. *Pain Reports*. 2022;7(3):e999. doi:10.1097/PR9.0000000000000999.

76. Sardi NF, Lazzarim MK, Guilhen VA, et al. Chronic sleep restriction increases pain sensitivity over time in a periaqueductal gray and nucleus accumbens dependent manner. *Neuropharmacology*. 2018;139:52–60.

77. King CD, Goodin B, Kindler LL, et al. Reduction of conditioned pain modulation in humans by naltrexone: An exploratory study of the effects of pain catastrophizing. *Journal of Behavioral Medicine*. 2013;36(3):315–327.

78. Pertovaara A, Kemppainen P, Johansson G, Karonen S-L. Ischemic pain nonsegmentally produces a predominant reduction of pain and thermal sensitivity in man: A selective role for endogenous opioids. *Brain Research*. 1982;251(1):83–92.

79. Sprenger C, Bingel U, Büchel C. Treating pain with pain: Supraspinal mechanisms of endogenous analgesia elicited by heterotopic noxious conditioning stimulation. *Pain*. 2011;152(2):428–439.

80. Eichhorn N, Treede R-D, Schuh-Hofer S. The role of sex in sleep deprivation related changes of nociception and conditioned pain modulation. *Neuroscience*. 2018;387:191–200. doi:10.1016/j.neuroscience.2017.09.044.

81. Iacovides S, George K, Kamerman P, Baker FC. Sleep fragmentation hypersensitizes healthy young women to deep and superficial experimental pain. *Journal of Pain*. 2017;18(7):844–854. doi:10.1016/j.jpain.2017.02.436.

82. Lee YC, Lu B, Edwards RR, et al. The role of sleep problems in central pain processing in rheumatoid arthritis. *Arthritis & Rheumatology.* 2013;65(1):59–68.

83. Paul-Savoie E, Marchand S, Morin M, et al. Is the deficit in pain inhibition in fibromyalgia influenced by sleep impairments? *Open Rheumatology Journal.* 2012;6:296.

84. Petrov ME, Goodin BR, Cruz-Almeida Y, et al. Disrupted sleep is associated with altered pain processing by sex and ethnicity in knee osteoarthritis. *Journal of Pain.* 2015;16(5):478–490.

85. Laverdure-Dupont D, Rainville P, Renancio C, Montplaisir J, Lavigne G. Placebo analgesia persists during sleep: An experimental study. *Progress in Neuro-Psychopharmacology & Biological Psychiatry.* 2018;85:33–38.

86. Laverdure-Dupont D, Rainville P, Montplaisir J, Lavigne G. Changes in rapid eye movement sleep associated with placebo-induced expectations and analgesia. *Journal of Neuroscience.* 2009;29(38):11745–11752.

87. Chouchou F, Chauny JM, Rainville P, Lavigne GJ. Selective REM sleep deprivation improves expectation-related placebo analgesia. *PLoS ONE.* 2015;10(12):e0144992.

88. Colloca L. The placebo effect in pain therapies. *Annual Review of Pharmacology and Toxicology.* 2019;59: 191.

89. Colloca L. Good and poor sleepers: In search of critical determinants of placebo analgesic effects. In: Luana Colloca, Jason Noel, Patricia Franklin, Chamindi Seneviratne, eds. *3rd International Conference of the Society for Interdisciplinary Placebo Studies (SIPS)* "Frontiers Media SA"; 2021:128. doi:10.3389/978-2-88971-003-4

90. Colloca L, Wang Y, Martinez PE, et al. OPRM1 rs1799971-COMT rs4680-FAAH rs324420 genes interact with placebo procedures to induce hypoalgesia. *Pain.* 2019; 160(8):1824.

91. Zahari Z, Ibrahim MA, Musa N, Tan SC, Mohamad N, Ismail R. Sleep quality and OPRM1 polymorphisms: A cross-sectional study among opioid-naive individuals. *Brazilian Journal of Pharmaceutical Sciences.* 2018;54(01). https://doi.org/10.1590/s2175-979020 18000117217

92. Kosek E, Rosen A, Carville S, et al. Lower placebo responses after long-term exposure to fibromyalgia pain. *Journal of Pain.* 2017;18(7):835–843.

93. Fillingim RB. Individual differences in pain: understanding the mosaic that makes pain personal. *Pain.* 2017;158(Suppl 1):S11.

94. Roth T, Roehrs T. Insomnia: Epidemiology, characteristics, and consequences. *Clinical Cornerstone.* 2003;5(3):5–15.

95. Coghill RC. Individual differences in the subjective experience of pain: New insights into mechanisms and models. *Headache.* 2010;50(9):1531–1535.

96. Edwards RR. Individual differences in endogenous pain modulation as a risk factor for chronic pain. *Neurology.* 2005;65(3):437–443.

97. Girardeau G, Lopes-Dos-Santos V. Brain neural patterns and the memory function of sleep. *Science.* 2021;374(6567):560–564.

98. Laverdure-Dupont D, Rainville P, Montplaisir J, Lavigne G. Relief expectation and sleep. *Annual Review of Neuroscience.* 2010;21(5):381–395.

99. Chouchou F, Dang-Vu TT, Rainville P, Lavigne G. The role of sleep in learning placebo effects. *International Review of Neurobiology.* 2018;139:321–355.

100. Lavigne GJ, Nashed A, Manzini C, Carra MC. Does sleep differ among patients with common musculoskeletal pain disorders? *Current Rheumatology Reports.* 2011;13(6):535–542.

101. Tang NK, Goodchild CE, Sanborn AN, Howard J, Salkovskis PM. Deciphering the temporal link between pain and sleep in a heterogeneous chronic pain patient sample: A multilevel daily process study. *Sleep.* 2012;35(5):675–687a.

102. Frange C, Hachul H, Hirotsu C, Tufik S, Andersen ML. Temporal analysis of chronic musculoskeletal pain and sleep in postmenopausal women. *Journal of Clinical Sleep Medicine.* 2019; 15(2):223–234.
103. Finan PH, Buenaver LF, Runko VT, Smith MT. Cognitive-behavioral therapy for comorbid insomnia and chronic pain. *Sleep Medicine Clinics.* 2014;9(2):261–274.
104. McCrae CS, Williams J, Roditi D, et al. Cognitive behavioral treatments for insomnia and pain in adults with comorbid chronic insomnia and fibromyalgia: Clinical outcomes from the SPIN randomized controlled trial. *Sleep.* 2019;42(3):zsy234.
105. Smith MT, Finan PH, Buenaver LF, et al. Cognitive-behavioral therapy for insomnia in knee osteoarthritis: A randomized, double-blind, active placebo-controlled clinical trial. *Arthritis & Rheumatology.* 2015;67(5):1221–1233.
106. Lami MJ, Martínez MP, Miro E, et al. Efficacy of combined cognitive-behavioral therapy for insomnia and pain in patients with fibromyalgia: A randomized controlled trial. *Cognitive Therapy and Research.* 2018;42(1):63–79.
107. Vitiello MV, McCurry SM, Shortreed SM, et al. Cognitive-behavioral treatment for comorbid insomnia and osteoarthritis pain in primary care: The lifestyles randomized controlled trial. *Journal of the American Geriatrics Society.* 2013;61(6):947–956.
108. Frange C, Naufel MF, Andersen ML, et al. Impact of insomnia on pain in postmenopausal women. *Climacteric.* 2017;20(3):262–267.
109. Tay DKL, Pang KP. Clinical phenotype of South-East Asian temporomandibular disorder patients with upper airway resistance syndrome. *Journal of Oral Rehabilitation.* 2018;45(1):25–33.
110. Mun CJ, Weaver KR, Hunt CA, et al. Pain expectancy and positive affect mediate the day-to-day association between objectively measured sleep and pain severity among women with temporomandibular disorder. *Journal of Pain.* 2022;23(4):669–679.
111. Okusogu C, Wang Y, Akintola T, et al. Placebo hypoalgesia: racial differences. *Pain.* 2020;161(8):1872–1883.
112. Olson EM, Akintola T, Phillips J, et al. Effects of sex on placebo effects in chronic pain participants: A cross-sectional study. *Pain.* 2021;162(2):531–542.
113. Wang Y, Chan E, Dorsey SG, Campbell CM, Colloca L. Who are the placebo responders? A cross-sectional cohort study for psychological determinants. *Pain.* 2022;163(6):1078–1090. doi:10.1097/j.pain.0000000000002478.
114. Sanders AE, Greenspan JD, Fillingim RB, Rathnayaka N, Ohrbach R, Slade GD. Associations of sleep disturbance, atopy, and other health measures with chronic overlapping pain conditions. *Journal of Oral & Facial Pain and Headache.* 2020;34:s73–s84.
115. Sinclair A, Wieckiewicz M, Ettlin D, Junior R, Guimarães AS, Gomes M, Meira E Cruz M. Temporomandibular disorders in patients with polysomnographic diagnosis of sleep bruxism: A case-control study. *Sleep Breath.* 2022;26(2):941–948. doi:10.1007/s11325-021-02449-2.
116. Marshansky S, Mayer P, Rizzo D, Baltzan M, Denis R, Lavigne GJ. Sleep, chronic pain, and opioid risk for apnea. *Progress in Neuro-Psychopharmacology & Biological Psychiatry.* 2018;87(Pt B):234–244. doi:10.1016/j.pnpbp.2017.07.014.
117. Herrero Babiloni A, Beetz G, Bruneau A, et al. Multitargeting the sleep-pain interaction with pharmacological approaches: A narrative review with suggestions on new avenues of investigation. *Sleep Medicine Reviews.* 2021;59:101459.
118. Choi S, Huang BC, Gamaldo CE. Therapeutic uses of cannabis on sleep disorders and related conditions. *Journal of Clinical Neurophysiology.* 2020;37(1):39–49.
119. Winiger EA, Hitchcock LN, Bryan AD, Cinnamon Bidwell L. Cannabis use and sleep: Expectations, outcomes, and the role of age. *Addictive Behaviors.* 2021;112:106642.

120. Tang NK, Goodchild CE, Salkovskis PM. Hybrid cognitive-behaviour therapy for individuals with insomnia and chronic pain: A pilot randomised controlled trial. *Behaviour Research and Therapy.* 2012;50(12):814–821.

121. Herrero Babiloni A, Beetz G, Tang NKY, et al. Towards the endotyping of the sleep-pain interaction: A topical review on multitarget strategies based on phenotypic vulnerabilities and putative pathways. *Pain.* 2021;162(5):1281–1288.

3.2
Placebo effects in cough

Ronald Eccles

Introduction

Cough is one of the most common and disturbing symptoms, and leading cough researchers in a comprehensive review of treatments have concluded "that cough remains a significant unmet medical need."[1] This chapter will discuss the physiology of cough, how it is under some voluntary control, and how it is susceptible to the placebo effects of treatments. The components of placebo effects on cough will be discussed, and a unique property of cough medicines (i.e., that they are mostly viscous, sapid syrups) will be highlighted. Placebo effects of cough medicines is both a gift and a problem to clinicians, as it makes all cough medicines effective but confounds the clinical trials on new cough medicines.[2] This chapter will discuss the mechanisms of cough and the importance of placebo effects in cough medicines and clinical trials.

Cough

Cough is an essential protective mechanism that serves to guard the airway from accidental entry of food and fluid, and which also clears the airway of irritants and excessive mucus.[3] Cough is a readily recognized respiratory phenomenon, just like sneeze, but when it comes to defining different causes and types of coughs "the semantics of cough is a mess with no conformity."[4] Cough can be defined as a "Forced expiratory maneuver usually against a closed glottis and associated with a characteristic sound."[5] Cough is associated with many different conditions: voluntary cough, refractory chronic cough, acute cough associated with the common cold, asthmatic cough, and cough associated with tuberculosis or lung cancer, for example, but all these different causes of cough are readily recognizable by the lay person or clinician as "cough." In this chapter, reference to *cough* will be mainly discussed in terms of literature related to studies on acute cough associated with the common cold and chronic refractory cough.

Mechanisms of cough

Cough is under voluntary control, and cough can be readily inhibited, for example, in the theater when cough is controlled during a tense scene but there is much coughing during the period of applause. However, the early literature always referred to the "cough reflex" and did not mention voluntary control of cough.[6] This may be because early research was performed on anesthetized animals rather than humans. Our present understanding of cough is that most cough is under voluntary control[7] and that cough associated with diseases such as the common cold,[8] and cough caused by inhalation of irritants such as capsaicin, can be voluntarily inhibited.[9] For example, voluntary inhibition of cough was studied in 79 patients with acute cough associated with the common cold, and patients could suppress cough for up to 20 minutes before breaking point when they coughed.[8] "The subjects who reached a breaking point had a greater baseline frequency of cough and a greater symptom severity score, and they also felt more feeble, clumsy, sad and antagonistic than the group which did not reach a breaking point. The subjects who reached a breaking point had significantly greater scores for the psychology parameter of obsessional symptoms than the group which did not reach a breaking point."[8] Suppression of cough induced by inhalation of capsaicin was studied in 24 healthy volunteers, and 21 out of 24 subjects were able to suppress cough completely on inhalation of this pepper-like irritant.[9]

Cough can only occur during consciousness,[7] and that cough is inhibited during sleep[10,11] and with general anesthesia.[12] Aspiration of food or fluid into the airway causes stimulation of sensory nerves in the larynx and trachea and a sudden reflex cough mediated through the brainstem cough control center. Cough associated with diseases of the airway, such as the common cold or bronchitis, is associated with a sensation of irritation mediated through higher centers in the brain, such as the cerebral cortex. This sensation initiates a sometimes-overwhelming urge to cough, forcing the typically voluntary response to become involuntary.[7] Placebo effects on cough are likely to be via an influence on the urge to cough and voluntary cough.

Cough associated with diseases of the airways is initiated by a sensation of irritation and an "urge to cough," which can be quantified by subjective scores.[13] Although cough can be shown to be inhibited by voluntary control, the urge to cough from a sensation of irritation may become an overwhelming urge that causes an involuntary cough.[7]

Components of placebo effects in cough medicines

The efficacy of any cough medicine is determined by two components: firstly, the efficacy of a pharmacological medicine such as codeine, and secondly the magnitude of placebo effects of the medicine. When discussing placebo effects, it is important to distinguish between the "perceived placebo effect" and the "true placebo effect." This distinction was first put forward by Ernst in 1995[14] and later applied to cough medicines.[15] A diagram illustrating the different components of the placebo effects in cough medicines is shown in Figure 3.2.1. The perceived placebo effect is the total response to a placebo treatment, and this is made up of three components as illustrated in Figure 3.2.1.

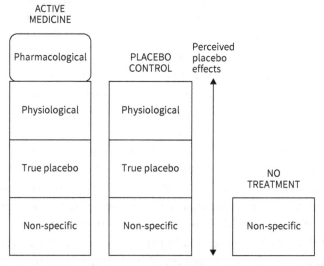

Figure 3.2.1 Four components of couch medicine efficacy.
Efficacy of a cough medicine can be considered as involving four components: *pharmacological*, related to efficacy of the active ingredient; *physiological*, related to sweetness and demulcent effects of a syrup; *true placebo*, related to the belief and expectation of the patient about the efficacy of the medicine; *nonspecific*, related to factors such as natural recovery of the patient. The total efficacy of placebo treatment is the *perceived placebo effect*, and this includes the *true placebo* and *nonspecific effects*. The magnitude of the *true placebo effects* can only be determined by using a no-treatment group to determine the magnitude of the *nonspecific effects*, owing to, for example, natural recovery.

Physiological effect

The physiological effect of a cough treatment is a component of the perceived placebo effects that is unique to cough medicines and has been previously discussed by Eccles.[2,15] Most cough medicines are sweet viscous syrups, and the physiological effect of a cough medicine is caused by stimulation of salivation to give a soothing demulcent effect, and by the sweetness, which may cause release of endogenous opioids in the brainstem area and inhibit cough.[16] Cough medicines are traditionally formulated as sweet viscous syrups, and honey has been used for centuries as treatment for cough.[16,17] Sweet tastes are pleasant and rewarding, and Eccles[16] proposed that the sweet taste of cough medicines may act as an antitussive by causing the release of endogenous opioids in an area of the brain (tractus solitarius of brainstem) that is involved in the control of cough. Since opioids such as morphine and codeine have been used as antitussives, it was proposed that the endogenous release of opioids by sweet taste would result in an antitussive effect.[16] Sucrose and other sweet-tasting substances have been shown to have analgesic actions in infants, and that a sweet taste modulates the generation of endogenous opioids.[18] The antitussive effect of a sweet taste has been demonstrated for cough induced by inhalation of capsaicin,[19] and in this study a sweet taste inhibited cough while a bitter taste had no effect. Potential mechanisms for the antitussive effect of sweet taste are shown in Figure 3.2.2. The rostral area of the solitary nucleus acts as a relay for gustatory fibers of the X, IX, and VII cranial nerves, and the caudal area is concerned with cardiorespiratory control and the initiation of cough,[20,21] but these areas overlap, and it is possible that gustatory information may influence cough as illustrated in Figure 3.2.2. Sweet taste may also be interpreted by higher centers as pleasant and rewarding, and this may result in a placebo effects as illustrated in Figure 3.2.2. The antitussive effects of sweet taste pose some interesting questions; is this a physiological effect as proposed by Eccles[16] or is it a true placebo effect? Does a true placebo effect become a physiological effect when explained in terms of neurophysiology and neurotransmitters, such as endogenous opioids?

Nonspecific effects

"Nonspecific" effects are often described as placebo responses and are mainly related to natural recovery, and regression of symptom measurements toward the mean, which is why it is so important to include a placebo arm in clinical

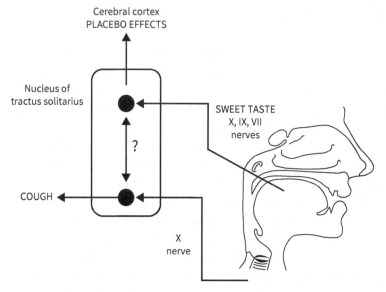

Figure 3.2.2 Gustatory effects on cough.
Gustation is mediated by branches of the VII (facial) IX (glossopharyngeal) and X (vagus) cranial nerves that supply the taste buds of the tongue. These gustatory fibers relay in the nucleus of the tractus solitarius that also serves as the first relay for the X cranial nerves that mediate the cough reflex. It is proposed that there may be some interaction between gustatory and cough pathways maybe by the generation of endogenous opioids which have antitussive actions. The rewarding effects of a sweet taste may also influence higher centers and cause a psychological placebo effects.

trials. Specifically, patients may recover from a disease during the course of the trial, and this recovery is unrelated to any pharmacological effect of a medicine.

True placebo effects

The true placebo effect is the phenomenon that is primarily under discussion in this book, and it only forms one component of the perceived placebo effects. The placebo phenomenon was first described in clinical trials, but interest in this phenomenon has progressed to a psychosocial model that incorporates a general interaction of the patient to their environment and how they respond to psychological mechanisms such as conditioning, expectation, reward, and anxiety reduction, and how these can be modulated by desire, motivation, and memory.[22] The magnitude of the true placebo effects can only be determined in a clinical trial if a "no-treatment" group is included to control for any non-specific effects such as natural recovery from disease, as discussed below.

Magnitude of placebo effects in cough

A review article explored eight clinical trials and reported that up to 85% of the efficacy of cough medicines in treatment of acute cough is due to placebo effects.[15] However, the reported placebo effects in this study is the "perceived placebo effect," and this consists of three components: the true placebo effects, physiological effects, and the nonspecific effects such as natural recovery. In a condition such as acute cough associated with the common cold it is to be expected that there will be natural recovery over a few days, and if the study is conducted for that length of time, then most of the perceived placebo effects will be due to natural recovery. As mentioned above, in order to get a better measure of the true placebo effects associated with a cough medicine, it is necessary to include a no-treatment group in the study. Any change in cough measured in the no-treatment group will be due to nonspecific effects such as natural recovery and likely, statistical effects such as regression to the mean. However, clinical trials rarely include a no-treatment group in the design and to date only one laboratory study with a no-treatment group has been performed on patients with cough.[23] Fifty-four patients with acute cough associated with the common cold were randomly assigned to receive treatment (a placebo capsule) or no treatment, with 27 in each group. In this study the placebo treatment consisted of a capsule containing vitamin E, which over the short duration of the measurement period (15 minutes) would not have been absorbed to have any effect on cough. Unlike a syrup, the capsule would not have any physiological effects contributing to the perceived placebo effects such as stimulation of salivation or sweet taste. The no-treatment group only took a sip of water to control the water ingested in the placebo group when swallowing the capsule. Cough frequency over a 15-minute period in the no-treatment group was reduced by 7%, which could be related to a demulcent effect of ingesting water, whereas there was a 49% reduction in cough frequency in the placebo treatment group (perceived placebo effects). The very large reduction in cough frequency (49%) over the short period of 15 minutes is unlikely to be due to any natural recovery, and it allows a measure of the magnitude of the "true placebo effects." Subtraction of the no-treatment effect on cough (7% reduction in cough frequency) from the perceived placebo effect on cough (49% reduction in cough frequency) allows calculation of the true placebo effects as a 42% reduction in cough frequency. Statistical effects such as regression to mean would be expected to be seen in both the no-treatment group and the placebo group and, therefore, cannot explain the very large *true* placebo effects seen in this study. Also, there would be no physiological effect associated with ingestion of a capsule. The study also reported that placebo treatment increased the duration of time that patients were able to voluntarily suppress their cough.

What is the magnitude of the placebo effects in cough clinical trials? Acute cough associated with the common cold declines over a period of days because of natural recovery, and this decline in cough could be mistakenly interpreted as placebo effects in a clinical trial. In order to obtain a measure of placebo effects in clinical trials on acute cough it is necessary to look at studies with measurements of cough over a few hours so that any natural recovery from cough will be minimal. A search of the literature for acute cough clinical trials that used a single dose of placebo treatment and measured changes in cough over a few hours found six suitable studies, and these are listed in Table 3.2.1 in which the change in cough measure recorded in the placebo arm of the study as a percentage change from baseline. Five of the studies used a placebo capsule, which would not elicit any demulcent or physiological effects. One study[24] used a sweet syrup as placebo, which would have had some demulcent and sweetness effects as described above, but the magnitude of the reduction in cough in this study (44%), as shown in Table 3.2.1, is comparable with that observed in the studies using a placebo capsule (28%–52%).[25-27] These studies give a measure of perceived placebo effects in acute cough clinical trials. Because of the short duration of the studies there is little time for natural recovery. It is important to note that resting in a quiet room for cough recording over a few hours could alleviate cough, and there is also the possibility of regression to a mean value for cough as the patients were selected for the trials on the basis that they had a high level of cough. However, the mean placebo effects of 44% reduction in cough frequency in these six studies is similar to the 42% reduction in cough reported as a true placebo effect by Lee et al.[23]

The measures of the placebo effects in clinical trials on cough discussed above all relate to acute cough associated with the common cold, and there may be differences in placebo effects in different disease states such as chronic cough and asthma. However, large placebo effects on the symptom of cough have been reported in clinical trials on chronic cough,[28] and a large placebo effect is likely to be seen in all disease states that cause cough.

Table 3.2.1 Magnitude of placebo effects in acute cough clinical trials
The change in cough measure recorded in the placebo arm of the study is calculated as a percentage change from the baseline measure of cough.

Placebo Medication	Time to Cough Measurement	Cough Measure	Placebo Responses	Patients	Source
Sweet syrup	150 min	Frequency of cough	44% reduction in cough frequency	45 treated with placebo	24
Capsule	90–120 min	Cough bouts	44% reduction in cough bouts	108 patients in total	25 (study 1)
Capsule	90–120 min	Cough bouts	28% reduction in cough bouts	134 patients in total	25 (study 2)
Capsule	90–120 min	Cough bouts	41% reduction in cough bouts	209 patients in total	25 (study 3)
Capsule	90 min	Cough frequency	50% reduction in cough frequency	34 treated with placebo	26
Capsule	180 min	Cough frequency	52% reduction in cough frequency	22 treated with placebo	27

Placebo effects confound clinical trials on new cough medicines

Placebo effects can confound research on antitussive medicines, as the response to placebo treatment may be so great as to make it very difficult to demonstrate any pharmacological activity of an antitussive medicine.[2] Placebo effects in clinical trials may also confound studies because of unblinding owing to side effects of the active medicine.[28] The issues concerning clinical trials on new antitussive medicines have recently been reviewed by Eccles.[28] ATP (adenosine triphosphate) is believed to act as an inflammatory mediator and cause chronic cough, and some new antitussive medicines act as ATP antagonists and are believed to reduce the frequency and severity of chronic cough.[29] The issue with using ATP antagonists as antitussives is that they also interfere with the sensation of taste. ATP has a major role in the sensation of taste as an excitatory transmitter between taste buds and gustatory sensory nerves, as first described in studies on rats,[30] and later apparent in human studies on ATP antagonists as antitussives.[29] Clinical trials on antitussive ATP antagonists have reported taste-related side effects such as hypogeusia and dysgeusia, and the investigators have expressed concerns that these side effects have unblinded the studies.[31–33]

The blinding of patients as regards which treatment they are taking in a double-blind placebo controlled clinical trial is a key element of the trial design. If patients recognize that they are taking an active medicine because they experience side effects, then they will have a greater expectancy that the treatment will benefit their cough than those patients in the placebo arm of the trial. This unblinding of the trial will unbalance the placebo effects in the two arms of the trial and make the trial more closely resemble an open-treatment versus no-treatment comparison, rather than the intended double-blind active treatment versus placebo comparison.[28,34]

The presence of side effects with a test medicine makes it difficult to separate the pharmacological efficacy of the medicine from placebo effects because of unblinding. In a recent study by Smith et al., 81% of patients taking a 50 mg dose of ATP antagonist reported a taste-related side effect.[31] The incidence of taste-related side effects was dose dependent (10% for 7.5 mg; 49% for 20.0 mg; and 81% for 50.0 mg) with significant antitussive action of the ATP antagonist only found at the 50 mg dose, which had the highest incidence of taste- related side effects.[31]

Unblinding of patients in clinical trials is not restricted to the side effects of an active medicine, as if the medicine is very effective patients will be aware of the benefit, and this could also unblind and unbalance the placebo effects in each arm of the trial. Moscucci et al.[35] discussed the issues related to unblinding in clinical trials as regards the side effects or efficacy of a medicine and concluded that no matter how trials may be designed the maintenance of blinding is difficult, and, therefore, the blinding should be checked to rule out or to quantify bias. However, since the problem of partial unblinding seems unresolvable, the results of a double-blind clinical trial should not be discarded even if there is some unblinding.[35]

The powerful placebo effects of over-the-counter cough medicines

Cough medicines available over the counter (OTC) from the pharmacy or supermarket for the treatment of cough can be considered very powerful placebo treatments. There is some doubt about the efficacy of the pharmacological ingredients in OTC cough medicines, and Schroeder and Fahey[36] state that "Over the counter cough medicines for acute cough cannot be recommended because there is no good evidence for their effectiveness." There may be doubt about the pharmacological efficacy of OTC cough medicines, but a case can be made that these medicines provide relief of cough from placebo effects rather than a pharmacological effect and, therefore, can be recommended as treatments.

The first cough medicines used hundreds of years ago contained honey as a placebo but over time, strong flavors such as lemon, menthol, and capsicum were used to enhance the sensory impact of the medicines and, therefore, increase placebo effects. Placebo effects of a cough medicine are related to the patients' expectations and beliefs about the efficacy of the medicine.[37,38] Expectations and beliefs of efficacy associated with an OTC cough medicine will be related to many different factors such as advertising of the medicine on media such as television and magazines, claims on the package about efficacy, belief about a well-known brand of medicine, price of the medicine, and recommendations from well-known personalities and from friends. However, a major component of the placebo effects will occur when the patient pours out a spoonful or small cup of the medicine and ingests the medicine. The color, viscosity, and sensory impact of the medicine will reinforce the expectation and belief in the medicine. A very viscous, strongly colored medicine with a powerful taste will indicate to the patient that they are taking a powerful medicine. Cough medicines available OTC are complex mixtures of excipients (e.g., affect, odor, viscosity, color, and taste of a medicine), and a recent review has highlighted the role of over 100 excipients in cough medicines.[39] The pharmacological component of cough medicines, such as dextromethorphan or guaifenesin, could be more easily and more cheaply delivered to the patient as a white tablet or capsule rather than as a complex syrup, but all OTC cough medicines are formulated as viscous sapid syrups, often with large amounts of sugars or artificial sweeteners. Over centuries of use, patients have come to expect a cough medicine to be formulated as a powerful tasting syrup. The first cough medicines were derived from foods such as honey, and beverages such as cider or vinegar, and modern cough medicines contain excipients that are the same as those used in the food and beverage industries to provide powerful tastes and smell.[39]

The composition of a modern OTC cough medicine is illustrated in Figure 3.2.3. The pharmacological effect of the medicine is due to the inclusion of guaifenesin, an expectorant medicine. Placebo effects of the medicine is due to 15 different excipients included in the medicine. The excipients cause placebo effects by influencing the sensory effect of the medicine as regards smell, taste, color, viscosity, and other sensory effects. Levomenthol will give the

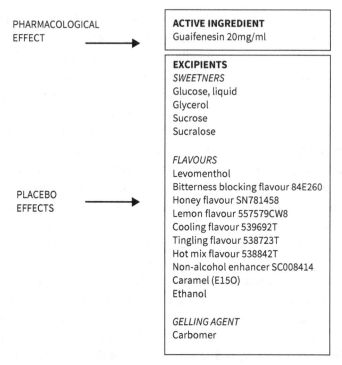

PHARMACOLOGICAL
EFFECT →

ACTIVE INGREDIENT
Guaifenesin 20mg/ml

EXCIPIENTS
SWEETNERS
Glucose, liquid
Glycerol
Sucrose
Sucralose

FLAVOURS
Levomenthol
Bitterness blocking flavour 84E260
Honey flavour SN781458
Lemon flavour 557579CW8
Cooling flavour 539692T
Tingling flavour 538723T
Hot mix flavour 538842T
Non-alcohol enhancer SC008414
Caramel (E150)
Ethanol

GELLING AGENT
Carbomer

PLACEBO
EFFECTS →

Figure 3.2.3 List of ingredients of modern over-the-counter cough medicine (Benylin Mucus Cough Max Honey & Lemon Flavor 100 mg/5 ml syrup), as detailed in summary of product characteristics of medicine.
The ingredients contain one pharmacological agent, guaifenesin, and 15 excipients that impart color, flavor, smell, and sensations to enhance placebo effects.

medicine a distinctive smell. Honey, lemon, and sweeteners will enhance the taste. Caramel, with give a brown color. Carbomer and glycerol will increase viscosity. Cooling, tingling, and hot mix excipients, and alcohol, will provide other sensations apart from taste. Overall, the 15 excipients provide a strong sensory impact to enhance placebo effects.

Conclusive remarks

There is a great need for new cough medicines to treat patients with chronic cough, and clinical trials on new treatments for chronic cough such as ATP antagonists have been confounded by large placebo effects seen in these trials.[2] However, powerful placebo medicines have been developed for the treatment of acute cough, formulated as sapid syrups. The complex mixture of excipients seen in modern OTC cough medicines available to the public demonstrates how the formulation of these medicines is primarily aimed at enhancing the sensory effect of these medicines, and, thus, at enhancing placebo effects. With cough being subject to large placebo effects, it seems reasonable that in the future, more research should be conducted on harnessing the placebo as a powerful treatment for all forms of cough, while we wait for any breakthrough in its pharmacological treatment.

References

1. Dicpinigaitis PV, Morice AH, Birring SS, et al. Antitussive drugs: Past, present, and future. *Pharmacological Reviews*. 2014;66(2):468–512.
2. Eccles R. The powerful placebo effect in cough: Relevance to treatment and clinical trials. *Lung*. 2020;198(1):13–21.
3. Fuller RW, Jackson DM. Physiology and treatment of cough. *Thorax*. 1990;45:425–430.
4. Chung KF, Bolser D, Davenport P, Fontana G, Morice A, Widdicombe J. Semantics and types of cough. *Pulmonary Pharmacology and Therapeutics*. 2009;22(2):139–142.
5. Morice AH, Fontana GA, Belvisi MG, et al. ERS guidelines on the assessment of cough. *European Respiratory Journal*. 2007;29(6):1256–1276.
6. May AJ, Widdicombe JG. Depression of the cough reflex by pentobarbitone and some opium derivatives. *British Journal of Pharmacology and Chemotherapy*. 1954;9(3):335–340.
7. Lee PC, Cotterill-Jones C, Eccles R. Voluntary control of cough. *Pulmonary Pharmacology and Therapeutics*. 2002;15(3):317–320.
8. Hutchings HA, Eccles R, Smith AP, Jawad MS. Voluntary cough suppression as an indication of symptom severity in upper respiratory tract infections. *European Respiratory Journal*. 1993;6(10):1449–1454.
9. Hutchings HA, Morris S, Eccles R, Jawad MS. Voluntary suppression of cough induced by inhalation of capsaicin in healthy volunteers. *Respiratory Medicine*. 1993;87(5):379–382.
10. Power JT, Stewart IC, Connaughton JJ, et al. Nocturnal cough in patients with chronic bronchitis and emphysema. *American Review of Respiratory Disease*. 1984;130(6):999–1001.
11. Lee KK, Birring SS. Cough and sleep. *Lung*. 2010;188(Suppl 1):S91–S94.
12. Nishino T, Hiraga K, Yokokawa N. Laryngeal and respiratory responses to tracheal irritation at different depths of enflurane anesthesia in humans. *Anesthesiology*. 1990;73(1):46–51.
13. Davenport PW. Urge-to-cough: what can it teach us about cough? *Lung*. 2008;186 Suppl 1:S107–S111.
14. Ernst E, Resch KL. Concept of true and perceived placebo effects. *British Medical Journal*. 1995;311:551–553.
15. Eccles R. The powerful placebo in cough studies? *Pulmonary Pharmacology and Therapeutics*. 2002;15(3):303–308.
16. Eccles R. Mechanisms of the placebo effect of sweet cough syrups. *Respiratory Physiology & Neurobiology*. 2006;152(3):340–348.
17. Kuropatnicki AK, Kłósek M, Kucharzewski M. Honey as medicine: Historical perspectives. *Journal of Apicultural Research*. 2018;57(1):113–118.
18. Bueno M, Yamada J, Harrison D, et al. A systematic review and meta-analyses of nonsucrose sweet solutions for pain relief in neonates. *Pain Research and Management*. 2013;18(3):153–161.
19. Wise PM, Breslin PA, Dalton P. Effect of taste sensation on cough reflex sensitivity. *Lung*. 2014;192(1):9–13. doi:10.1007/s00408-013-9515-z.

20. Martin J. *Neuroanatomy Text and Atlas.* Elsevier; 1988.

21. Cutsforth-Gregory JK, Benarroch EE. Nucleus of the solitary tract, medullary reflexes, and clinical implications. *Neurology.* 2017;88(12):1187–1196.

22. Benedetti F, Amanzio M. Mechanisms of the placebo response. *Pulmonary Pharmacology and Therapeutics.* 2013;26(5):520–523.

23. Lee PC, Jawad MS, Hull JD, West WH, Shaw K, Eccles R. The antitussive effect of placebo treatment on cough associated with acute upper respiratory infection. *Psychosomatic Medicine.* 2005;67(2):314–317.

24. Eccles R, Morris S, Jawad M. Lack of effect of codeine in the treatment of cough associated with acute upper respiratory tract infection. *Journal of Clinical Pharmacy and Therapeutics.* 1992;17(3):175–180.

25. Parvez L, Vaidya M, Sakhardande A, Subburaj S, Rajagopalan TG. Evaluation of antitussive agents in man. *Pulmonary Pharmacology.* 1996;9(5–6):299–308.

26. Freestone C, Eccles R. Assessment of the antitussive efficacy of codeine in cough associated with common cold. *Journal of Pharmacy and Pharmacology.* 1997;49(10):1045–1049.

27. Lee PCL, Jawad MS, Eccles R. Antitussive efficacy of dextromethorphan in cough associated with acute upper respiratory tract infection. *Journal of Pharmacy and Pharmacology.* 2000;52(9):1137–1142.

28. Eccles R. Placebo and side effects confound clinical trials on new antitussives. *Lung.* 2021;199(4):319–326.

29. Dicpinigaitis PV, McGarvey LP, Canning BJ. P2X3-receptor antagonists as potential antitussives: Summary of current clinical trials in chronic cough. *Lung.* 2020;198(4):609–616.

30. Bo X, Alavi A, Xiang Z, Oglesby I, Ford A, Burnstock G. Localization of ATP-gated P2X2 and P2X3 receptor immunoreactive nerves in rat taste buds. *Neuroreport.* 1999;10(5):1107–1111.

31. Smith JA, Kitt MM, Morice AH, et al. Gefapixant, a P2X3 receptor antagonist, for the treatment of refractory or unexplained chronic cough: A randomised, double-blind, controlled, parallel-group, phase 2b trial. *Lancet Respiratory Medicine.* 2020;8(8):775–785.

32. Morice AH, Kitt MM, Ford AP, Tershakovec AM, Wu WC, Brindle K, Thompson R, Thackray-Nocera S, Wright C. The effect of gefapixant, a P2X3 antagonist, on cough reflex sensitivity: A randomised placebo-controlled study. *European Respiratory Journal.* 2019;54(1):1900439. doi:10.1183/13993003.00439-2019.

33. Smith JA, Kitt MM, Butera P, Smith SA, Li Y, Xu ZJ, Holt K, Sen S, Sher MR, Ford AP. Gefapixant in two randomised dose-escalation studies in chronic cough. *European Respiratory Journal.* 2020;55(3):1901615. doi:10.1183/13993003.01615-2019.

34. Colagiuri B. Participant expectancies in double-blind randomized placebo-controlled trials: Potential limitations to trial validity. *Clinical Trials.* 2010;7(3):246–255.

35. Moscucci M, Byrne L, Weintraub M, Cox C. Blinding, unblinding, and the placebo effect: An analysis of patients' guesses of treatment assignment in a double-blind clinical trial. *Clinical Pharmacology and Therapeutics.* 1987;41(3):259–265.

36. Schroeder K, Fahey T. Systematic review of randomised controlled trials of over the counter cough medicines for acute cough in adults. *British Medical Journal (Clinical Research Ed).* 2002;324(7333):329–331.

37. Brown WA. Expectation, the placebo effect and the response to treatment. *Rhode Island Medical Journal (2013).* 2015;98(5):19–21.

38. Evans D. *Placebo: The Belief Effect.* Harper Collins; 2003.

39. Eccles R. What is the role of over 100 excipients in over the counter (OTC) cough medicines? *Lung.* 2020;198(5):727–734.

3.3

Learned immune responses

How associations affect immunity

Stefanie Hölsken, Manfred Schedlowski, Martin Hadamitzky,
and Laura Heiss-Lückemann

Introduction

Learning experiences shape our behavior. This comes as no surprise to anyone who has ever touched a hot stove: they will avoid this painful experience in the future. What we learned from the early experiments by Pavlov and coworkers, however, was that learning not only shapes overt behavior but also affects physiological processes. In their most famous experiment in dogs, the sound of a bell was associated with the salivary response.[1] Maybe an even more stunning though less well-known work demonstrated that in guinea pigs the same associative learning process was able to link the effects of a pharmacological agent to tactile sensations, culminating in leukocyte production when guinea pigs where subsequently scratched on the belly.[2]

Several experimental studies in the early to mid-twentieth century reported behaviorally conditioned alterations of immune functions (e.g., conditioned leukocytosis in humans and dogs), revealing that similar rules to those applicable to conditioned physiological reflexes also apply to immune responses.[2] However, these studies were almost completely discontinued due to methodological issues, vague and partly inconsistent outcomes, and in particular because of the insufficient knowledge regarding the connection between the brain and the peripheral immune functions prevailing at that time. The interest in the phenomenon of behaviorally conditioned immune responses revitalized in 1975, when Robert Ader and Nicholas Cohen published a pioneering study demonstrating the behaviorally conditioned suppression of antibody titers in rats.[3] This approach simultaneously set the stage for the research field of psychoneuroimmunology.

Acknowledging the existence of behaviorally conditioned immune responses raises the question of their benefit for the organism. Following an evolutionary perspective, Pavlovian conditioning enables the organism to avoid consuming a harmful food or liquid by linking a certain sensation, such as its smell or look, with the physiological response the food or liquid elicits. This concept is known as conditioned taste aversion (or avoidance) and is not restricted to hunter gatherer societies but can still be seen nowadays when we get sick from ingesting spoiled food or drink. At the same time, the conditioned immune response allows the body to quickly counter the sickening agent by anticipatory immune reactions.[2]

The underlying neurobiological and psychological mechanisms responsible for the phenomenon of behaviorally conditioned immune responses have been increasingly better understood during the last few decades. This knowledge offers a range of possibilities to exploit these learned pharmacological effects in clinical conditions to optimize current treatment regimens for the patients' benefit.[4] In addition to the patients' expectation, behavioral conditioning is assumed to be one of the major mechanisms underlying the placebo (and nocebo) effect. In this chapter, we provide an overview of experimental approaches that have especially targeted conditioned placebo effects in the context of immune mediated diseases, illustrating their potential application in the clinical context (see Figure 3.3.1, as well as Tables 3.3.1 and 3.3.2). We further elaborate on the supposed mechanisms and critically acknowledge open questions and necessary future research activities.

Allergy

Allergic diseases provide a valuable opportunity for the study of placebo effects, as they appear to be highly susceptible to placebo interventions. Placebo effects rates in clinical allergen immunotherapy trials are reported to be as high as 77%, making pharmacological research in this area quite challenging.[5] This observation also raises the question of how far placebo effects play a role in the occurrence of allergic symptoms in the first place. The earliest—and arguably most regularly cited—account of an allergic reaction being subject to conditioning effects is that of a woman allergic to roses who suffered from an asthma attack after being confronted with an artificial rose.[6] Over the years, more reliable approaches have shown that this phenomenon can also be induced experimentally. A small laboratory study in the 1950s showed an impressive case of context conditioning. By simply being exposed to the same context in which they had previously suffered from an asthma attack, two patients experienced asthmatic symptoms in the absence of any allergen.[7] Similar experimental results could be observed in guinea pigs, where

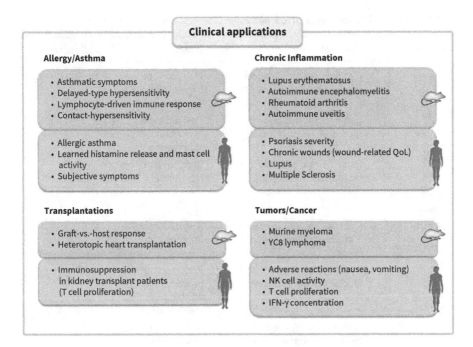

Figure 3.3.1 Clinical relevance of learned immune responses.
The potential clinical applicability of learned immune responses has been tested
in several disease conditions, such as allergy and asthma, chronic inflammation,
transplantations, and tumors and cancer, in experimental rodent models (yellow) and
human volunteers and patients (green).
Abbreviations: QoL, quality of life; IFN, Interferon.

asthmatic symptoms were elicited by conditioning allergens to auditory
stimuli or a certain context.[2] Together, these findings in humans and animals
led to the assumption that asthma, at least in some cases, may be a "learned"
disease or response. Later on, paradigms were aimed at pairing allergens with
specific taste or odor stimuli, with observed symptoms such as increased his-
tamine release upon re-exposure to the taste or odor.[8]

Later studies showed that not only the allergen itself, but also
antihistaminergic drugs, can be paired with a gustatory stimulus, thereby
dampening the allergic response. A preclinical model of contact hypersensitivity in rats found reduced leukocyte infiltration in the challenged skin after
administration of cyclosporine A (CsA) and, more importantly, after presentation of saccharin which had previously been presented together with
CsA.[9] Similar results were reported in humans, with studies documenting
a reduction in subjective rhinitis symptom scores and skin prick test results
induced by mere expectation.[10] However, the immunological response

Table 3.3.1 Clinical relevance of learned immune responses in animals

Disease	Protocol	Effect	Source
Allergy	Cyclophosphamide injection + saccharin solution (taste)	Delayed-type hypersensitivity response	50, 51
	Lithium chloride injection + saccharin solution (taste)	Delayed-type hypersensitivity suppression	52
	Cyclosporine A injection + saccharin solution (taste)	Reduced leukocyte infiltration	9
Autoimmune diseases			
Arthritis	Cyclophosphamide injection + saccharin/vanilla solution (taste)	Reduced arthritic inflammation	21
	Cyclosporine A injection + saccharin solution (taste)	Reduced lymphocyte proliferation/ inhibition of arthritic inflammation	23
	Cyclosporine A injection + saccharin solution (taste)	Reduced lymphocyte proliferation/ inhibition of arthritic inflammation	22
Encephalo- myelitis	ALA (alpha lipoic acid) + saccharin solution (taste)	Reduced disease severity	25
Lupus	Cyclophosphamide injection + saccharin solution (taste)	Reduced rate of autoimmune disease progression	53
Uveitis	Cyclosporine A injection + saccharin solution (taste)	Reduction in IL-2, IFN-γ, and IL-17 production	26
Cancer	Cyclophosphamide injection + saccharin solution (taste)	Reduced of plaque-forming cell antibody response	54
	Poly(I:C) injection + camphor smell (odor)	Increased survival of tumor-bearing mice	55, 56
	DBA/2 spleen cells as alloantigen + camphor smell (odor)	Elevated cytotoxic T-lymphocyte response to YC8 tumor/increased survival rate	57, 58
Transplantation	Cyclophosphamide injection + saccharin solution (taste)	Reduction of a graph vs. host response	59, 60
	Cyclosporine A injection + saccharin solution (taste)	Prolonged survival time of heterotopically transplanted heart allografts	44, 61, 62
Depression	Ketamine injection + chocolate (taste) and blue light conditions (visual)	Reduction of depressive-like behavior	63

Table 3.3.2 Clinical relevance of learned immune responses in humans

Disease	Protocol	Effect	Source
Allergy	Allergen solution: D. pteronyssinus and D. farinae + blue-colored water with methyl anthranylate and benzaldehyde (taste, smell)	Increased mast cell tryptase levels in nasal lavage fluid	64
	Desloratadine + green-colored strawberry milk with lavender oil (taste, smell)	Reduction in skin prick test responses, lower percentage of activated basophile granulocytes	10, 11
	Seasonal grass mix + benzaldehyde (smell)	Increased histamine release	8
Autoimmune diseases			
Multiple sclerosis	Cyclophosphamide + anise-flavored syrup (taste)	Reduced leukocyte numbers	29
Lupus	Cyclophosphamide + cod liver oil and rose perfume (taste, smell)	Alleviated symptoms	28
Psoriasis	Acetonide triamcinolone + environmental cues (*partial reinforcement* → medication every other day)	Reduced glucocorticoid doses and symptoms	14
Transplantation	Cyclosporine A/tacrolimus + green-colored strawberry milk with lavender oil (taste, smell)	Reduced T cell functions compared to baseline kinetics under routine drug intake	30

reflected by basophil activation was inhibited through the conditioning process only.[11] More recently, the effects of antihistaminergic drugs were found to be enhanced by the open administration of said drugs—as opposed to a regimen in which patients do not know whether they have received a drug or a placebo—as well as by prior learning experiences with the specific medication.[12]

Inflammatory skin diseases and wounds

Similarly, inflammatory skin conditions are mediated to a significant degree by psychological factors and are therefore susceptible to placebo interventions.[13] Robert Ader and colleagues applied the idea of learned immune responses to a sample of patients suffering from psoriasis, a chronic inflammatory skin disease.[14] In this study, up to three quarters of the administrations of cortico-steroid drugs were replaced by the administration of an identical looking placebo. This so-called partial reinforcement strategy, where the administration of a placebo pill is only reinforced by the drug at certain intervals or ratio of time, led to outcomes in one subgroup of patients comparable to the standard treatment with just a fraction of the medication required. Across dermato-logical conditions, itch is one of the most prevalent symptoms. A range of studies in animals, healthy volunteers, and patients showed that itching and scratching can be elicited by several of the mechanisms known to underlie the nocebo effect, including conditioning, verbal suggestion, and social learning.[15] While findings from healthy volunteers also indicate similar pla-cebo effects on experimentally induced itch (i.e., alleviation of itch[16,17]), a pu-tative application in dermatological patients needs to be investigated.

Chronic wounds also present substantial constraints to the patients' quality of life and are possibly a relevant target for placebo interventions. An exper-imental manipulation involving verbal suggestions was found to improve patients' wound-related quality of life but not the actual duration of wound healing.[18] These results were mirrored by a study in healthy participants with experimentally induced wounds that found no effects of the application of a placebo gel combined with positive verbal suggestions for wound healing.[19]

Autoimmune diseases and organ transplantation

Dose reduction of immunosuppressive medication is of high clinical rel-evance, as these drugs are associated with severe side effects and toxicity.[20] Paradigms of taste-immune associative learning commonly pair the admin-istration of an immunosuppressive drug such as CsA or cyclophosphamide with a distinct gustatory stimulus. The possibilities this approach offers for the treatment of autoimmune diseases were first documented in preclinical rodent models, reflected by reduced inflammatory symptoms[21] and reduced lymphocyte proliferation[22,23] in a model of rheumatoid arthritis, or by a reduced rate of disease progression in a model of lupus erythematosus.[24] Similar procedures have proven efficient at dampening symptomatology in preclinical models of encephalomyelitis and uveitis.[25,26] Some promising studies also document a successful translation of behaviorally conditioned immunosuppression to humans. Parallel to findings from healthy human subjects,[27] one study demonstrated the behaviorally conditioned alleviation of symptoms in a single lupus patient,[28] as well as in patients suffering from multiple sclerosis, where a learned reduced leukocyte number was reported.[29]

Treatment with immunosuppressive drugs is a prerequisite to prevent the rejection of transplanted organs. By pairing cyclophosphamide or CsA with saccharin, reductions in graph versus host response, as well as a prolonged survival time of heterotopically transplanted heart allografts could be documented in preclinical rodent models.[2] In humans, a study with renal transplant patients who had been treated with a standard immunosuppressive regimen of calcineurin inhibitors (CsA or tacrolimus) employed a modified taste-immune conditioning paradigm.[30] During retrieval, re-exposure to the taste stimulus significantly reduced T cell proliferative capacity in comparison to the baseline kinetics of T cell functions under routine medication. This proof-of-concept study in humans provides a basis for designing conditioning protocols that could be employed as a supportive therapy in clinical settings.

Cancer

The possibility of exploiting behaviorally conditioned immunopharmacological responses as a supportive approach to target tumor development and metastasis has already been demonstrated in early preclinical animal models. Pairing different drugs or alloantigens frequently used in cancer treatment with gustatory or odor stimuli was found to be efficient at reducing plaque-forming cell responses, as well as at elevating the cytotoxic T-lymphocyte response, thereby increasing the overall survival of tumor-bearing mice.[2] However, so far, no drug conditioning trials have been performed in humans, although a similar regimen like the one used in renal transplant patients[30] would provide a safe option to test this much-needed translation from preclinical models. Nocebo effects already play a role in cancer treatment when it comes to unwanted side effects. For instance, conditioned nausea that occurs frequently in patients upon re-entering the context where chemotherapy was received reflects the obvious problem in this clinical field.[31] Moreover, the occurrence of conditioning is not only reflected by subjectively reported symptoms. Several studies compared blood samples collected at home (i.e., in a neutral setting) with those collected in the clinic (i.e., after re-evocation of the conditioning context, but prior to the actual treatment). Importantly, in the following analysis of plasma cytokines, reduced natural killer (NK) cell activity, T cell proliferation, and interferon (IFN)-γ concentrations were measured in the clinic samples.[32] Such findings suggest that placebo research may open new ways to improve current treatments for cancer, both when it comes to reducing necessary medication dosages as well as to managing side effects.

Mechanisms of behaviorally conditioned immune responses

Encoding detailed immunological information is an evolutionary advantage for every organism since it can prevent threats and may predict uncertain environments by adaptive behavior. Thus knowledge related to the mechanisms of behaviorally conditioned immune responses has relevant implications in the field of health care.

Central mechanisms

The central nervous system synchronizes the immune functions and neuroendocrine responses, while these two systems are further controlled by cognitive and emotional processes. In this regard, several brain areas such as the hypothalamus, the insular cortex (IC), the amygdala, and the brainstem, have been implicated in the regulation of neural-immune interactions. However, one of most important structures, essential for mediating immune learning, is the IC. Specific immune-related information is stored in this structure and neuronal ensembles in this region can acquire and retrieve immune information.[33] While lesion studies indicated that the IC is involved in conditioned taste aversion, as well as in conditioned immunosuppression during acquisition and retrieval, the amygdala seems to recognize the input of visceral information necessary at acquisition time.[34,35] In contrast, the ventromedial nucleus of the hypothalamus appears to participate within the output pathway essential for evoking the behaviorally conditioned immune response.[36]

Peripheral mechanisms

In immune conditioning-paradigms, the brain perceives changes in the peripheral immune system induced by the pharmacological drug used as an unconditioned stimulus (US) via two afferent pathways (Figure 3.3.2). On the one hand, the signals are transmitted through a systemic/humoral branch, where neuroendocrine or immune messengers such as cytokines can reach the brain via the circumventricular organs or cerebral vasculature.[37] On the other hand, information is transmitted neuronally via the vagus nerve. In this context, vagotomy has been shown to culminate in a dysfunction of many behavioral responses and autonomic reflexes induced by immunomodulators.[38]

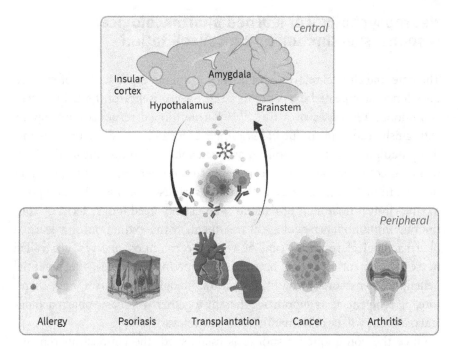

Figure 3.3.2 Schematic overview of neural regions involved in conditioned (learned) immunological responses.

The CS (saccharin) is perceived via neural afferences during the acquisition phase, while the unconditioned stimulus (immunomodulatory drug) can reach the brain via the central nervous system immune-sensing capacities, or the circumventricular organs. Important structures for mediating the input of visceral immune information required at acquisition time are the insular cortex and the amygdala. At retrieval, the insular cortex together with hypothalamic relays (e.g., ventromedial, lateral hypothalamic nucleus) and sympathetic peripheral mechanisms seem to form at least one major pathway, enabling the brain to modify immunological effects in the context of conditioning.

However, it is still unknown, whether and to what extent these afferent pathways are also activated during learned immunosuppression.[39]

On the efferent arm, the conditioned immune response seems to be mediated via the sympathetic innervation of lymphoid organs such as spleen and lymph nodes. The involvement of noradrenaline and beta-adrenoceptors expressed on immune competent cells[34] was more recently confirmed during immune conditioning with CsA, as continuous application of the beta-adrenoceptor antagonist nadolol exerted attenuating effects on inflammatory disease progression.[23] However, the precise peripheral mechanisms responsible for decreased proliferative T cell capacity or suppressed cytokine production during conditioning are still unclear and need further investigation.[40]

Neuropsychology of learned pharmacological responses: extinction and reconsolidation

The potential clinical relevance of learned immune responses has often been questioned as repeated exposure to a CS in the absence of the US weakens conditioned responses over time.[41,42] If conditioned responses are rapidly extinguished and only inducible as a single event and only short-term lasting, this paradigm can still be utilized as a valuable tool to investigate the bidirectional communication between the brain and peripheral immune functioning. In that case, however, it cannot be seriously considered as an option for the clinical treatment of patients who usually need longer term or continuous immunopharmacological treatment. If the extinction of a learned pharmacological response can, however, be modified or even controlled by reinforcement strategies or memory-updating processes, the potential benefits of behaviorally conditioned immunological responses, and, therefore, placebo effects as supportive therapy together with basic pharmacological regimens will be of tremendous clinical relevance.[43]

Once the conditioned response is established, the connection remains stable. As soon as the conditioned stimulus is presented, however, the memory trace is reactivated for a certain period of time. Within this so-called reconsolidation window, the memory trace becomes temporarily susceptible for modification and can be disrupted or strengthened. This state is termed *memory reconsolidation*. However, it is well-known that repeated re-exposure to the CS in absence of the US during this phase of transient lability destabilizes conditioned memory traces and facilitates extinction.

Importantly, it has been shown that low or subeffective doses of the US administered in close temporal proximity (inside the "reconsolidation window") to the CS at retrieval, generate a persistence of conditioned responses.[2] Although the mechanisms of this phenomenon are largely unknown, it is suggested that the presentation of such reminders cues partially replicate an encoding experience, thereby enabling memories to be distorted or strengthened. The extinction of conditioned immunosuppressive responses ceased in rats[44,45] and humans[42] when immunomodulatory drugs (cyclosporine A or Rapamycin) were administered as sub- or low-therapeutic doses (reminder cue) together with the CS during retrieval.

Differentially, partial reinforcement strategies of Pavlovian conditioning refer to the expression of "dose-extension."[2,46] In this procedure, only a portion of the responses or CS presentations is followed by a reinforcer (i.e., US) implying that "medication" and the attendant cues (CS) are therapeutically reinforced on some occasions but not on others.[47] In most cases of partial reinforcement, resistance to the extinction of the conditioned response is greater since the response is intermittently rather than consistently paired with reinforcement.[48] Taken together, these different learning strategies might be promising options for transferring our knowledge of immunomodulatory conditioning research into clinical practice.

Conclusions

A prominent hypothesis states that patient expectations mediated via verbal suggestion, context factors or social learning processes primarily affect subjective outcomes such as pain experience or mood. Objective symptoms, however, such as immune functions, are hypothesized to be shaped primarily by associative learning experiences (i.e., behavioral conditioning processes).[49] The phenomenon of behaviorally conditioned immunological responses has been identified and studied for over 100 years. Our growing understanding of the bidirectional communication between the brain and peripheral immune functions, as well as the neuropsychological mechanisms of associative learning and memory, provides several fascinating challenges and opportunities (see Box 3.3.1) with which we can make optimal use of this still-understudied phenomenon of behaviorally conditioned immune responses. A major challenge is to further analyze the mechanisms steering these learned

---

BOX 3.3.1 Open questions

- Can "physiological" parameters only be shaped by behavioral conditioning, or do we just need other paradigms?
- Can we find ways of avoiding extinction of learned immunopharmacological responses that work in daily clinical routine?
- Does the concept of conditioning drug responses apply to all types of medication thereby sharing a common physiological mechanism?
- Which learning protocols, including partial reinforcement or memory updating, induce the most effective learned immune responses for which compounds?
- To what extent do "context cues" (e.g., pills, syringes, environment cues, medication boxes, and medical devices) serve as conditioned stimuli sufficient to induce the desired conditioned immune responses?
- Are unwanted drug side effects also behaviorally conditioned?
- How do conditioning and conscious expectation interact in shaping placebo responses?

responses in immune functions, which in turn will form the basis to exploit these mechanisms in clinical practice for the patients' benefit.

Acknowledgments

This work was funded by center grants of the German Research Foundation (Deutsche Forschungsgemeinschaft, DFG) project number 316803389 - SFB 1280 (TP A18 to M.H. and M.S.) and project number 422744262 - TRR 289 (TP A12 to M.S.).

References

1. Pavlov IP, Anrep GV. *Conditioned Reflexes*. Oxford University Press; 1927.
2. Hadamitzky M, Luckemann L, Pacheco-Lopez G, Schedlowski M. Pavlovian conditioning of immunological and neuroendocrine functions. *Physiological Reviews*. 2020;100(1):357–405. http://doi:10.1152/physrev.00033.2018
3. Ader R, Cohen N. Behaviorally conditioned immunosuppression. *Psychosomatic Medicine*. 1975;37(4):333–340.
4. Enck P, Bingel U, Schedlowski M, Rief W. The placebo response in medicine: Minimize, maximize or personalize? *Nature Reviews Drug Discovery*. 2013;12(3):191–204. http://doi:10.1038/nrd3923
5. Pfaar O, Agache I, Bergmann KC, et al. Placebo effects in allergen immunotherapy: An EAACI Task Force position paper. *Allergy*. 2020;76(3):629–647. http://doi:10.1111/all.14331
6. Mackenzie JN. The production of the so-called "rose cold" by means of an artificial rose, with remarks and historical notes. *American Journal of the Medical Sciences*. 1886;91(181):45.
7. Dekker E, Pelser HE, Groen J. Conditioning as a cause of asthmatic attacks: A laboratory study. *Journal of psychosomatic Research*. 1957;2(2):97–108. http://doi:10.1016/0022-3999(57)90015-6
8. Barrett JE, King MG, Pang G. Conditioning rhinitis in allergic humans. *Annals of the New York Academy of Sciences*. 2000;917(1):853–859. http://doi:10.1111/j.1749-6632.2000.tb05451.x
9. Exton MS, Elferst A, Jeong W-Y, Bull DF, Westermann J, Schedlowski M. Conditioned suppression of contact sensitivity is independent of sympathetic splenic innervation. *American Journal of Physiology Endocrinology and Metabolism*. 2000;279(4):R1310–R1315.
10. Vits S, Cesko E, Benson S, et al. Cognitive factors mediate placebo responses in patients with house dust mite allergy. *PLoS ONE*. 2013;8(11):e79576. http://doi:10.1371/journal.pone.0079576
11. Goebel MU, Meykadeh N, Kou W, Schedlowski M, Hengge UR. Behavioral conditioning of antihistamine effects in patients with allergic rhinitis. *Psychotherapy and Psychosomatics*. 2008;77(4):227–234. http://doi:10.1159/000126074
12. Solle A, Worm M, Benedetti F, Bartholomaus ST, Schwender-Groen L, Klinger R. Targeted use of placebo effects decreases experimental itch in atopic dermatitis patients: A

randomized controlled trial. *Clinical Pharmacology and Therapeutics*. 2021;110(2):486–497. http://doi:10.1002/cpt.2276

13. Sondermann W, Reinboldt-Jockenhofer F, Dissemond J, Pfaar O, Bingel U, Schedlowski M. Effects of patients' expectation in dermatology: Evidence from experimental and clinical placebo studies and implications for dermatologic practice and research. *Dermatology*. 2021: 237(6):857–871. doi:10.1159/000513445.

14. Ader R, Mercurio MG, Walton J, et al. Conditioned pharmacotherapeutic effects: A preliminary study. *Psychosomatic Medicine*. 2010;72(2):192–197. http://doi:10.1097/PSY.0b013 e3181cbd38b

15. Meeuwis SH, van Middendorp H, van Laarhoven AIM, van Leijenhorst C, Pacheco-Lopez G, Lavrijsen APM, Veldhuijzen DS, Evers AWM. Placebo and nocebo effects for itch and itch-related immune outcomes: A systematic review of animal and human studies. *Neuroscience and Biobehavioral Reviews*. 2020 Jun;113:325–337. doi:10.1016/j.neubiorev.2020.03.025.

16. Darragh M, Chang JW, Booth RJ, Consedine NS. The placebo effect in inflammatory skin reactions: The influence of verbal suggestion on itch and weal size. *Journal of Psychosomatic Research*. 2015;78(5):489–494. http://doi:10.1016/j.jpsychores.2015.01.011

17. van Laarhoven AI, Vogelaar ML, Wilder-Smith OH, et al. Induction of nocebo and placebo effects on itch and pain by verbal suggestions. *Pain*. 2011;152(7):1486–1494. http://doi:10.1016/j.pain.2011.01.043

18. Jockenhofer F, Knust C, Benson S, Schedlowski M, Dissemond J. Influence of placebo effects on quality of life and wound healing in patients with chronic venous leg ulcers. *Journal der Deutschen Dermatologischen Gesellschaft*. 2020;18(2):103–109. http://doi:10.1111/ddg.13996

19. Vits S, Dissemond J, Schadendorf D, et al. Expectation-induced placebo responses fail to accelerate wound healing in healthy volunteers: Results from a prospective controlled experimental trial. *International Wound Journal*. 2015;12(6):664–668. http://doi:10.1111/iwj.12193

20. Bosche K, Weissenborn K, Christians U, et al. Neurobehavioral consequences of small molecule-drug immunosuppression. *Neuropharmacology*. 2015;96:83–93. http://doi:10.1016/j.neuropharm.2014.12.008

21. Klosterhalfen W, Klosterhalfen S. Pavlovian conditioning of immunosuppression modifies adjuvant arthritis in rats. *Behavioral Neuroscience*. 1983;97(4):663–666. http://doi:10.1037//0735-7044.97.4.663

22. Klosterhalfen S, Klosterhalfen W. Conditioned cyclosporine effects but not conditioned taste aversion in immunized rats. *Behavioral Neuroscience*. 1990;104(5):716–724.

23. Lückemann L, Stangl H, Straub RH, Schedlowski M, Hadamitzky M. Learned immunosuppressive placebo response attenuates disease progression in a rodent model of rheumatoid arthritis. *Arthritis & Rheumatology*. 2020;72(4):588–597. http://doi:10.1002/art.41101

24. Ader R, Cohen N. Behaviorally conditioned immunosuppression and murine systemic lupus erythematosus. *Science*. 1982;215(4539):1534–1536.

25. Jones RE, Moes N, Zwickey H, Cunningham CL, Gregory WL, Oken B. Treatment of experimental autoimmune encephalomyelitis with alpha lipoic acid and associative conditioning. *Brain, Behavior, and Immunity*. 2008;22(4):538–543. https://doi.org/10.1016/j.bbi.2007.10.017

26. Bauer D, Busch M, Pacheco-Lopez G, et al. Behavioral conditioning of immune responses with cyclosporine A in a murine model of experimental autoimmune uveitis. *Neuroimmunomodulation*. 2017;24(2):87–99. http://doi:10.1159/000479185

27. Goebel MU, Trebst AE, Steiner J, et al. Behavioral conditioning of immunosuppression is possible in humans. *FASEB Journal*. 2002;16(14):1869–1873. http://doi:10.1096/fj.02-0389com

28. Olness K, Ader R. Conditioning as an adjunct in the pharmacotherapy of lupus erythematosus. *Journal of Developmental & Behavioral Pediatrics.* 1992;13(2):124–125.
29. Giang DW, Goodman AD, Schiffer RB, et al. Conditioning of cyclophosphamide-induced leukopenia in humans. *Journal of Neuropsychiatry and Clinical Neurosciences.* 1996;8(2):194–201.
30. Kirchhof J, Petrakova L, Brinkhoff A, et al. Learned immunosuppressive placebo responses in renal transplant patients. *Proceedings of the National Academy of Sciences USA.* 2018;115(16):4223–4227. http://doi:10.1073/pnas.1720548115
31. Stockhorst U, Enck P, Klosterhalfen S. Role of classical conditioning in learning gastrointestinal symptoms. *World Journal of Gastroenterology.* 2007;13(25):3430–3437. http://doi:10.3748/wjg.v13.i25.3430
32. Stockhorst U, Spennes-Saleh S, Korholz D, et al. Anticipatory symptoms and anticipatory immune responses in pediatric cancer patients receiving chemotherapy: Features of a classically conditioned response? *Brain, Behavior, and Immunity.* 2000;14(3):198–218. http://doi:10.1006/brbi.1999.0581
33. Koren T, Yifa R, Amer M, et al. Insular cortex neurons encode and retrieve specific immune responses. *Cell.* 2021;184(24):5902–5915e17. http://doi:10.1016/j.cell.2021.10.013
34. Riether C, Kavelaars A, Wirth T, et al. Stimulation of beta(2)-adrenergic receptors inhibits calcineurin activity in CD4(+) T cells via PKA-AKAP interaction. *Brain, Behavior, and Immunity.* 2011;25(1):59–66. http://doi:10.1016/j.bbi.2010.07.248
35. Schiller M, Ben-Shaanan TL, Rolls A. Neuronal regulation of immunity: Why, how and where? *Nature Reviews Immunology.* 2021;21(1):20–36. http://doi:10.1038/s41577-020-0387-1
36. Pacheco-Lopez G, Niemi MB, Kou W, Harting M, Fandrey J, Schedlowski M. Neural substrates for behaviorally conditioned immunosuppression in the rat. *Journal of Neuroscience.* 2005;25(9):2330–2337. http://doi:10.1523/jneurosci.4230-04.2005
37. Quan N, Banks WA. Brain-immune communication pathways. *Brain, Behavior, and Immunity.* 2007;21(6):727–35. http://doi:10.1016/j.bbi.2007.05.005
38. Chavan SS, Pavlov VA, Tracey KJ. Mechanisms and therapeutic relevance of neuroimmune communication. *Immunity.* 2017;46(6):927–942. http://doi:10.1016/j.immuni.2017.06.008
39. Pacheco-Lopez G, Doenlen R, Krugel U, et al. Neurobehavioural activation during peripheral immunosuppression. *International Journal of Neuropsychopharmacology.* 2013;16(1):137–149. http://doi:10.1017/S1461145711001799
40. Lückemann L, Unteroberdorster M, Kirchhof J, Schedlowski M, Hadamitzky M. Applications and limitations of behaviorally conditioned immunopharmacological responses. *Neurobiology of Learning and Memory.* 2017;142:91–98. http://doi:10.1016/j.nlm.2017.02.012
41. Berman DE, Dudai Y. Memory extinction, learning anew, and learning the new: Dissociations in the molecular machinery of learning in cortex. *Science.* 2001;291(5512):2417–2419. http://doi:10.1126/science.1058165
42. Albring A, Wendt L, Benson S, et al. Preserving learned immunosuppressive placebo response: Perspectives for clinical application. *Clinical Pharmacology and Therapeutics.* 2014;96(2):247–255. http://doi:10.1038/clpt.2014.75
43. Schedlowski M, Enck P, Rief W, Bingel U. Neuro-bio-behavioral mechanisms of placebo and nocebo responses: Implications for clinical trials and clinical practice. *Pharmacological Reviews.* 2015;67(3):697–730. http://doi:10.1124/pr.114.009423
44. Exton MS, Schult M, Donath S, et al. Conditioned immunosuppression makes subtherapeutic cyclosporin effective via splenic innervation. *American Journal of Physiology.* 1999;276(6):R1710–R1717.

45. Luckemann L, Hetze S, Horbelt T, Jakobs M, Schedlowski M, Hadamitzky M. Incomplete reminder cues trigger memory reconsolidation and sustain learned immune responses. *Brain, Behavior, and Immunity.* 2021;95:115–121. http://doi:10.1016/j.bbi.2021.03.001

46. Colloca L, Enck P, DeGrazia D. Relieving pain using dose-extending placebos: A scoping review. *Pain.* 2016;157(8):1590–1598. http://doi:10.1097/j.pain.0000000000000566

47. Doering BK, Rief W. Utilizing placebo mechanisms for dose reduction in pharmacotherapy. *Trends in Pharmacological Sciences.* 2012;33(3):165–172. http://doi:10.1016/j.tips.2011.12.001

48. Harris JA, Bouton ME. Pavlovian conditioning under partial reinforcement: The effects of nonreinforced trials versus cumulative conditioned stimulus duration. *Journal of Experimental Psychology: Animal Learning and Cognition.* 2020;46(3):256–272. http://doi:10.1037/xan0000242

49. Benedetti F, Pollo A, Loplano L, Lanotte M, Vighetti S, Rainero I. Conscious expectation and unconscious conditioning in analgesic, motor, and hormonal placebo/nocebo responses. *Journal of Neuroscience.* 2003;23(10):4315–4323.

50. Bovbjerg D, Cohen N, Ader R. Behaviorally conditioned enhancement of delayed-type hypersensitivity in the mouse. *Brain, Behavior, and Immunity.* 1987;1(1):64–71.

51. Roudebush RE, Bryant HU. Conditioned immunosuppression of a murine delayed type hypersensitivity response: Dissociation from corticosterone elevation. *Brain, Behavior, and Immunity.* 1991;5(3):308–317.

52. Kelley KW, Dantzer R, Mormede P, Salmon H, Aynaud JM. Conditioned taste aversion suppresses induction of delayed-type hypersensitivity immune reactions. *Physiology and Behavior.* 1985;34(2):189–193.

53. Ader R, Cohen N. Behaviorally conditioned immunosuppression and murine systemic lupus erythematosus. *Science.* 1982;215:1534–1536.

54. Bovbjerg D, Kim YT, Siskind GW, Weksler ME. Conditioned suppression of plaque-forming cell responses with cyclophosphamide: The role of taste aversion. *Annals of the New York Academy of Sciences.* 1987;496:588–594.

55. Ghanta V, Hiramoto RN, Solvason B, Spector NH. Influence of conditioned natural immunity on tumor growth. *Annals of the New York Academy of Sciences.* 1987;496:637–646.

56. Ghanta VK, Hiramoto RN, Solvason HB, Spector NH. Neural and environmental influences on neoplasia and conditioning of NK activity. *Journal of Immunology.* 1985;135(2):848s–852s.

57. Hiramoto RN, Hiramoto NS, Rish ME, Soong SJ, Miller DM, Ghanta VK. Role of immune cells in the Pavlovian conditioning of specific resistance to cancer. *International Journal of Neuroscience.* 1991;59(1-3):101–17.

58. Ghanta VK, Hiramoto NS, Soong SJ, Hiramoto RN. Conditioning of the secondary cytotoxic t-lymphocyte response to YC8 tumor. *Pharmacology Biochemistry and Behavior.* 1995;50(3):399–403.

59. Bovbjerg D, Ader R, Cohen N. Behaviorally conditioned suppression of a graft-versus-host response. *Proceedings of the National Academy of Sciences USA.* 1982;79:583–585.

60. Bovbjerg D, Ader R, Cohen N. Acquisition and extinction of conditioned suppression of a graft-vs-host response in the rat. *Journal of Immunology.* 1984;132:111–113.

61. Hadamitzky M, Bösche K, Wirth T, et al. Memory-updating abrogates extinction of learned immunosuppression. *Brain, Behavior, and Immunity.* 2016;52:40–48. http://doi:10.1016/j.bbi.2015.09.009

62. Grochowicz PM, Schedlowski M, Husband AJ, King MG, Hibberd AD, Bowen KM. Behavioral conditioning prolongs heart allograft survival in rats. *Brain, Behavior, and Immunity.* 1991;5(4):349–356.

63. Krimmel SR, Zanos P, Georgiou P, Colloca L, Gould TD. Classical conditioning of antidepressant placebo effects in mice. *Psychopharmacology (Berl)*. 2020;237(1):93–102. http://doi:10.1007/s00213-019-05347-4

64. Gauci M, Husband AJ, Saxarra H, King MG. Pavlovian conditioning of nasal tryptase release in human subjects with allergic rhinitis. *Physiology and Behavior*. 1994;55(5):823–825. http://doi:10.1016/0031-9384(94)90066-3

3.4

Placebo effects in sports performance and exercise outcomes

Jacob B. Lindheimer, Chris Beedie, and John S. Raglin

Introduction

The legitimacy of placebo effects has been a subject of debate throughout much of the history of modern Medicine, swinging from acceptance to outright rejection. Among its most ardent proponents is Henry Beecher,[1] who described placebo effects as "powerful" in his review of intervention studies, reporting that an average of 35% of patients benefited from placebos. But others have criticized the quality of this and subsequent placebo research, contending that the placebo effect is entirely illusory, the result of an additional motivational incentive or of one or more nonspecific effects such as regression toward the mean or remission of symptoms.[2]

While placebo research is now well established in Sports and Exercise research, a considerable degree of doubt yet exists among many working in these disciplines. This is in part due to the overlap between placebo effects and related sports and exercise phenomena such as motivation, emotion regulation, and social facilitation, each of which have at times been proposed as explanations for placebo effects, despite the challenges associated with disentangling their interrelationships.

These and other concerns have likely contributed to the dearth of placebo research on Sports and Exercise published prior to the year 2000. Since then, research in Sports and Exercise has become sufficiently well developed to warrant the publication of systematic reviews in 2009, 2015, and 2019,[3-5] a consensus statement signed by 19 authors from 11 countries in 2018,[6] and a subsequent special edition of the *European Journal of Sport Science* in 2020.[7]

It should be emphasized that we use the terms *sports* and *exercise* specifically. In discussing *sports*, we refer to physical activity that is competitive, structured, rule-governed, and organized, with good examples being netball, track and field, and triathlon. In this case, performance is the outcome of interest. In discussing *exercise*, we refer to physical activity that is done for health reasons rather than competitively, as well as for active commuting or enjoyment: for example, jogging, yoga, or weight-lifting. In this case, the psychological benefit of physical activity is the outcome of interest. This chapter will focus on research conducted within the academic field of Sports and Exercise Science, despite some interesting research having been published beyond that field in, for example, Psychology and Neuroscience.[8-10]

Placebo effects in sports performance

Sports performance is characterized by the pursuit of high levels of physical and mental function as well as by rigorous measurement, thus Sports provides a very rich environment for researchers interested in investigating the placebo phenomenon.

Sports as a rich environment for placebo research

Very often, the winning (or losing) margins in sports are tiny and can be measured as low as 0.1% of the total performance time. In this context, placebo effects—which research demonstrates can be in the region of 1%–3%—could make the difference between winning and losing. Athletes train for many years to achieve relatively small improvements in performance and will commonly pursue any potentially viable route to performance enhancement, even those that may be dubious. They are, therefore, often willing and highly motivated participants in research, with both the experimental environment and associated research findings being meaningful to many. Further, in considering experimental research, many athletes are habituated to laboratory-like conditions through their day-to-day physical training regimes, as well as performance analysis tests, and especially in the case of elite sportspeople, many are able to produce close to identical performances in numerous experimental trials, facilitating the reliable estimation of intervention effects. Even beyond the laboratory in field research, ecologically valid but nonetheless rule-governed and standardized sports environments often provide a high level of control over variables; running tracks and swimming pools, for example, are constrained environments in which athletes tend to perform over set distances at relatively consistent intensities and speeds and in line with the dictates of the sport.

Placebo effects are still far from embraced in Sports Science and practice

None of the above should be construed as evidence that placebo effects have been widely embraced by Sports Science researchers and practitioners. For example, while placebo effects have been described as a "relatively new consideration and area of research"[11] (p. 26), its status has been equally disputed. In some Sports Science research textbooks,[12] placebo effects have been attributed to *nonspecific effects*, even though improvements in sports performance deviate not toward but *away* from the mean. For example, in a study of experimental pain in which placebo ultrasound therapy is administered following experimental pain induction, should pain be reduced by comparison with baseline as the result of the placebo treatment, the researcher is always faced with the reality that acute pain tends to reduce with time. Counter to this, in an experimental study of human performance in which caffeine is administered and in which the athlete performs to a higher level than at baseline, such an argument is moot: an athlete suddenly performing 3% better than predicted is not so easily explained. The placebo effect has also been described as: "an imaginary improvement in performance"[13] (p. 218) and not unexpectedly, textbooks in Sports research[14,15] and even Sports Psychology[15] often neglect to even describe placebo effects. There is a sense in which Sports Science, with the goal of observing, explaining, and applying factors that enhance human physical performance, rejects the contribution of placebo effects, preferring to attribute improvements to more acceptable and well-defined sports phenomena such as motivation and confidence. Sports Science, like Psychology, has long been sharply divided along subdisciplinary lines including Physiology, Psychology, Medicine, Nutrition, and Biomechanics. While one study of the placebo effect might fall between these disciplinary boundaries, another might cross one or more of them, meaning that research findings relating to the placebo effect in sports can struggle to find a natural home within a single Sports Science subdiscipline.

This relative neglect of the placebo effect in Sports Medicine becomes more problematic given that in the previous 2 decades, research has substantiated the contribution of the placebo effect to established medical treatments for a range of clinical conditions and identified the neurobiological pathways underlying many of these benefits.[16] While this evidence comes largely from medical studies, there is—as this chapter attests—a nascent body of research in Sports Science and Sports Science research substantiating the contribution of the placebo effect to the benefits associated with many sports' performance products and techniques,[4] and a smaller but equally compelling line

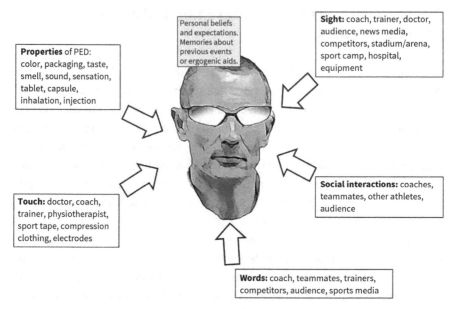

Personal beliefs and expectations. Memories about previous events or ergogenic aids.

Properties of PED: color, packaging, taste, smell, sound, sensation, tablet, capsule, inhalation, injection

Sight: coach, trainer, doctor, audience, news media, competitors, stadium/arena, sport camp, hospital, equipment

Touch: doctor, coach, trainer, physiotherapist, sport tape, compression clothing, electrodes

Social interactions: coaches, teammates, other athletes, audience

Words: coach, teammates, trainers, competitors, audience, sports media

Figure 3.4.1 A model of the psychosocial milieu in sport.[19] PED, performance enhancing drug.

of research has revealed the contribution of placebo effects to psychological benefits stemming from physical exercise.[17] Yet placebo effects remain disregarded or mired in outdated definitions and models in much Exercise and Sports research.[17,18]

How Sports research differs from medical research

There are, of course, significant differences between placebo research in Medicine and Sports. Primary among these is the focus on target populations with very different characteristics (i.e., patients vs. athletes) and desired experimental outcomes (i.e., reduced illness vs. improved performance). It has been argued however that despite these differences, similar processes and mechanisms underlie placebo effects in medicine and sport.[6,19] For example, as with medical research, the results of Sports studies[20] indicate that the physical characteristics of placebos including color and form (e.g., pill or capsule) often influence their efficacy. Medical research has also demonstrated that the efficacy of placebos is also influenced by the characteristics of the environment in which they are administered, as well as the status and behavior of the provider. The role of the psychosocial milieu[21] has been incorporated into most contemporary medical definitions and models of placebo effects, and it has been recently modified for sports settings (see Figure 3.4.1). In addition, Sports researchers have proposed an updated definition of the *placebo effect* that integrates these findings, describing it as: "the simulation of a proven ergogenic aid within a psychosocial context"[19] (p. 4).

Methods and findings of Sports research

A closer look at findings in Sports indicates that studies have generally adopted a deceptive expectancy paradigm in which verbal and contextual cues aim to lead the athlete to believe that they will receive a scientifically proven and legal *ergogenic aid* (literally a work-enhancing substance often in the form of a sports supplement), when in fact they receive a biologically inert substance. This approach contrasts with the conditioning paradigm often used in other disciplines in which a biologically active substance is administered in a run-in period and then deceptively replaced with a placebo for the experimental trial. Research in Sports is often conducted on relatively small yet homogeneous samples and in controlled laboratory or sports competition conditions. Further, research in Sports has often reported standard measures of Sports and Exercise Physiology, such as changes in heart rate, ventilation, oxygen uptake and blood lactate in response to receipt of a placebo. Findings using the expectancy approach in sports indicate that:

- The administration of a placebo described as an ergogenic aid can significantly enhance sports performance in numerous sports contexts. A recent systematic review of 32 studies involving 1,513 participants reported small but significant effects for both placebo ($d = 0.36$) and nocebo ($d = 0.37$) treatments.[4]
- A placebo can enhance performance by a magnitude not dissimilar to that associated with the real substance (e.g., caffeine) with improvements of close to 3% on performance observed in deceptive "high-dose caffeine" conditions.[22]
- Improvements in performance associated with the administration of a placebo might be evident in the absence of the increase in physiological work that would normally accompany this effect: for example, power output was increased in the absence of a concomitant increase in oxygen uptake, heart rate, and blood lactate.[23]

- A deceptively administered placebo can enhance performance in a dose-response manner with an expected high dose associated with greater improvement in performance than an expected low dose.[23]
- Athletes actively calculate and calibrate their effort in line with their expectations of an ergogenic aid, specifically that athletes calculate the chances of having received a "real ergogenic aid and calibrate their pacing strategy accordingly."[23]
- Effects of a placebo and a real drug such as caffeine are additive (and that real ergogenic aids are less effective if the athlete does not know that they have ingested them). Specifically, when athletes in repeated measures balanced placebo design were given placebo and informed it was caffeine, effects on performance were equivalent to the condition in which they were administered real caffeine believing that they had received no treatment. However, when they were openly administered caffeine, the placebo and biological effects of caffeine were additive.[22]
- People who use ergogenic aids are more likely to respond to a placebo than those who do not. In a large-scale placebo intervention study using a between-subjects design, a relationship between intention to use sports supplements and performance following the deceptive administration of a placebo was observed. Performance worsened by −1.10% ± 0.30% compared to baseline for participants not intending to use supplements, worsened by −0.64 ± 0.43% among those who were undecided about supplement use, but improved by 0.19 ± 0.24% among those participants intending to use supplements.[24]
- Open-label placebos can enhance sports performance. In a study of female competitive cyclists, open-placebo improved time-to-completion in a time-trial (TT) event (P = 0.039, 103.6 ± 5.0 vs. 104.4 ± 5.1 s, −0.7 ± 1.8 s, −0.7 ± 1.7%) and mean power output (P = 0.01, 244.8 ± 34.7 vs. 239.7 ± 33.2, +5.1 ± 9.5 W) during the TT. Individual data analysis showed that 11 individuals improved; 13 remained unchanged; and 4 worsened their performance with open-label placebos. Heart rate, ratings of perceived exertion, and blood lactate were not different between sessions (all P > 0.05). Positive expectation did not appear necessary to induce performance improvements, suggesting unconscious processes occurred, although the authors indicated that a lack of improvement appeared to be associated with a lack of belief.[25]
- Experiencing a placebo effect of an ergogenic aid, or even receiving education about the prevalence and mechanisms of placebo effects, might reduce an athlete's likelihood of using legal and illegal sports drugs.[26] For example, a group of elite UK athletes (N = 169; 56% male, age = 18.2 ±

0.4yrs) attended a 1-hour educational session on the placebo effect, which introduced participants to the role expectations and prior experiences (conditioning) play in the effectiveness of performance-enhancing drugs. Participants completed measures of performance-enhancing drug use pre- and 1-week postintervention, with data suggesting that participants were less likely to use performance-enhancing drugs following the intervention ($p < .001$, d = 0.42).[27]

While research in Sports to date has been relatively atheoretical, in terms of application, researchers have encouraged practitioners to capitalize on the placebo component of treatments[28] while at the same time drawing attention to the ethical and practical pitfalls associated with the indiscriminate use of placebos, perhaps most saliently in the context of complementary and alternative Sports Medicine.[29]

Sports researchers have also acknowledged the significant and largely unexplored overlap between many sports processes—including but not limited to social facilitation, emotion regulation, and coach-athlete trust—and placebo effects.[28,30] It has also been noted that nocebo effects are not only frequently observed in sports[31] but might even be more common in sports than placebo effects[24] (a reasonable observation is that it is probably easier to disrupt an athlete's performance using a nocebo intervention or inadvertent nocebo than it is to enhance it by using a placebo). In fact, it has been speculated that in many situations in sports, the manifestation of placebo effects might be little more than the reduction of nocebo effects. Although that proposal awaits experimental verification, it is lent some support by anecdotal data indicating that while a placebo intervention appears to improve performance, athletes often describe the mechanism as a reduction in one or more negative perceptual processes such as anxiety, fatigue, or pain.[3,23]

Sports and placebo research

Research over the last 20 or so years has supported the idea that the placebo effect is certainly a factor in sports performance. This is probably of little surprise to those who understand the mechanisms of the placebo effects and the strong likelihood that those mechanisms extend beyond the health context.

However, little programmatic research has been conducted in Sports, and future research needs to not only demonstrate the effect of a placebo on performance and perhaps some physiological correlates of these effects, but should also aim to identify the neurobiological mechanisms of these effects and by doing so begin to tease apart placebo effects and other sports phenomenon such as social facilitation and motivation. As suggested in a recent consensus statement,[6] researchers in Sports should seek to adopt research methods that:

a. Effectively elucidate the role of the brain in mediating the effects of treatments and interventions.
b. Factor for and/or quantify placebo effects that could explain a percentage of interindividual variability in response to treatments and intervention.

Perhaps the most promising specific line of research into application in Sports at present lies in the use of placebos to help athletes themselves better understand these mechanisms, and the extension of that better understanding into antidrug interventions and policies in Sports. While this idea has been supported by a number of experts,[6,32,33] it is perhaps best illustrated in an interview with an ex-professional cyclist in 2005—and reported in part in a subsequent scientific paper—who described how he was administered what he thought was an illegal drug, how he experienced one of the best performances of his life as the result, only to be informed subsequently by his team that he had been administered a placebo. He indicated that following this experience he was determined that he would never again cross the ethical line into using drugs because he realized that the improved performance was a result of his brain and not the capsule.[34]

Placebo effects in exercise

Numerous mechanisms have been proposed to explain placebo effects in exercise, these ranging from cognitive, such as distraction and self-esteem, to physiological, such as increased oxygen supply to the brain, to neurobiological, such as increases in brain-derived neurotrophic factor.

Psychological outcomes of exercise

Psychological outcomes of exercise and/or physical activity have been documented in the scientific literature for over 30 years.[35] The effects of exercise have become increasingly important to health in a world in which mental illness is becoming a major challenge for health agencies. The relationship between exercise and depression is perhaps a good case in point. The World Health Organization describes depression as the largest contributor to global disability, with over 300 million people affected by the condition. They estimate that prevalence has increased by over 18% in the 10 years to 2015.[36] The treatment of depression is, therefore, a serious challenge. Drugs are associated with relatively low effectiveness, with a failure rate as high as 50% in clinical trials,[37] with psychological treatments equally problematic: for example, effects for cognitive behavioral therapy are small to moderate when compared to care-as-usual or placebo.[38]

But depression is also associated with physical inactivity, with exercise reported to reduce the risk of depression by 17% in studies adjusting the odds for potential covariates and 41% in those studies that did not.[39] Findings from meta-analytic reviews of randomized trials in the Exercise and Mental Health literature report significant effect size estimates for exercise in psychological and perceptual variables including depression, fatigue, and pain.[40-42] However, concerns have been raised about methodologies employed in studies of exercise and mental health in relation to the potential influence of placebo effects.[5,43,44] Foremost among these is the inability to perform double-blind studies. Unlike pharmacological interventions in which the vehicles used to deliver the treatment and placebo are identical (e.g., capsule, fluid, and injection), it is generally regarded to be problematic if not impossible to truly blind participants to receiving exercise in research settings.

The challenges of placebo exercise

To date, little progress has been made in developing a valid exercise placebo that mirrors every aspect of exercise except the "active ingredients." The limitations of continuing to use weak methodologies are significant. Given the wide variability in response to nearly all treatments for mental health and given research that demonstrates substantial placebo effects in drug treatments, for example,[45-48] understanding placebo effects might explain some variability in response to exercise and from there how expectation might be enhanced toward better clinical outcomes is important. This is especially the case given that many patients (and practitioners) hold negative expectations about the effectiveness of exercise in treating mental health.

Meta-analytic review of the literature

With these shortcomings in mind, Lindheimer and colleagues quantified placebo effects in psychological outcomes of exercise training studies in a meta-analysis of randomized controlled trials that included an exercise treatment, control, and placebo arm ($n = 9$).[5] In this case, a *placebo condition* was defined as "an intervention that was not generally recognized as efficacious, that lacked adequate evidence for efficacy, and that has no direct pharmacological, bio-chemical, or physical mechanism of action according to the current standard of knowledge" (p. 695). After estimating placebo effects by aggregating the standardized mean difference between placebo and control groups from each study (Hedges' $d = 0.20$), placebo effects were subtracted from the observed effect of exercise (Hedges' $d = 0.37$), and the authors concluded that the effect of exercise training on psychological responses (Hedges' $d = 0.17$) was less than half of the observed effect of exercise after accounting for placebo effects.

Measuring and manipulating expectations in exercise studies

Research has consistently demonstrated the role of expectations as a psychological mechanism of placebo effects,[49] and it follows that placebo effects are more likely to occur in participants who expect that exercising will result in a certain psychological response (e.g., "exercise will improve my mood") compared to those who do not. Measuring self-reported expectations should not be viewed as a surrogate for a placebo condition, but this practice can help explain variability in psychological responses to exercise. Taking this suggestion one step further, experimental manipulation of expectations via verbal suggestion,[50] film clips,[51] and reading standardized scripts[52] can provide insight into the magnitude of their contribution to treatment responses to exercise. More recently, Colloca and colleagues have demonstrated the value of conditioned placebo and nocebo effects in the context of perceptual responses to exercise.[53] Common across all of these studies is the idea that placebo and nocebo effects can be studied without traditional placebo treatments, a concept that is germane to advancing the understanding of their effect on psychological responses to exercise.

Summary and future directions in exercise research

Presently, the best empirical estimate of the influence of placebo effects on psychological responses to exercise is that they explain over half of the therapeutic effects. Nevertheless, the overall understanding of placebo and nocebo effects in psychological responses to exercise has lagged behind other scientific disciplines. One key sign of this disparity is the lack of awareness among Exercise researchers that psychological mechanisms of placebo and nocebo effects (e.g., expectations, conditioning, and social observation) can be used to infer the contribution of placebo effects to treatment responses. To bridge this interdisciplinary knowledge gap, a greater emphasis should be placed on determining which existing models that have been successfully used by other fields to study placebo and nocebo mechanisms best translate to studies of psychological responses to exercise.[53]

Further, despite compelling evidence that expectations are a central mechanism of placebo effects, few Exercise studies consider the expectations of their research participants and even fewer consider the possibility that some people may have negative expectations. Characterizing baseline expectations for psychological outcomes of exercise should be routinely practiced in Exercise research. Importantly, questionnaires with item phrasing and scales that allow a respondent to indicate expectations for either positive *or* negative changes should be used rather than those with inherent biases toward only measuring expectations for desirable outcomes.[54] Moreover, administering these instruments at multiple timepoints in studies that use experimental manipulations to alter expectations would allow researchers to begin cataloging which types of expectancy modification procedures are most effective in Exercise research.

Finally, the role of nocebo effects in Exercise research is virtually untouched as the extant data on nocebo effects and their respective mechanisms in psychological responses to exercise can be traced to a handful of studies.[52,53] This line of research requires further attention and may have particularly important implications for explaining interindividual variability in how healthy and clinical populations respond negatively to exercise. Taking these above considerations together (i.e., translating existing placebo and nocebo models to Exercise research, improving the measurement and reporting of expectations, and increasing research on the role of nocebo effects in exercise) would go a long way toward advancing the understanding of placebo and nocebo effects in psychological responses to exercise (Figure 3.4.2).

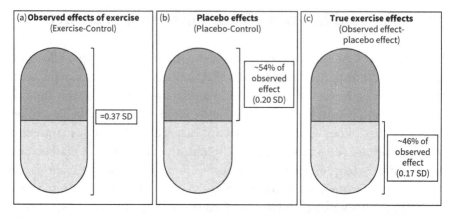

Figure 3.4.2 Distinguishing treatment effects from placebo effects and nonspecific effects requires the inclusion of a placebo and no-treatment control group. Panel A shows the observed effects of exercise, which are estimated by comparing the change in the exercise group to the control group. Panel B shows placebo effects, which are estimated by comparing the change in the placebo group to the control group. Panel C shows that the true effects of exercise can be estimated by subtracting placebo effects from the observed effects of exercise. In a meta-analysis of nine randomized controlled studies that included an exercise, placebo, and control group, approximately half of the observed effects of exercise on psychological outcomes were attributed to placebo effects.[5]

References

1. Beecher HK. The powerful placebo. *Journal of the American Medical Association.* 1955;159(17):1602–1606. http://doi:10.1001/jama.1955.02960340022006
2. Kienle GS, Kiene H. The powerful placebo effect: Fact or fiction? *Journal of Clinical Epidemiology.* 1997;50(12):1311–1318.
3. Beedie C, Foad A. The placebo effect in sports performance: A brief review. *Sports Medicine.* 2009;39(4):313–329. http://doi:10.2165/00007256-200939040-00004
4. Hurst P, Schipof-Godart L, Szabo A, Raglin J, Hettinga F, Roelands B, Lane A, Foad A, Coleman D, Beedie C. The Placebo and Nocebo effect on sports performance: A systematic review. *European Journal of Sport Science.* 2020 Apr;20(3):279–292. doi:10.1080/17461391.2019.1655098.
5. Lindheimer JB, O'Connor PJ, Dishman RK. Quantifying the placebo effect in psychological outcomes of exercise training: A meta-analysis of randomized trials. *Sports Medicine.* 2015;45(5):693–711. http://doi:10.1007/s40279-015-0303-1
6. Beedie C, Benedetti F, Barbiani D, Camerone E, Cohen E, Coleman D, Davis A, Elsworth-Edelsten C, Flowers E, Foad A, Harvey S, Hettinga F, Hurst P, Lane A, Lindheimer J, Raglin J, Roelands B, Schiphof-Godart L, Szabo A. Consensus statement on placebo effects in sports and exercise: the need for conceptual clarity, methodological rigour, and the elucidation of neurobiological mechanisms. *European Journal of Sport Science.* 2018;18(10):1383–1389. doi:10.1080/17461391.2018.1496144.

7. Beedie C, Hettinga F. *Introduction to the Special Edition on the Placebo Effect in Sport and Exercise.* Taylor & Francis; 2020.

8. Benedetti F, Barbiani D, Camerone E. Critical life functions: Can placebo replace oxygen? *International Review of Neurobiology.* 2018;(138):201–218. doi:10.1016/bs.irn.2018.01.009.

9. Pollo A, Carlino E, Benedetti F. The top-down influence of ergogenic placebos on muscle work and fatigue. *European Journal of Neuroscience.* 2008;28(2):379–388. http://doi:10.1111/j.1460-9568.2008.06344.x

10. Benedetti F, Pollo A, Colloca L. Opioid-mediated placebo responses boost pain endurance and physical performance: Is it doping in sport competitions? *Journal of Neuroscience.* 2007;27:11934–11939.

11. Castell LM, Stear SJ, Burke LM. *Nutritional Supplements in Sport, Exercise and Health: An AZ Guide.* Routledge; 2015.

12. Hodges NJ, Williams AM. *Skill Acquisition in Sport: Research, Theory and Practice.* 3rd ed. Routledge; 2019.

13. Baitsch H, Bock HE, Bolte M, Bokler W, Heidland HW, Lotz F. *The Scientific View of Sport: Perspectives, Aspects, Issues.* Springer Science & Business Media; 2012.

14. Atkinson M. *Key Concepts in Sport and Exercise Research Methods.* Sage; 2011.

15. Jones I. *Research Methods for Sports Studies.* Routledge; 2022.

16. Benedetti F, Mayberg HS, Wager TD, Stohler CS, Zubieta J-K. Neurobiological mechanisms of the placebo effect. *Journal of Neuroscience.* 2005;25(45):10390.

17. Lindheimer JB, Szabo A, Raglin JS, Beedie C. Advancing the understanding of placebo effects in psychological outcomes of exercise: Lessons learned and future directions. *European Journal of Sport Science.* 2020;(3):326–337. doi:10.1080/17461391.2019.1632937.

18. Beedie C, Benedetti F, Barbiani D, Camerone E, Lindheimer J, Roelands B. Incorporating methods and findings from neuroscience to better understand placebo and nocebo effects in sport. *European Journal of Sport Science.* 2020;20(3):313–325.

19. Raglin J, Szabo A, Lindheimer JB, Beedie C. Understanding placebo and nocebo effects in the context of sport: A psychological perspective. *European Journal of Sport Science.* 2020;20(3):293–301.

20. Trojian TH, Beedie CJ. Placebo effect and athletes. *Current Sports Medicine Reports.* 2008;7(4):214–217. http://doi:10.1249/JSR.0b013e31817ed050

21. Benedetti F. Placebo and the new physiology of the doctor-patient relationship. *Physiological Reviews.* 2013;93(3):1207–1246. http://doi:10.1152/physrev.00043.2012

22. Foad AJ, Beedie CJ, Coleman DA. Pharmacological and psychological effects of caffeine ingestion in 40-km cycling performance. *Medicine & Science in Sports & Exercise.* 2008;40(1):158–165. http://doi:10.1249/mss.0b013e3181593e02

23. Beedie C, Stuart E, Coleman D, Foad A. Placebo effects of caffeine on cycling performance. *Medicine & Science in Sports & Exercise.* 2006;38(12):2159–2164. http://doi:10.1249/01.mss.0000233805.56315.a9

24. Hurst P, Foad AJ, Coleman D, Beedie C. Athletes intending to use sports supplements are more likely to respond to a placebo. *Medicine & Science in Sports & Exercise.* 2017;49(9):1877–1883.

25. Saunders B, Saito T, Klosterhoff R, et al. "I put it in my head that the supplement would help me": Open-placebo improves exercise performance in female cyclists. *PLoS ONE.* 2019;14(9):e0222982.

26. Hurst P. *The Placebo and Nocebo Effect in Sport: Intentions, Attitudes and Beliefs Towards Sport Supplements and Banned Performance Enhancing Substances.* Canterbury Christ Church University (United Kingdom); 2018.

27. Hurst P, Foad A, Coleman D, Beedie C. An educational placebo effect intervention reduces the likelihood of athletes using performance enhancing drugs. presented at: Society for

Interdisciplinary Placebo Studies (SIPS) conference on placebo studies; 2017; Lieden, Netherlands.

28. Beedie C, Foad A, Hurst P. Capitalizing on the placebo component of treatments. *Current Sports Medicine Reports*. 2015;14(4):284–287. http://doi:10.1249/JSR.0000000000000172

29. Beedie C, Whyte G, Lane AM, et al. "Caution, this treatment is a placebo. It might work, but it might not": Why emerging mechanistic evidence for placebo effects does not legitimise complementary and alternative medicines in sport. *British Journal of Sports Medicine*. 2017;52:817–818.

30. Davis A, Hettinga F, Beedie C. You don't need to administer a placebo to elicit a placebo effect: Social factors trigger neurobiological pathways to enhance sports performance. *European Journal of Sport Science*. 2020;(3):302–312. doi:10.1080/17461391.2019.1635212.

31. Beedie C, Coleman DA, Foad AJ. Positive and negative placebo effects resulting from the deceptive administration of an ergogenic aid. *International Journal of Sport Nutrition and Exercise Metabolism*. 2007;17(3):259–269.

32. McClung M, Collins D. "Because I know it will!": Placebo effects of an ergogenic aid on athletic performance. *Journal of Sport & Exercise Psychology*. 2007;29(3):382–394.

33. Maganaris CN, Collins D, Sharp M. Expectancy effects and strength training: Do steroids make a difference? *Sport Psychologist*. 2000;14(3):272–278.

34. Beedie C. Placebo effects in competitive sport: Qualitative data. *Journal of Sports Science and Medicine*. 2007;6(1):21–28.

35. Raglin JS. Exercise and mental health. *Sports Medicine*. 1990;9(6):323–329. http://doi:10.2165/00007256-199009060-00001

36. WHO. *Depression and Other Common Mental Disorders: Global Health Estimates*. World Health Organization; 2017.

37. Khan A, Mar KF, Brown WA. The conundrum of depression clinical trials: One size does not fit all. *International Clinical Psychopharmacology*. 2018;33(5):239–248. http://doi:10.1097/YIC.0000000000000229

38. Cuijpers P, Cristea IA, Karyotaki E, Reijnders M, Huibers MJH. How effective are cognitive behavior therapies for major depression and anxiety disorders? A meta-analytic update of the evidence. *World Psychiatry*. 2016;15(3):245–258. http://doi:10.1002/wps.20346

39. Schuch FB, Vancampfort D, Firth J, et al. Physical activity and incident depression: A meta-analysis of prospective cohort studies. *American Journal of Psychiatry*. 2018;175(7):631–648. http://doi:10.1176/appi.ajp.2018.17111194

40. Cooney GM, Dwan K, Greig CA, Lawlor DA, Rimer J, Waugh FR, McMurdo M, Mead GE. Exercise for depression. *Cochrane Database of Systematic Reviews*. 2013;(9):CD004366. doi:10.1002/14651858.CD004366.pub6.

41. Searle A, Spink M, Ho A, Chuter V. Exercise interventions for the treatment of chronic low back pain: A systematic review and meta-analysis of randomised controlled trials. *Clinical Rehabilitation*. 2015;29(12):1155–1167.

42. Puetz TW, Herring MP. Differential effects of exercise on cancer-related fatigue during and following treatment: A meta-analysis. *American Journal of Preventive Medicine*. 2012;43(2):e1–e24.

43. Ojanen M. Can the true effects of exercise on psychological variables be separated from placebo effects? *International Journal of Sport Psychology*. 1994;25(1):63–80.

44. Szabo A. Acute psychological benefits of exercise: Reconsideration of the placebo effect. *Journal of Mental Health*. 2013;22(5):449–455.

45. Kirsch I, Sapirstein G. Listening to Prozac but hearing placebo: A meta-analysis of antidepressant medication. *Prevention & Treatment*. 1998;1(2):Article 2a. https://doi.org/10.1037/1522-3736.1.1.12a

46. Lichtigfeld FJ, Gillman MA. Possible role of the endogenous opioid system in the placebo response in depression. *International Journal of Neuropsychopharmacology.* 2002;5(1):107–108. http://doi:10.1017/S1461145701002735

47. Mitsikostas DD, Mantonakis L, Chalarakis N. Nocebo in clinical trials for depression: A meta-analysis. *Psychiatry Research.* 2014;215(1):82–86. https://doi.org/10.1016/j.psychres.2013.10.019

48. Rutherford BR, Wall MM, Brown PJ, et al. Patient expectancy as a mediator of placebo effects in antidepressant clinical trials. *American Journal of Psychiatry.* 2017;174(2):135–142. http://doi:10.1176/appi.ajp.2016.16020225

49. Finniss DG, Kaptchuk TJ, Miller F, Benedetti F. Biological, clinical, and ethical advances of placebo effects. *Lancet.* 2010;375(9715):686–695.

50. Lindheimer JB, O'Connor PJ, McCully KK, Dishman RK. The effect of light-intensity cycling on mood and working memory in response to a randomized, placebo-controlled design. *Psychosomatic Medicine.* 2017;79(2):243–253.

51. Mothes H, Leukel C, Jo H-G, Seelig H, Schmidt S, Fuchs R. Expectations affect psychological and neurophysiological benefits even after a single bout of exercise. *Journal of Behavioral Medicine.* 2017;40(2):293–306.

52. Kwan BM, Stevens CJ, Bryan AD. What to expect when you're exercising: An experimental test of the anticipated affect–exercise relationship. *Health Psychology.* 2017;36(4):309.

53. Colloca L, Corsi N, Fiorio M. The interplay of exercise, placebo and nocebo effects on experimental pain. *Scientific Reports.* 2018;8(1):1–11.

54. Lindheimer JB, Szabo A, Raglin JS, Beedie C, Carmichael KE, O'Connor PJ. Reconceptualizing the measurement of expectations to better understand placebo and nocebo effects in psychological responses to exercise. *European Journal of Sport Science.* 2020;20(3):338–346.

3.5

Nocebos in migraine

Implications for clinical research and practice

Dimos D. Mitsikostas

Introduction

The clinical course and treatment outcome of a medical condition are not exclusively associated with the pathophysiology of the condition or to the biological or physical mechanisms of action of the therapeutic interventions. Additional environmental, random, or patient's idiosyncratic variables are also involved in modifying the outcome. Thus, to identify the authentic natural history of a medical condition that is attributable to the causative pathophysiology exclusively, long-lasting longitudinal observational studies with repeated measurements including a large number of participants with the medical condition in question are essential. Similarly, to assess the effect size of a potential treatment attributed to the mechanism of action of the treatment exclusively, testing in parallel with an inert treatment is crucial. This inert treatment (e.g., an agent, a manipulation or intervention) is called a *placebo*. Inert agents are also administered in humans to induce negative outcomes in order to investigate their underlying mechanisms. These agents, or interventions that cause unfavorable outcomes although their active components lack this potential, are called *nocebos*. The *nocebo effect* refers to the negative outcomes recorded after treatment application that are not attributable to the treatment's mechanism of action, but to negative expectations and a person's experience.

As with placebos, nocebo responses contribute to clinical research and daily practice enormously affecting the treatment outcomes, the natural history of medical conditions, and treatment related adverse event (AE) experiences significantly.[1] *Nocebo* refers to a set of symptoms that are related to either a negative expectation that a medical treatment will most likely harm (effect), to spontaneous worsening of the symptoms, or even to random comorbidities (response). There are different terms that refer to specific conditions related to placebo or nocebo administration or application (e.g., the *nocebo* or the trigger for a reaction, most often a medical treatment; *nocebo effect*, which refers to negative expectation for the health outcome; and *nocebo response*, which includes all bad outcomes after an inert agent administration).[2,3]

In clinical practice and research, when treating physicians or clinical investigators inform patients or trial participants about the safety data of the offered treatment, or the treatment in testing, they report the potential risk to experience an AE in fact. This represents a nocebo application verbally, which triggers nocebo effects naturally (e.g., negative expectations) resulting in nocebo responses (e.g., AEs). Unfavorable outcomes can be due to patients' negative expectations with consequences for treatment adherence and treatment resistance. Correspondingly, by presenting the treatment's efficacy data (= placebo administration verbally) one can induce placebo effects. Thus, although not on purpose, but rather unavoidably, both placebo and nocebo responses are induced in daily practice[4] and in clinical trials,[5] and being more prevalent and powerful in pain conditions.[6]

There is good evidence that placebo and nocebo effects are associated with release of neuropeptides including opioids, endocannabinoids, dopamine, oxytocin, and vasopressin, among others.[1,7,8] Genetic factors are also implicated (e.g., polymorphisms in the dopamine, opioid, and endocannabinoid genes).[9–11] The neuropeptide and receptor systems associated with placebo and nocebo effects are also implicated in the hypothalamic-pituitary-adrenal system, pain processing, mood control, and limbic system, which is why placebo and nocebo effects are enhanced in pain conditions and modulated by anxiety- and depression-like states and personality trends.[12,13]

Among pain conditions, primary headaches are the most prevalent and disabling medical conditions along with low back pain.[14] Migraine affects more than one billion people worldwide and is associated with a significant disability causing substantial effects not only on those immediately affected but also on their environment.[15] Chronic primary headaches, particularly chronic migraine, are highly comorbid with anxiety- and depression-like conditions,[16] further increasing the occurrence of placebo and nocebo phenomena. Like in other medical conditions, placebo responses modulate treatment effects for headaches favorably, yet nocebo responses unfavorably, limiting treatment outcomes and adherence, resulting in headache refractoriness and chronification.

In this chapter, we aim to summarize current evidence for the prevalence of nocebo responses in clinical trials for treatment of migraine and other primary headaches, focusing primarily on the prophylactic ones that share increased risks for low adherence.

Nocebo responses in trials for migraine

Nocebo responses in trials for migraine are attributable to the nocebo effects plus a set of other factors (e.g., the natural history of the medical condition in question). In clinical trials for the symptomatic treatment of migraine, the proportion of participants who experienced any AE in the placebo arms is smaller than those observed in clinical trials for the prophylaxis of migraine. These aspects are described in detail below.

Symptomatic treatment

There are two meta-analyses focused on AEs recorded in the placebo arms of randomized controlled trials (RCTs) for the symptomatic treatment of migraine.[17,18] The first one estimated that 21% (95% CI 12%–30%) of participants treated with placebo in the trials for the acute treatment of migraine with triptans reported at least one AE. The authors classified these AEs into three classes: migraine-related AEs (e.g., nausea, photophobia, and phonophobia), drug-related AEs (e.g., chest pressure), and nonspecific or coincidental AEs (e.g., sleep disturbance). Consequently, the AEs in the placebo arms were most likely related either to the treatment or to the condition in test.[17]

Another meta-analysis revealed that 18.5% (95% CI 14.90%–22.23%) of placebo-treated participants in trials for symptomatic migraine treatment with all acute antimigraine reported at least one AE.[18] In trials with triptans, this proportion was 20.93% (95% CI 16.46%–25.78%). However, the proportion of patients treated with a placebo who discontinued treatment because of AEs were only 0.36%, indicating that nocebo outcomes in trials for symptomatic treatment of migraine were not sufficiently powerful.

This proportion was similar (0.39%) in the third meta-analysis for nocebos in migraine trials, by Amanzio and colleagues.[19] In this study, the investigators studied the AEs after placebo in trials testing NSAIDs, triptans, or anticonvulsants in migraine and found that the AEs recorded mirrored the AEs expected of the active medication tested (e.g., chest symptoms in trials with triptans), suggesting that nocebo responses in migraine trials arose from patients' distrust.[19] Nocebo responses did not change by the condition tested and were similarly prevalent among trials for migraine and cluster headache in symptomatic treatment.[18]

Preventive treatment

Data for prevention of migraine are coming from those three above-mentioned meta-analyses as well. In addition, there is a meta-analysis for the prevalence of nocebo responses in trials with monoclonal antibodies targeting the *Anti-Calcitonin Gene-Related Peptide* (anti-CGRP mAbs).[20] By polling participants in trials for migraine prevention with oral drugs and botulinum toxin A (BOTA), 42.78% (95% CI 34.73%–51.36%) of participants treated with the placebo experienced at least one AE and 4.75% (95% CI 3.28%–6.49%) discontinued treatment because of AEs. Nocebo response rates did not vary with the drug tested, with headache type, but in studies with BOTA, the dropout ratio was significantly greater than in any other prophylactic treatment [0.92% (95% CI 0.20–2.16%)], reflecting participants' greater positive expectations for the treatment, along with the route and the frequency of drug administration,[18] as high placebo responses in these trials confirm.[21] As in trials with symptomatic treatments, Amanzio and colleagues[19] found that AEs in the placebo-treated participants mirrored drug-related AEs recorded in the active arms of trials.[22]

In the more recent and larger clinical trials with anti-CGRP mAbs, pooled analysis revealed that the proportion of placebo-treated participants who achieved the 50% responder rate (placebo responses) was 32.7% (95% CI 28.6%–37.0%) in anti-CGRP mAbs versus 24.4% (95% CI 20.5%–28.5%) in trials with topiramate in episodic migraine (EM).[20] The proportion of dropouts attributable to AEs in placebo-treated participants (nocebo responses) was 1.9% (95% CI 1.4%–2.6%) in anti-CGRP mAbs versus 9.9% (95% CI 7.7%–12.3%) in topiramate trials. In chronic migraine (CM), the 50% placebo responder rate was 23.6% (95% CI 11.2%–38.8%) in anti-CGRP mAbs trials versus 36.4% (95% CI 32.6%–39.3%) in trials with BOTA.[21] The nocebo dropout response in anti-CGRP mAbs and BOTA trials was 1.4% (95% CI 0.8%–2.1%) and 0.9 (95% CI 0.3%–1.7%), respectively. The incidence of nocebo responses (any AE experienced in the placebo arms) was 60% (95% CI 57.9%–62.1%) in EM and 51.1% (95% CI 38.1%–64.2%) in CM trials with anti-CGRP mAbs, and the incidence of severe AEs was 1.8% (95% CI 1.3%–2.5%) for EM and 1.1% (95% CI 0.6%–1.7%) for CM trials of anti-CGRP mAbs. In trials for CM no significant differences regarding the placebo and nocebo responses were observed between the anti-CGRP mAbs and BOTA. Thus, with anti-CGRP mAbs, nocebo responses were more prevalent in trials with EM versus CM. The lower nocebo responses along with the high placebo responses of anti-CGRP mAbs in EM undoubtedly reflect an advantage over traditional oral preventive treatments for migraine.[20]

Nocebo-prone behaviors in outpatients with migraine

The Q-No is a specific questionnaire that has been developed to detect nocebo-prone behaviors.[23] It is a self-administered questionnaire that predicts potential nocebo behavior in outpatients seeking neurological consultation. The Q-No predicts nocebo response with 71.7% specificity, 67.5% sensitivity, and 42.5% positive predictive value.[23] Using this questionnaire, 514 individuals attending Headache Centers in Athens, Greece, were interviewed to collect their preferences for antimigraine treatment options to investigate whether their preferences were related to nocebo-prone behaviors. Of all participants, 56.6% scored more than 15 in the Q-No questionnaire, indicating potential nocebo behaviors that contributed significantly to their treatment choices. More specifically, participants who scored more than 15 in the Q-No questionnaire preferred to use daily external neurostimulation over daily drug treatment (OR = 1.6; 95% CI 1.1–2.3; $p < 0.05$) for headache prevention. They also preferred to use acute neurostimulation for symptomatic headache treatment over drugs (OR = 1.7; 95% CI 1.1–2.5, $p = 0.008$).[24] Thus, individuals with headache and nocebo-prone behaviors tend to avoid drugs and prefer the use of external devices for treatment, which is in harmony with the suspicion and the fear that characterize nocebo phenomenon.

Factors influencing nocebo responses

Stratified analyses in the above-mentioned meta-analyses of the trials for migraine treatment revealed that nocebo responses are significantly rarer in:

(1) Chronic versus EM.[20]
(2) Acute versus prophylactic drug treatments.[18]
(3) Trials with nonsteroidal anti-inflammatory drugs versus triptans.[19]
(4) Injectable (including the novel prophylactic treatments with monoclonal antibodies targeting the calcitonin gene related peptide and botulinum toxin A) versus traditional oral prophylactic antimigraine treatments.[18,20]

Nocebo and placebo responses are recorded in parallel in migraine tests (i.e., the more AEs recorded in the active part and the more frequent placebo responses, the more widespread the nocebo responses are, either as an AE experience or as an AE withdrawal).[18,19,20]

The AEs recorded by placebo-treated participants mirror the AEs of the drug in test, suggesting that expectancies may drive nocebo effects as part of the overall responses.[19,20] No data are available to account for potential influences related to sex, age, health disparities, and comorbidities including mood disorders.

Conclusions

Migraine is usually treatable but because of safety and tolerability reasons, available preventive treatments often have limited success. Some of those headache sufferers who do not adhere to the treatment because of AEs are powered by nocebos.[25] Recent evidence on the nocebo phenomenon in pharmaceutical treatment of migraine revealed that one out of five participants, treated with a placebo in clinical trials for the symptomatic treatment of migraine, experienced any AE, but the proportion of participants who discontinued treatment because of AEs is less than 1%. In clinical trials for the prophylaxis of migraine, half of the participants treated with a placebo experienced an AE, and 1 out of 20 discontinued treatments because of AEs. The available data for analysis showed that nocebo responses in clinical trials for migraine are significantly rarer in chronic versus EM, in acute versus prophylactic drug treatments, in trials with nonsteroidal anti-inflammatory drugs versus triptans, and in the injectable (including the novel prophylactic treatments with monoclonal antibodies targeting the calcitonin gene related peptide and botulinum toxin A) versus traditional oral prophylactic antimigraine treatments. Notably, nocebo responses are in line with placebo responses (e.g., the better are outcome in the placebo arm the higher the AEs being reported). In addition, the higher the AEs recorded in the active arm of the RCT, the wider the AEs recorded in the placebo-treated participants are (nocebo responses). Nocebo responses naturally exist in clinical practice, induced by the summary of product characteristic documents and/or leaflets of the drugs or internet information.

It would be important, therefore, to limit this phenomenon to increase treatment adherence, which is very low in migraine prophylaxis.[27] Several variables influence nocebo effects including expectation, conditioning, and observational learning.[28] Some of these are modifiable, and some are not. By taking care of the modifiable ones, treating physicians or clinical investigators have the chance to increase adherence and improve good outcomes in their practice or clinical science respectively. In this context appropriate delivery of safety information for the offered treatment is crucial[6] because people with migraine are very sensitive to tolerability issues, more than in other brain conditions (e.g., epilepsy).[29] Patients' education and close follow-up, along with positive suggestions and continuous support, increase patients' compliance and decrease nocebo effects and responses.

References

1. Colloca L, Barsky AJ. Placebo and nocebo effects. *New England Journal of Medicine.* 2020;382(6):554–561. http://doi:10.1056/NEJMra1907805
2. Mitsikostas DD, Blease C, Carlino E, et al.; European Headache Federation. European Headache Federation recommendations for placebo and nocebo terminology. *Journal of Headache and Pain.* 2020;21(1):117. http://doi:10.1186/s10194-020-01178-3
3. Evers AWM, Colloca L, Blease C, et al. Implications of placebo and nocebo effects for clinical practice: expert consensus. *Psychotherapy and Psychosomatics.* 2018;87(4):204–210. http://doi:10.1159/000490354
4. Hansen E, Zech N. Nocebo effects and negative suggestions in daily clinical practice—Forms, impact and approaches to avoid them. *Frontiers in Pharmacology.* 2019;10:77. http://doi:10.3389/fphar.2019.00077
5. Colloca L. The placebo effect in pain therapies. *Annual Review of Pharmacology and Toxicology.* 2019;59:191–211. http://doi:10.1146/annurev-pharmtox-010818-021542
6. Colloca L. Tell me the truth and I will not be harmed: Informed consents and nocebo effects. *American Journal of Bioethics.* 2017;17(6):46–48. http://doi:10.1080/15265 161.2017.1314057
7. Finniss DG, Kaptchuk TJ, Miller F, Benedetti F. Biological, clinical, and ethical advances of placebo effects. *Lancet.* 2010;375(9715):686–695. http://doi:10.1016/ S0140-6736(09)61706-2
8. Theodosis-Nobelos P, Filotheidou A, Triantis C. The placebo phenomenon and the underlying mechanisms. *Hormones (Athens).* 2021;20(1):61–71. http://doi:10.1007/s42 000-020-00243-5
9. Colloca L, Wang Y, Martinez PE, et al. OPRM1 rs1799971, COMT rs4680, and FAAH rs324420 genes interact with placebo procedures to induce hypoalgesia. *Pain.* 2019;160:1824–1834.
10. Hall KT, Loscalzo J, Kaptchuk TJ. Genetics and the placebo effect: The placebome. *Trends in Molecular Medicine.* 2015;21:285–294.
11. Wendt L, Albring A, Benson S, et al. Catechol-O-methyltransferase Val158Met polymorphism is associated with somatosensory amplification and nocebo responses. *PLoS ONE.* 2014;9(9):e107665.
12. Benedetti F, Amanzio M, Giovannelli F, Craigs-Brackhahn K, Shaibani A. Hypothalamic-pituitary-adrenal activity in adverse events reporting after placebo administration. *Clinical Pharmacology and Therapeutics.* 2021;110(5):1349–1357. http://doi:10.1002/cpt.2388
13. Benedetti F, Amanzio M, Rosato R, Blanchard C. Nonopioid placebo analgesia is mediated by CB1 cannabinoid receptors. *Nature Medicine.* 2011;17(10):1228–1230. http://doi:10.1038/nm.2435
14. GBD 2016 Disease and Injury Incidence and Prevalence Collaborators. Global, regional, and national incidence, prevalence, and years lived with disability for 328 diseases and injuries for 195 countries, 1990–2016: A systematic analysis for the Global Burden

of Disease Study 2016. *Lancet.* 2017;390(10100):1211–1259. http://doi:10.1016/S0140-6736(17)32154-2. Erratum in: *Lancet.* 2017;390(10106):e38.

15. Ashina M, Katsarava Z, Do TP, et al. Migraine: Epidemiology and systems of care. *Lancet.* 2021;397(10283):1485–1495. http://doi:10.1016/S0140-6736(20)32160-7

16. Mitsikostas DD, Thomas AM. Comorbidity of headache and depressive disorders. *Cephalalgia.* 1999;19(4):211–217. http://doi:10.1046/j.1468-2982.1999.019004211.x

17. Reuter U, Sanchez del Rio M, Carpay JA, Boes CJ, Silberstein SD; GSK Headache Masters Program. Placebo adverse events in headache trials: Headache as an adverse event of placebo. *Cephalalgia.* 2003;23:496–503.

18. Mitsikostas DD, Mantonakis LI, Chalarakis NG. Nocebo is the enemy, not placebo: A meta-analysis of reported side effects after placebo treatment in headaches. *Cephalalgia.* 2011;31(5):550–561. http://doi:10.1177/0333102410391485

19. Amanzio M, Corazzini LL, Vase L, Benedetti F. A systematic review of adverse events in placebo groups of anti-migraine clinical trials. *Pain.* 2009;146(3):261–269. http://doi:10.1016/j.pain.2009.07.010

20. Kokoti L, Drellia K, Papadopoulos D, Mitsikostas DD. Placebo and nocebo phenomena in anti- CGRP monoclonal antibody trials for migraine prevention: A meta-analysis. *Journal of Neurology.* 2020;267(4):1158–1170. http://doi:10.1007/s00415-019-09673-7

21. Frank F, Ulmer H, Sidoroff V, Broessner G. CGRP-antibodies, topiramate and botulinum toxin type A in episodic and chronic migraine: A systematic review and meta-analysis. *Cephalalgia.* 2021;41(11–12):1222–1239. http://doi:10.1177/03331024211018137

22. Benedetti F, Lanotte M, Lopiano L, Colloca L. When words are painful: Unraveling the mechanisms of the nocebo effect. *Neuroscience.* 2007;147:260–271.

23. Mitsikostas DD, Deligianni CI. Q-No: A questionnaire to predict nocebo in outpatients seeking neurological consultation. *Neurological Sciences.* 2015;36:379–381.

24. Mitsikostas DD, Belesioti I, Arvaniti C, et al.; Hellenic Headache Society. Patients' preferences for headache acute and preventive treatment. *Journal of Headache and Pain.* 2017;18(1):102. http://doi:10.1186/s10194-017-0813-3

25. Mitsikostas DD. Nocebo in headache. *Current Opinion in Neurology.* 2016;29(3):331–336. http://doi:10.1097/WCO.0000000000000313

26. Benedetti F, Pollo A, Lopiano L, Lanotte M, Vighetti S, Rainero I. Conscious expectation and unconscious conditioning in analgesic, motor, and hormonal placebo/nocebo responses. *Journal of Neuroscience.* 2003;23(10):4315–4323. http://doi:10.1523/JNEUROSCI.23-10-04315.2003

27. Hepp Z, Dodick DW, Varon SF, Gillard P, Hansen RN, Devine EB. Adherence to oral migraine-preventive medications among patients with chronic migraine. *Cephalalgia.* 2015;35(6):478–488. http://doi:10.1177/0333102414547138

28. Frisaldi E, Shaibani A, Trucco M, Milano E, Benedetti F. What is the role of placebo in neurotherapeutics? *Expert Review of Neurotherapeutics.* 2022;22(1):15–25. http://doi:10.1080/14737175.2022.2012156

29. Romoli M, Costa C, Siliquini S, et al. Antiepileptic drugs in migraine and epilepsy: Who is at increased risk of adverse events? *Cephalalgia.* 2018;38(2):274–282. http://doi: 10.1177/0333102416683925

3.6

Placebos, nocebos, and COVID-19

Society, science, and health care during the pandemic

Leonard Calabrese

Introduction: COVID-19 and its effects on science and society

Since the identification of the first case of infection with the virus SARS CoV-2, the global Coronavirus Disease 2019 (COVID-19) pandemic has disrupted the fabric of the entire planet in a way that has not been witnessed since World War II. It has been felt at the macro level with a 2-year toll of over a quarter of a billion cases, 5 million fatalities, and profound effects on the global economy and supply chains. On the micro level, the pandemic has caused individual suffering, social disruption, and, for many, personal loss. Collectively these influences have the potential to affect the population's positive and negative expectations regarding the clinical illness including the risk of death and yet undefined postinfection sequelae, and the benefits and risks of new and evolving therapies, as well as the promise and threats of preventive measures, particularly a new generation of vaccines. These factors and more make COVID-19 treatment and prevention a fertile ground for placebo and nocebo effects and investigation. These disruptive effects have also affected our institutions, causing political strife within national and local governments, exposing weaknesses and fragilities in how we acquire and appraise news, and exposing the power and frailties.[1] Most importantly and predictably, society has witnessed a profound erosion in our trust in science and its traditional role in illuminating rationale courses of action in times of uncertainty. Even the process of science has been disrupted with the tsunami-like pace and force of information both the lay and scientific comminutes attempt to discern. Since the first reports in January 2020, as demonstrated by a search of PubMed and MedrxIv, there have been over 250,000 papers published in peer reviewed publications, with an additional 25,000 in pre–peer reviewed formats. Even more mind-boggling is the fact that there are over five billion Google citations (often referred to as "gray literature") on COVID-19. This torrent of data and opinion has disrupted the linear flow of science (hypothesis generation, testing, reporting and iterative experimentation, and dissemination of science-based recommendations) to a state which can only be described at times as epistemic chaos. Even more alarming has been the shift in the attitudes, beliefs, and trust of large segments of our society regarding the value of science to provide the best evidence to guide us though times of evolving uncertainty. This attitudinal shift is not a new phenomenon and was elegantly described by the late Carl Sagan in his last book *The Demon Haunted World*.[2] Sagan asserted that lack of trust in science and the embrace of pseudoscience has been experienced in every age when there has been social disruption. In those times, as well as now, rationalism and scientific progress are eschewed in favor of irrational beliefs and pseudoscience, confounding development and acceptance of effective therapies (including vaccines), while embracing the use of unproven remedies based on popular beliefs. It is against this background of COVID-19-induced unrest and uncertainty, with its potential influences on social anxiety within the general population, that we will consider the implications, opportunities, and challenges for the field of placebo and nocebo science.

COVID-19 pathogenesis: natural history and clinical sequelae

In order to consider the potential impact of placebo and nocebo effects stemming from the COVID-19 pandemic, a basic understanding of the clinical and immunopathogenic disease course after infection with SARS CoV-2 is necessary (Figure 3.6.1).[3] *Stage 1* refers to the encounter of a healthy individual with SARS CoV-2 and the engagement of the innate immune response (the early warning system within the integrated immune response). It is important to note that during the incubation phase, which generally lasts 3–5 days, the virus is replicating but the patient remains asymptomatic. In the majority of patients, innate defenses are unable to contain the virus, and patients progress to Stage 2: adaptive responses of both humoral and cellular immunity, often with the development of mild-to-moderate symptoms characteristic of a respiratory tract infection. For most individuals the disease ends at Stage 2: the majority of infected individuals remain asymptomatic or pauci-symptomatic with mild disease.[4] In an unfortunate minority (influenced by risk factors noted in the figure), the disease progresses to Stage 3: a hyperinflammatory phase largely driven by a dysregulated immune response and often requiring critical care and respiratory support. This phase

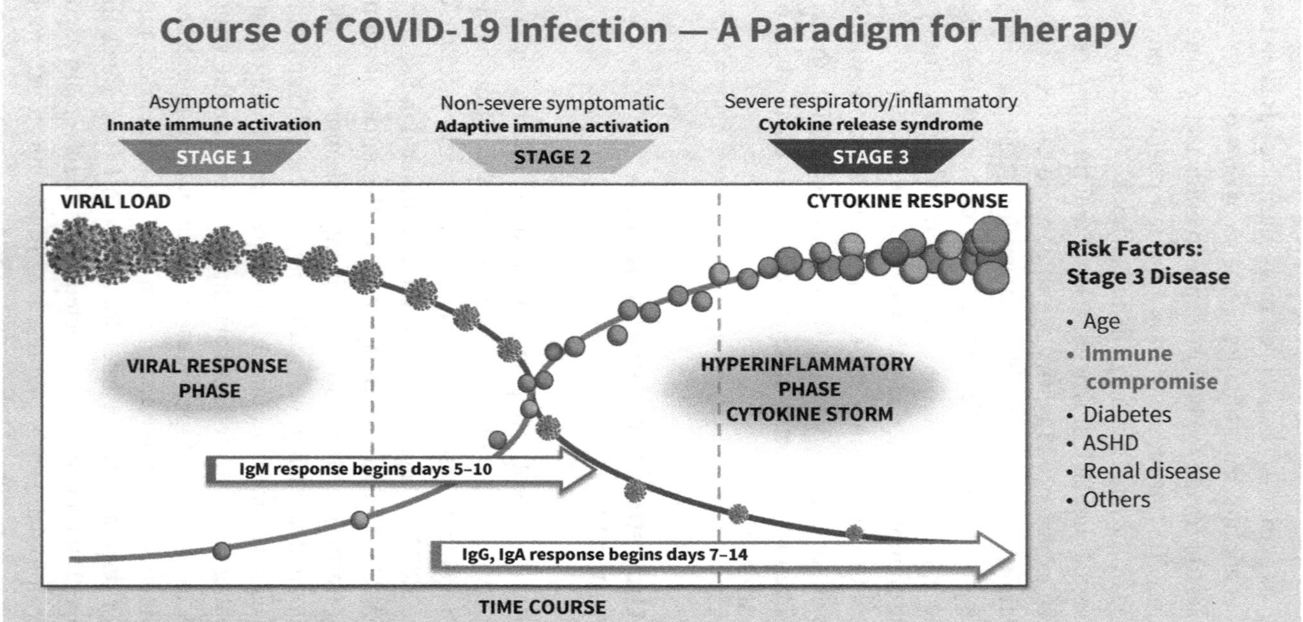

ASHD = arteriosclerotic heart disease; Ig = immunoglobulin.
Calabrese LH. *Cleve Clin J Med.* 2020;87(7):389–393.

Figure 3.6.1 This figure provides an overview of the clinical course of COVID-19 disease, highlighting the different stages, immune responses, and the potential for long-lasting symptoms in some individuals. Understanding these stages is crucial for the management and care of COVID-19 patients.

can be fatal in 1%–2% of infected individuals.[5] Following the acute phase of COVID-19 disease—regardless of whether patients experience a biphasic (Phase 1 and 2) or triphasic (Phases 1 through 3) illness—recovery is experienced over a variable time course in the majority of patients. A growing concern regarding infection with SARS CoV-2 is the recognition of the persistence or recrudescence of symptoms long after the acute phases of the infection are over. This phenomenon has been given several names, including long COVID or post–acute sequelae of SARS CoV-2 infection (PASC). While lacking a uniform definition, *long COVID* generally refers to symptoms that persist beyond 30 days and frequently persist to 180 days or longer.[6] It is estimated to occur in up to one in three COVID patients.

Each stage of the COVID-19 disease carries unique implications for placebo and nocebo effects from the process of being diagnosed to recovery and/ or sequelae.

Long COVID

Among all sequelae from COVID-19 infection, long COVID will likely become both the greatest public health problem in the foreseeable future, as well as the greatest opportunity and challenge for the field of placebo and nocebo science. In terms of scope alone, the data are staggering: as of January 2022, the US Centers for Disease Control and Prevention estimates over 150 million Americans have been infected with SARS CoV-2, and (conservatively) an estimated 10%–15% may develop long COVID, totaling somewhere between 15 and 22 million individuals in the United States alone.[7] The disorder itself has no clearly delineated consensus definition and no diagnostic tests; it is associated with a myriad of unknowns, making it easier to describe clinically than to understand pathogenically. Thus, the syndrome of long COVID is surrounded by both misery and mystery and is a logical target for the investigation of nocebo effects.

In terms of its clinical spectrum long COVID is vast, with one meta-analysis describing over 50 long-term effects, including fatigue, mental fogginess, viscero-somatic pain, autonomic dysfunction, and dyspnea.[8] Epidemiologically, the disease is more common in females and older aged individuals, and is more frequently observed following more severe forms of COVID-19 illness, but it can be seen following mild and possibly even asymptomatic infection.[9] In many ways it is not dissimilar from other poorly understood disorders of a postinfective nature such as myalgic encephalomyelitis (ME/CFS) and post Lyme disease,[10] which are also within the realm of medically unexplained disorders. Collectively, patients with long COVID and related postinfectious disorders are frequently dismissed by clinicians who lack understanding of these conditions and often ascribe them to the realm of psychosomatic illnesses arising as a result of anxiety.[10] Even now, 2 full years into the pandemic, there is no way to predict how long recovery takes nor, indeed, what proportion of patients with long COVID will actually recover. These uncertainties only add to the deep concerns surrounding the disorder. In the early phases of the pandemic, little attention from the medical establishment was given to long COVID, but thankfully, through a combination of patient advocacy and a massive funding effort of 1.1 billion dollars by the National Institutes of Health, there is now a strong push to unravel long COVID at all levels.[11]

From a pathogenesis perspective, there is no clear or predominant theory of the cause of long COVID, but many hold biologic plausibility including underlying comorbidities (physical and/or psychologic), organ damage from acute infection, persistent and/or restricted viral replication, persistent immune activation and/or autoimmune responses, and unknown mechanisms. Most prominent among the putative mechanisms is aberrant immune activation, either from virally induced loss of self-tolerance with autoantibody formation or alternatively the untoward effects of persistent viral infection.[12] More recently work has begun to advance our understanding of the lingering neurological symptoms including loss of attention and concentration (i.e., brain fog), which are emblematic of long COVID, demonstrating in both a preclinical model of SARS CoV-2 infection, as well from analysis of human brain tissue that the neuropathology induced by this virus demonstrated numerous similarities to those found in cancer chemotherapy induced neuropathology which bears many clinical similarities ("chemo brain")[13] (see Box 3.6.1).[14] The role of premorbid disease sates and psychological and personality profiles are poorly understood but all-important considerations to fully understand the syndrome. Clearly a great deal of basic translational and clinical research is needed to address this impending public health challenge.

There are currently more unanswered questions than answers surrounding long COVID, which in itself contributes to giving the syndrome meaning. Once internalized, this meaning—surrounded by mystery and associated with great potential morbidity—may itself generate a nocebo effect, belying some of the many symptoms described in patients with long COVID. Thus, it is logical to investigate the role of nocebo effects in both etiopathogenesis as well as in long COVID's clinical expressions. Finally, the effects of a nocebo

---

BOX 3.6.1 Potential causes of long COVID

---

1. Unmasking of underlying comorbidities (physical and/or psychological)
2. Residual damage from acute infection
3. Persistent or restricted viral replication
4. Persistent immune activation and/or autoimmune response
5. Untoward neuropathological effects of SARS Co-V2
6. Unknown mechanisms

---

effect must be explored when considering therapies for a condition that is dominated by subjective symptoms (e.g., fatigue, brain fog, and pain) and lacks a diagnostic test or effective treatments.

Placebo and nocebo effects before and at time of infection

As mentioned above the majority of patients with COVID-19 disease experience asymptomatic or pauci-symptomatic illness and, in the absence of laboratory testing, may be unaware they were infected at all. Factors favoring a mild disease course include young age, good general health, and nonobese body habitus. The immunologic basis for those who experience severe disease is still incompletely understood, but nascent stages of chronic inflammation (possibly because of underlying disease or life style factors) may be contributory. Unproven, but meritorious of further research, are the influences of numerous acquired physiologic changes that all share some degree of chronic inflammation potentially brought on or exacerbated by COVID-19-related disruptions of the social matrix.[15] As noted above, the COVID-19 pandemic has been associated with not only an increase in psychological distress but a variety of physical disturbances in the general population, including sleep disorders, eating disorders, physical inactivity, circulatory disorders, and pain.[16-18] These physiologic disturbances in themselves have been linked to chronic low-grade inflammation, which is a known risk factor for more severe COVID-19 disease.

Nocebo effects on self-diagnosis of COVID-19

Diagnosis of the clinical syndrome of COVID-19 can be straightforward when accompanied by loss of smell or taste (anosmia and/or aguesia)—both of which have been relatively specific for infection with SARS CoV-2 in comparison to other respiratory viruses. However, these symptoms are absent in over 50% of patients[19] and have been anecdotally noted to be largely absent with COVID-19 arising from the most recent Omicron variant. For many, then, the clinical diagnosis by either a health care provider or by self-assessment are reliant on a rather nonspecific constellation of signs and symptoms shared by many other respiratory pathogens. Laboratory testing is limited in diagnostic accuracy; PCR is both the most sensitive and specific testing available, while rapid home test kits may suffer from reduced sensitivity, especially in patients with mild infection. Serum antibody tests are available to detect more remote cases by assessing reactivity to the nucleoprotein component of the virus; importantly, this component is not elicited by the vaccination process. Serum antibody testing is not widely performed; the results are often misinterpreted, and such testing also suffers from a lack of specificity with some evidence of cross reactivity to other coronaviruses which are frequently responsible for seasonal colds.[20] As a result, there is a contingency of individuals who have not undergone diagnostic testing for COVID-19 or who have had negative tests but yet have a strong belief that they are (or were) infected. There have been several analyses by a single group which has examined such a cohort to assess what psychological factors may favor the individual belief of COVID-19 infection.[21,22] In these studies, anxiety was the leading predictor of reporting COVID-like illness; a high level of conscientiousness personality trait was also independently associated with this belief. The authors concluded that these factors may contribute to patients over-reporting bodily experiences. A major limitation of this study is a lack of laboratory testing to confirm or refute evidence of actual infection, as the vast majority of patients responded that they had not undergone such testing.

Placebo and nocebo effects and long COVID

Thus far there is a lack of empirical data on the association of nocebo effect and long COVID, but there are strong reasons for questioning the potential for nocebo effects to influence the development and clinical expression of the syndrome. The nocebo effect (from the Latin "I harm") describes when a negative outcome occurs because of a belief that an intervention will cause harm; it is the opposite of the placebo effect. In support of this assertion is the fact that long COVID is enmeshed with numerous negative contextual factors that have arisen from the pandemic (e.g., severe illness and death, contagion, the effects of quarantine and lockdown, and changing scientific information). These factors have been associated with the rise in psychological morbidity including anxiety, depression and posttraumatic stress.[6] This is important because psychological morbidities may contribute to the development of long COVID, either causally or as amplifiers of the syndrome. Previous studies of postinfectious forms of chronic fatigue have identified numerous social, behavioral, cognitive, and emotional factors.[23] These factors will be important areas of study that we hope will provide some level of clarity about the pathogenesis of long COVID, its severity and durability. Studies of psychological cofactors in patients recovering from acute COVID-19 have revealed significant anxiety and depression in up to 30%–40% of individuals acutely, and evidence of anxiety, depression, and sleep disorders in at least one quarter at 6 months;[6] new onset psychiatric diseases have been observed in 18% of patients within the first 90 days of acute COVID-19.[24] Importantly many of these same psychological comorbidities have been linked to nocebo effects and responses.[25,26] Ultimately, as biomedical research begins to unravel long COVID's mysteries, it will likely be found not to arise from one common cause or pathway nor be one single disease. Rather it appears more likely that it may arise from numerous mechanisms and be frequently confounded by neuropsychological amplifiers with resultant nocebo effects.

In terms of placebo effects and long COVID, this too is relatively unexplored, and empiric data are currently lacking. Nevertheless, for patients with long COVID, the strategic use of the placebo effect by leveraging the practitioner-patient encounter is potentially important. There is growing scientific evidence that the placebo effect may alter patients' signs and symptoms, as neuroimaging studies have demonstrated that brain areas related to the mind and cognitive processing are involved in the neurobiological basis of the patient-practitioner interaction.[25,27] A practical approach and discussion of how to apply these findings in the daily care of patients with long COVID has recently been proposed; these recommendations for optimizing symptom management by leveraging the placebo effect are shown in Box 3.6.2.[28] Formal study of this approach in the management of long COVID and other similar postinfective disease states is urgently needed.

BOX 3.6.2 Six recommendations for leveraging the patient-clinician interaction to optimize symptom management in patients with COVID-19

- Treat the symptoms and causes while empathically understanding the patient's experience of sickness
- Recognize that the diagnosis itself of long COVID carries with it a strong personal dimension
- Validate patients' symptoms and expunge them of guilt
- Dispel patients' fears surrounding the diagnosis of long COVID
- Establish a genuine working relationship with the patient
- Find meaning and compassion in order to minimize burnout when facing a complex problem such as long COVID

General effects of the pandemic and nocebo effects

The emergence of a new and highly contagious virus, the authorization of new vaccine with a novel mechanism of action, and nocebo effects are the ingredients for a perfect storm with the ability to leave heretofore unheard-of levels of emotional and physical damage in its wake. It is axiomatic that cognitive and emotional factors (which are influenced by beliefs and psychological makeup) mediate the perceptive experience of the individual;[29] when these factors are negative, the risk for nocebo effects increases. This framework helps us understand how the COVID-19 pandemic has influenced the perceptive experience at both individual and societal levels. The notion that negative diagnoses can carry powerful nocebo or nocebo-like effects is widely recognized,[25] and it is clear that COVID-19 has profound negative meaning and thus carries such potential. The constellation of contagion, death, and economic strife gives rise to feelings of fear, loss, and estrangement. These feelings in turn form a basis for powerful nocebo effects that, it has been suggested, may contribute to a state of mass hysteria.[30] Under these circumstances it is not surprising that typical buffers, such as the words of trusted leaders or communications regarding the remarkable advances in scientific technology, have done little to assuage the negative meaning of COVID-19. Negative framing of accurate information can contribute to stress, with important neuropsychiatric implications.[26] Stress also occurs when accurate, appropriately framed public health messaging is necessarily changed based on shifting scientific information. Lastly, the effects of lockdowns and the resultant social isolation felt by virtually all individuals at one or more points in the pandemic have provided further stressors.[16,31] Data from the US Centers for Disease Control and Prevention reveal that two in five US adults said they were struggling with mental health issues, especially anxiety, depression, and/or substance use. Younger adults, racial/ethnic minorities, essential workers, and those with preexisting psychiatric conditions suffer the most.[32] The implications of these collective sources of stress and uncertainty provide fertile ground for nocebo effects at virtually all stages of the pandemic; a list of potential nocebo effects from "mass hysteria" to psychological morbidities with or without attendant physical symptoms (e.g., fatigue, pain, and mental fog), from self-reported acute COVID-19 in the absence of laboratory confirmation to long COVID in the absence of evidence of COVID-19.

Placebo and nocebo effects and vaccination practices and outcomes

The world is in a race to vaccinate rapidly as many individuals as possible; achieving this goal is viewed as the best single hope to mitigate the pandemic over the long term. While costs, resource allocation, and logistics cannot be over-emphasized as formidable problems in reaching universal vaccination, vaccine hesitancy and vaccine refusal are even larger obstacles in many areas—even in wealthy and advanced countries such as the United States. Vaccine hesitancy is an important public health problem to understand. Across numerus studies vaccine hesitancy (as opposed to vaccine refusal on religious or political grounds) has been linked to fear of adverse effects.[33] It is important and ironic that many of the adverse effects of vaccines may be caused by nocebo effects, as has been clearly demonstrated with COVID-19 vaccines. In the pivotal trial of the Pfizer m-RNA vaccine, conducted in 40,000 individuals, fatigue following the first shot was reported in 23% to 33%; headache in 18% to 34%; and myalgia in 8% to 11%, which may suggest evidence of the power of nocebo effects.[34] A systematic review of adverse effects (AEs) in COVID-19 vaccine trials in both active and placebo arms found that solicited adverse events, especially headache, fatigue, and myalgia were common in both the active and the placebo groups, and while more common in the active group, they were formidable in those receiving placebo and, interestingly, tended to occur more frequently in younger patients not on medications.[35] A recent meta-analysis of all published vaccine trials for COVID-19 in adults calculated that 75% of systemic AEs after the first dose and 52% of the adverse events after the second dose were nocebo responses.[36] Collectively these data strongly suggest that a substantial proportion of solicited AEs are not a result of the vaccine per se but are, in fact, nocebo effects. A reasonable interpretation would lead to endorsement of the expectancy theory, which, in other words, is the result of a self-fulfilling prophecy leading to nocebo effects. Another study of patients with autoimmune conditions examined vaccine hesitancy and found that it appeared to correlate with nocebo-prone behavior.[37] Unfortunately, despite remarkable progress in the science of vaccine development, there is at the same time increasing uncertainty among vaccine-hesitant and -resistant individuals, owing to a multitude of factors. These include the emergence of variants which now appear to escapee our original vaccines' effectiveness and in some minds represent a failure or breach of trust of science as opposed to complexities of an evolving viral pandemic. Further, changing messages surround scheduling and numbers of vaccines, and the likely need for future vaccines also can contribute to uncertainty, distrust, and fear among those who have been resistant or hesitant from the beginning. Recognizing the societal stresses associated with such uncertainty both now and in the future will be important in crafting messaging to encourage vaccine uptake. Strategies which address nocebo-prone behavior (e.g., assuaging fear with techniques such as positive framing and providing easy to understand education) may provide avenues to increase vaccine uptake and coverage both now and in the future.

Conclusions

The COVID-19 pandemic has revealed great stressors within our society and within individuals. The studies of placebo and nocebo effects have great relevance at all levels of the pandemic, from early phases of disease acquisition and recognition to post-COVID sequelae including long COVID. Lessons can be learned in the field of vaccinology by investigating these same domains in an effort to understand vaccine toxicity and increase vaccine coverage.

References

1. Cinelli M, Quattrociocchi W, Galeazzi A, et al. The COVID-19 social media infodemic. *Scientific Reports.* 2020;10(1):16598.
2. Sagan C. *The Demon-Haunted World: Science As a Candle in the Dark.* Random House; 1995.
3. Calabrese LH. Cytokine storm and the prospects for immunotherapy with COVID-19. *Cleveland Clinic Journal of Medicine.* 2020;87(7):389–393.

4. Fisman DN, Tuite AR. Asymptomatic infection is the pandemic's dark matter. *Proceedings of the National Academy of Sciences of the United States of America.* 2021;118(38):e2114054118. doi:10.1073/pnas.2114054118.

5. Berlin DA, Gulick RM, Martinez FJ. Severe Covid-19. *New England Journal of Medicine.* 2020;383(25):2451–2460. doi:10.1056/NEJMcp2009575.

6. Nalbandian A, Sehgal K, Gupta A, et al. Post-acute COVID-19 syndrome. *Nature Medicine.* 2021;27(4):601–615.

7. Phillips S, Williams MA. Confronting our next national health disaster —Long-haul Covid. *New England Journal of Medicine.* 2021;385(7):577–579.

8. Lopez-Leon S, Wegman-Ostrosky T, Perelman C, et al. More than 50 long-term effects of COVID-19: a systematic review and meta-analysis. *Scientific Reports.* 2021;11(1):16144.

9. Huang Y, Pinto MD, Borelli JL, Asgari Mehrabadi M, Abrahim HL, Dutt N, Lambert N, Nurmi EL, Chakraborty R, Rahmani AM, Downs CA. COVID symptoms, symptom clusters, and predictors for becoming a long-hauler: Looking for clarity in the haze of the pandemic. *Clinical Nursing Research.* 2022;31(8):1390–1398. doi:10.1177/10547738221125632.

10. Sigal LH. What is causing the "long-hauler" phenomenon after COVID-19? *Cleveland Clinic Journal of Medicine.* 2021;88(5):273–278.

11. Kennedy NA, Jones GR, Lamb CA, et al. British Society of Gastroenterology guidance for management of inflammatory bowel disease during the COVID-19 pandemic. *Gut.* 2020;69(6):984–990.

12. Knight JS, Caricchio R, Casanova JL, Combes AJ, Diamond B, Fox SE, Hanauer DA, James JA, Kanthi Y, Ladd V, Mehta P, Ring AM, Sanz I, Selmi C, Tracy RP, Utz PJ, Wagner CA, Wang JY, McCune WJ. The intersection of COVID-19 and autoimmunity. *Journal of Clinical Investigation.* 2021;131(24):e154886. doi:10.1172/JCI154886.

13. Fernández-Castañeda A, Lu P, Geraghty AC, et al. Mild respiratory COVID can cause multi-lineage neural cell and myelin dysregulation. *Cell.* 2022;185(14):2452–2468.e16. doi:10.1016/j.cell.2022.06.008.

14. Nath A. Long-haul COVID. *Neurology.* 2020;95(13):559–560.

15. Brodin P. Immune determinants of COVID-19 disease presentation and severity. *Nature Medicine.* 2021;27(1):28–33.

16. Colloca L, Thomas S, Yin M, Haycock NR, Wang Y. Pain experience and mood disorders during the lockdown of the COVID-19 pandemic in the United States: An opportunistic study. *Pain Reports.* 2021;6(3):e958.

17. Furman D, Campisi J, Verdin E, et al. Chronic inflammation in the etiology of disease across the life span. *Nature Medicine.* 2019;25(12):1822–1832.

18. Nieman DC. Coronavirus disease-2019: A tocsin to our aging, unfit, corpulent, and immunodeficient society. *Journal of Sport and Health Science.* 2020;9(4):293–301.

19. Antonelli M, Capdevila J, Chaudhari A, et al. Optimal symptom combinations to aid COVID-19 case identification: Analysis from a community-based, prospective, observational cohort. *Journal of Infection.* 2021;82(3):384–390.

20. Wang IE, Cooper G, Mousa SA. Diagnostic approaches for COVID-19 and its associated complications. *Diagnostics (Basel).* 2021;11(11):2071. doi:10.3390/diagnostics11112071.

21. Daniali H, Flaten MA. What psychological factors make individuals believe they are infected by coronavirus 2019? *Frontiers in Psychology.* 2021;12:667722.

22. Daniali H, Flaten MA. Experiencing COVID-19 symptoms without the disease: The role of nocebo in reporting of symptoms. *Scandinavian Journal of Public Health.* 2022;50(1):61–69. doi:10.1177/14034948211018385. Epub 2021 May 27.

23. Hulme K, Hudson JL, Rojczyk P, Little P, Moss-Morris R. Biopsychosocial risk factors of persistent fatigue after acute infection: A systematic review to inform interventions. *Journal of Psychosomatic Research.* 2017;99:120–129.

24. Taquet M, Dercon Q, Luciano S, Geddes JR, Husain M, Harrison PJ. Incidence, co-occurrence, and evolution of long-COVID features: A 6-month retrospective cohort study of 273,618 survivors of COVID-19. *PLoS Medicine*. 2021;18(9):e1003773.

25. Colloca L, Barsky AJ. Placebo and Nocebo Effects. *New England Journal of Medicine*. 2020;382(6):554–561.

26. Amanzio M, Howick J, Bartoli M, Cipriani GE, Kong J. How do nocebo phenomena provide a theoretical framework for the COVID-19 pandemic? *Frontiers in Psychology*. 2020;11:589884.

27. Schenk LA, Colloca L. The neural processes of acquiring placebo effects through observation. *Neuroimage*. 2020;209:116510.

28. Calabrese L, Colloca L. Long COVID-19 and the role of the patient-clinician interaction in symptom management. *Journal of Patient Experience*. 2022;9:23743735221077514. doi:10.1177/23743735221077514.

29. Benedetti F, Lanotte M, Lopiano L, Colloca L. When words are painful: Unraveling the mechanisms of the nocebo effect. *Neuroscience*. 2007;147(2):260–271.

30. Bagus P, Peña-Ramos JA, Sánchez-Bayón A. COVID-19 and the political economy of mass hysteria. *International Journal of Environmental Research and Public Health*. 2021;18(4):1376. doi:10.3390/ijerph18041376.

31. Torales J, O'Higgins M, Castaldelli-Maia JM, Ventriglio A. The outbreak of COVID-19 coronavirus and its impact on global mental health. *Indian Journal of Social Psychiatry*. 2020;66(4):317–320.

32. Czeisler M, Drane A, Winnay SS, et al. Mental health, substance use, and suicidal ideation among unpaid caregivers of adults in the United States during the COVID-19 pandemic: Relationships to age, race/ethnicity, employment, and caregiver intensity. *Journal of Affective Disorders*. 2021;295:1259–1268.

33. Rief W. Fear of adverse effects and COVID-19 vaccine hesitancy: Recommendations of the treatment expectation expert group. *JAMA Health Forum*. 2021;2(4):e210804. doi:10.1001/jamahealthforum.2021.0804.

34. Polack FP, Thomas SJ, Kitchin N, et al. Safety and efficacy of the BNT162b2 mRNA Covid-19 vaccine. *New England Journal of Medicine*. 2020;383(27):2603–2615.

35. Amanzio M, Mitsikostas DD, Giovannelli F, Bartoli M, Cipriani GE, Brown WA. Adverse events of active and placebo groups in SARS-CoV-2 vaccine randomized trials: A systematic review. *Lancet Regional Health Europe*. 2022;12:100253. doi:10.1016/j.lanepe.2021.100253.

36. Haas JW, Bender FL, Ballou S, et al. Frequency of adverse events in the placebo arms of COVID-19 vaccine trials: A systematic review and meta-analysis. *JAMA Network Open*. 2022;5(1):e2143955.

37. Fragoulis GE, Evangelatos G, Arida A, et al. Nocebo-prone behaviour in patients with autoimmune rheumatic diseases during the COVID-19 pandemic. *Mediterranean Journal of Rheumatology*. 2020;31(Suppl 2):288–294.

4

PLACEBOS AND NOCEBOS IN MENTAL ILLNESSES

This Section offers a comprehensive exploration of placebo effects and expectations within clinical interventions, shedding light on their underlying mechanisms and potential applications. By understanding and harnessing these phenomena, we can further enhance treatment outcomes and optimize healthcare practices. The first chapter presents a conceptual model that elucidates the contribution of placebo responses in antidepressant treatment. Factors such as expectancy and physician contact are highlighted as influential elements, and their manipulation holds the potential to optimize placebo responses in both pharmacotherapy research and clinical practice. Moving forward, the second chapter focuses on placebo and nocebo effects in depression, examining their mechanisms of action. The discussion revolves around the possibility that placebos could offer substantial benefits comparable to antidepressants, while avoiding medication side effects, with potential implications for clinical trial design. The role of participant expectations in cognitive training interventions takes center stage in the third chapter. While cognitive training has demonstrated improvements in cognition, the impact of expectations or placebo effects on these outcomes is examined to mitigate their influence or harness them to maximize intervention effectiveness. Lastly, the fourth chapter explores the transformation of placebos, particularly open-label placebos, from deceptive controls to a form of psychotherapy. It contemplates the integration of open-label placebos into psychotherapy and reflects on the possibilities and benefits that arise from this fusion.

4.1

A model of placebo responses in antidepressant clinical trials

Sigal Zilcha-Mano and Bret R. Rutherford

Historical background: placebo responses as nuisance, threat to drug development, and potential therapeutically

Major depressive disorder (MDD) is the leading cause of disability worldwide.[1] Antidepressant medication (ADM) is a commonly prescribed, effective treatment for MDD[2] that remedies dysfunctional activations in brain regions related to MDD. Yet it is also true that a substantial proportion of the response observed to clinical treatment with antidepressants is not due to specific effects of the medication (i.e., serotonin reuptake inhibition) but rather to nonspecific features of the treatment. Meta-analyses of placebo-controlled antidepressant trials show that medication response averages approximately 50%, whereas placebo response rates are typically 30%–35%.[3]

Substantial placebo responses generally have been viewed as a nuisance to be eliminated in pharmacologic research and clinical practice. Historically, the patient variables explored as predictors of placebo responses were histrionic traits, such as suggestibility, which were in general not considered desirable traits for an individual to possess. In addition, prevailing models construed the therapeutic action of ADM as being incremental, delayed (i.e., after 4 weeks), and persistent,[4] as opposed to the "abrupt" and transient pattern of response associated with a placebo.[4] This contrast between "true drug" effects and placebo responses conceptualized the latter in pejorative terms that did not lead investigators to take up placebo responses as a phenomenon worthy of serious scientific investigation.

In addition, the high magnitude of placebo responses relative to medication response posed significant challenges to new drug development and led to methodological changes in clinical trials aimed at minimizing placebo response. Increasing numbers of failed trials have made developing psychiatric medications progressively more time-consuming and expensive.[5] These considerations led several large pharmaceutical companies to reduce or discontinue research and development on medications for brain disorders. Moreover, media coverage of failed trials has been used as a platform for critiques of the pharmaceutical industry and questioning the efficacy of antidepressants, which may have the dangerous public health consequence of dissuading patients with depression from accessing treatment.

Newer data suggested a need to revisit previous assumptions and question whether placebo responses in fact represented true, durable change in a patient's depression. Meta-analyses of clinical trial data reported similar time courses of response by medication- and placebo-treated patients.[6] Findings suggested that one-third of all patients, irrespective of whether they received a placebo or ADM, showed sudden symptom improvements, which were often sustained over time.[7] Data-driven approaches further suggested that most individuals receiving antidepressant medication do not show a more distinct pattern of early treatment symptomatic change than do those receiving a placebo.[8] Rather than being restricted to suggestible individuals, it was appreciated that most any individual is capable of experiencing placebo responses.[9]

Most importantly, insights into the neuroscience of placebo effects led to increased interest in placebo effects as tools to understand both the pathophysiology of specific disorders such as depression and the mechanisms of brain regulatory systems across disorders.[10] For example, studies of placebo analgesia[11] found that the anticipation of pain relief was associated with activations in orbitofrontal, dorsolateral prefrontal, parietal, and pregenual anterior cingulate cortices, which modulated activity in parts of the insula, thalamus, and cingulate cortex associated with pain,[11] possibly by potentiating pain-related opioid release.[12] Such top-down modulation underlying expectancy effects was supported by further research in both pain and depression.[13] The possibility arose of harnessing these internal self-regulatory capacities as a means of safely optimizing therapeutic outcomes.

A model of placebo effects in antidepressant clinical trials

It is heuristically useful to differentiate placebo *responses*, which refer to the directly observable treatment responses occurring among individuals randomly assigned to placebo in a clinical trial, from placebo *effects*, which represent a conceptual cause of placebo responses. Specifically, a *placebo effect* can be defined as a genuine effect of a substance or procedure upon a target disorder that is not due to the inherent powers of the substance or proce-dure.[14] From that definition it is apparent that clinical trials comprise many sources of placebo responses that are not attributable to placebo effects (see Figure 4.1.1).

For example, individuals with MDD may experience spontaneous improve-ment and worsening unrelated to the study procedures.[15] Patients with MDD typically experience symptoms for several months prior to seeking treat-ment.[16] Those who choose to enroll in a clinical trial during a time of peak symptomatology may experience alleviation in the precipitating stressors and a natural waning of symptoms. A meta-analysis of acute symptom changes among participants in wait-list control conditions in psychotherapy studies re-ported an average improvement of four Hamilton Rating Scale for Depression (HRSD) points over a mean follow-up duration of 10 weeks. This magnitude of change is approximately 33% of the average improvement occurring with medication treatment and 40% of the improvement seen with placebo admin-istration in clinical trials.[17]

In addition, clinical trials contain sources of bias and error inherent in measuring depressive symptoms. Regression to the mean is a statistical phe-nomenon occurring when repeated measurements associated with random error are made on the same individual over time.[18] Regression to the mean

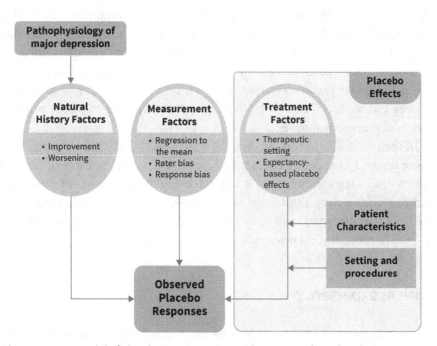

Figure 4.1.1 A model of placebo responses in antidepressant clinical trials.

poses a problem at the group level in clinical trials because a threshold depression severity score is set as an inclusion criterion, and some enrolled participants in the study have true means below this threshold. Rater bias occurs when an individual's rating of symptom severity in an antidepressant clinical trial is influenced by underlying beliefs or motivations with respect to the treatments under study.[19] Conversely, response biases on the part of participants occur when respondents choose the responses that they perceive to be the most socially desirable or that is favored by the clinicians in a research study.[20]

True placebo effects contrast with these sources of placebo responses that either are unrelated to study procedures (i.e., natural history) or do not involve true change in a patient's depression (i.e., rater bias and regression to the mean). First, taking a pill believed to be an effective treatment for depression may generate an expectancy of improvement in a patient, which may directly influence medication response[21–22] or lead to symptom reduction via positive behavioral changes (e.g., improved compliance). Second, medications are provided in the context of therapeutic contacts with doctors and other research staff that possess many elements in common with supportive psychotherapy.[23] Patients are given diagnoses and psycho-education to explain their symptoms. They regularly meet with research staff who listen to their experiences and are encouraged to have faith in the potential effectiveness of the treatment. Each clinic visit in an antidepressant randomized controlled trial (RCT) amounts to an additional "dose" of these therapeutic factors that may influence medication response. In the case of patients assigned to a placebo, expectancy of improvement, positive behavioral change, and the therapeutic contacts provided during clinic visits (in combination with natural history factors and measurement error) are hypothesized to be the primary causes of placebo responses.

In the remainder of this chapter, we review recent research on patient expectancy and therapeutic contact with providers as mechanisms of placebo effects in antidepressant trials. We synthesize findings based on meta-analyses indirectly indicating the effects of expectancy and therapeutic contact, as well as RCTs designed to directly investigate their effects. We conclude with implications for clinical practice and future research.

Patient expectancy

A growing body of literature suggests that a significant portion of the improvement observed in clinical trials is due to active neurobiological processes related to expectancy.[24] *Expectation* and *expectancy* are interchangeable terms referring to an individual's beliefs about future events. In the context of antidepressant clinical trials, they refer to expectations about the outcome of treatment and to how a patient estimates the probabilities associated with various future scenarios, including anticipated positive or negative effects of treatment.[24] Patients entering treatment have an outcome expectation based on their understanding of the treatment offered, their own illness, and experiences with past treatments. *Expectancy* is a dynamic construct that may change during the course of treatment as a function of many factors, such as the patient's therapeutic alliance with the physician, initial treatment benefits or side effects, and the severity of the patient's illness.

Several studies tested the association between expectancy and outcome in antidepressant trials and found that higher expectancy was associated with better treatment outcome.[25-27] Meta-analyses suggest that antidepressant response rates are higher in open-label studies, where patients are certain of receiving an active drug, compared to placebo-controlled RCTs, in which their chances of receiving an active drug are lower. Rutherford et al.[21] conducted a systematic analysis of clinical trials of antidepressants for MDD in adults. In the 48 placebo-controlled and 42 comparator trials examined, the odds of being classified as a responder to medication in comparator trials were 1.8 times higher than the odds of being classified as a responder in placebo-controlled trials, and the odds of being classified as a remitter to medication in comparator trials were 1.5 times higher than the odds of being classified as a remitter in placebo-controlled trials. In a sample of patients with late life depression, Sneed et al.[28] found the odds of being classified as responder in comparator trials were nearly two times higher than the odds of responding in the placebo-controlled trials.

Interestingly, whereas patient expectancy strongly influences response rates to medication and placebos in depressed adults, it appears to be less important in the treatment of children and adolescents with depression. Specifically, a meta-analysis based on data derived from nine open, four active comparator, and 18 placebo-controlled studies of antidepressants for children and adolescents with depressive disorders suggests that no significant difference in medication response emerged between comparator and placebo-controlled studies.[29] One explanation of these findings is that generating treatment expectancies requires relatively advanced cognitive capacities, as well as receiving a detailed information disclosure, neither of which may be the case among children in pediatric depression trials.

Just as increasing patient expectancy of benefit may contribute to symptom improvement, decreasing expectancy of benefit may result in a corresponding symptom worsening. A nocebo effect of expectancy in antidepressant trials has been documented as well.[30] Specifically, among adults with MDD responding to a 12-week open treatment, randomization to continued fluoxetine or a placebo for an additional year, resulted in a nocebo effect. The possibility of receiving a placebo following 12 weeks of open fluoxetine was associated with significant symptoms worsening. These results suggest that treatment changes may have influenced patients' expectancies of improvement, which in turn affect their depressive symptoms.

Causal evidence for expectancy effects and their neural mechanisms

Expectancy must be experimentally manipulated to determine whether it causally influences treatment outcome. Searching for a method to effectively manipulate expectancy in an ethical manner, researchers have sought to manipulate therapist style (e.g., optimistic, neutral, and pessimistic), but this approach was not found to be successful in manipulating patients' expectancy and outcome.[31] Our group has developed a methodology to experimentally manipulate expectancy effects prospectively by randomizing individuals to a high-expectancy group (open trial with a 100% chance of receiving an antidepressant medication) versus a low-expectancy group (placebo-controlled trial, where the chances of receiving medication are lower).[32] Using this approach, it is feasible to manipulate expectancy in young adults. Depressed individuals randomly assigned to high-expectancy conditions experience more symptomatic improvement than those in the low-expectancy condition.[33] This finding indicates that despite receiving the identical antidepressant medication, being treated by the same study clinicians, and visiting the same treatment site, depressed individuals who knew they were receiving antidepressant medication improved on average six points more on the HRSD (indicative of a large and clinically significant change) than individuals receiving the exact same drug who were aware they had a chance of receiving a placebo. The difference between antidepressant medication outcomes under high- versus low-expectancy conditions was greater in magnitude than the typically observed differences between drug and placebo responses in antidepressant trials, testifying to the powerful influence of expectancy manipulation.

To understand the neural mechanisms by which expectancy affects MDD, a recent study employed an antidepressant trial design capable of manipulating outcome expectancies with integrated functional magnetic resonance imaging (fMRI).[34] Following the expectancy manipulation, significant differences between the high- versus low-expectancy conditions were found in neural activation changes in the amygdala as well as in superior temporal gyrus, insula, and thalamus. The findings support a mediation model according to which activation in the left amygdala decreased significantly in the high- versus low-expectancy condition in response to sad emotional faces. The reduced left amygdala activation, in turn, was a significant predictor of decreased depressive symptoms, and the mediation model was significant. These findings suggest that therapeutic modulation of amygdala activity may be an important pathway by which patient outcome expectancy influences depressive symptoms. The findings are consistent with another study investigating the neural correlates of response to a 1-week placebo lead-in phase and the association of placebo responses during lead-in with response to brief antidepressant treatment and pointing to the important role of the amygdala.[35]

Integrating such findings with studies of placebo analgesia, it appears that treatment expectancies, instantiated in activations within prefrontal cortex regions (PFC) critical for the cognitive regulation of emotion, may function by modulating the activity subcortical areas such as the amygdala, nucleus accumbens (NAcc), and insula, which are important for appraising the aversive or rewarding properties of stimuli.[36] There is now evidence to suggest that a PFC-amygdala pathway linked to negative emotional experience and a PFC-NAcc/ventral striatum pathway linked to positive emotional experience may constitute top-down modulatory pathways by which expectancies exert their effects.

As an indirect test of this model, a recent study evaluated neurocognitive predictors of expectancy effects in depressed older adults. Older adults with MDD are a population of great interest in identifying moderators of expectancy-based placebo effects because by virtue of brain aging, they exhibit variability in cognitive (e.g., memory and executive function) and neural (e.g., integrity of frontostriatal tracts, white matter hyperintensities) markers that may be highly relevant to expectancy. Consistent with this possibility, we recently used a combined moderators approach in a population of older adults.[37] We were able to identify a subpopulation of older adults with MDD who benefited from expectancy manipulation: those individuals with intact executive functioning (enabling reappraising responses based on the new expectancy-related information arriving) as well as less reduced integrity of the frontostriatal tract (enabling the modulation of limbic and striatal structures).

The therapeutic context and doctor-patient interaction as a source of placebo effects

Meta-analyses suggest that, irrespective of assignment to a medication or a placebo, more visits with the treating physician may result in significantly greater symptom reduction. Posternak and Zimmerman[6] investigated the influence of therapeutic contact frequency on antidepressant and placebo responses in 41 RCTs of antidepressants for MDD. They calculated the change in HRSD scores observed over the first 6 weeks of treatment in patients assigned to either antidepressant medication or a placebo, comparing studies having six weekly assessments to those having five and four assessments. A cumulative therapeutic effect of additional follow-up visits on placebo responses was found: between weeks 2 and 6, patients with weekly visits improved 4.24 HRSD points, while those with one fewer visit improved 3.33 points, and those with two fewer visits improved 2.49 points. The presence of additional visits explained approximately 50% of the symptom change observed between weeks 2 and 6 among patients receiving a placebo. This was true to a lesser extent for participants receiving active medication, in whom the effect of this increased therapeutic contact was approximately 50% less than in the placebo group. Subsequent meta-analyses have reported convergent findings and extended these results to both children and adolescents with depression,[29] depressed older adults,[38] and individuals with anxiety disorders.[39]

The quantity of therapeutic contact with health care staff provided in a clinical trial has major implications for detecting a signal of effect between antidepressant medication and a placebo. Rutherford et al.[38] reported in antidepressant trials for late life depression a significant treatment assignment by visits interaction, whereby increased visit frequency dramatically decreased the average difference between the medication and placebo arms. For a 12-week placebo-controlled study, providing six clinic visits resulted in an average medication response rate of 51.7% and placebo response rate of 39.5%. Intensifying supportive care from 6 to 10 visits over 12 weeks resulted in a reduction of the average medication/placebo difference from 12.2% to 0.4%. While these analyses are suggestive of a relationship between visit frequency and treatment outcome, they leave unclear whether it is the amount of contact with health care staff itself that is the therapeutic factor leading to increased medication and placebo responses or whether visit frequency is a marker for more specific aspects of the doctor-patient interaction.

Direct support of the importance of a strong therapeutic doctor-patient relationship in antidepressant trials comes from studies assessing the associations between measures of the *therapeutic relationship*, most commonly defined as the working alliance, and treatment outcome.[40] The *working alliance* is commonly defined as the emotional bond established in the therapeutic dyad, and the agreement between the two about the goals of therapy and the tasks necessary to achieve them.[41] Downing and Rickels[42] were among the first to speculate that nonpharmacologic factors, such as the doctor-patient bond, might affect medication and placebo responses. The first data were reported in Krupnick et al.'s[43] analysis of the Treatment of Depression Collaborative Research Program (TDCRP), in which early and mean therapeutic alliance ratings were found to predict imipramine and placebo responses. More recent findings suggest that the alliance served as a common factor in the antidepressant medication condition but functioned as an active specific ingredient mostly in the placebo condition.[44]

Causal evidence for therapeutic contact effects and their mechanisms

To infer causality regarding its effect, visit frequency must be manipulated. An ongoing study randomly assigned patients to research frequency management (weekly study visits) versus community frequency management (monthly study visits), and double-blind escitalopram versus placebo. To the best of our knowledge, this is the first study to directly examine the effect of the manipulation of visit frequency on medication and placebo responses. Preliminary findings suggest that increasing visit frequency results in greater treatment response across drug and placebo conditions but that the effect of more frequent study visits is particularly important for placebo responses. The average difference in HRSD between research frequency management and community frequency management for those receiving medication was 3.8 points, while the average difference for those receiving placebo 11.7 points. Based on behavioral coding of the sessions, as well as automatic coding of patient and physician movement and acoustic, further analyses test whether the therapeutic alliance and supportive techniques mediate visit frequency effects, and whether these nonpharmacologic factors have stronger effects in placebo responses than in medication responses. The study has the potential to improve clinical recommendations regarding best-practice clinical management techniques. At present, clinical management techniques follow the Fawcett et al.[45] manual, which is based mainly on clinical intuition. The study has the potential to provide up-to-date, empirically established guidelines for the use of each technique.

Patient characteristics bearing on the magnitude of placebo effects

Identifying clinical and demographic characteristics of placebo versus medication responders has been one of the main aims of placebo research in the last decades. Brown et al.[46] initially identified short episode duration, few previous episodes, good response to previous antidepressant treatment, and low overall symptom severity as key determinants of increased placebo responses.

Weimer et al.[9] conducted a comprehensive review of 31 meta-analyses and systematic reviews of more than 500 randomized placebo-controlled trials in various areas of psychiatry to identify consistent moderators across studies. Based on their review, only one patient disease characteristic was found to be consistently linked to increased placebo responses: low baseline severity of symptoms.

Going beyond a single moderator, which is expected to explain the heterogeneity between individuals who respond to a placebo and those that do not, researchers have combined moderators. By combining multiple weak moderators into a single stronger one of the expectancy effect a clinically useful index emerges. A combined moderator can amplify the effects of weaker, individual moderators. Moreover, each individual moderator alone may provide conflicting treatment indications for a given individual.

Our group has recently demonstrated the benefits of combining different moderators for the purpose of identifying older adults with MDD who may respond to a placebo.[46] Using a machine-learning approach capable of evaluating the contributions of multiple predictor variables, we found that the greatest signal detection between the medication and the placebo in favor of medication was in patients with fewer years of education (≤ 12) who suffered from a longer duration of depression since their first episode (>3.47 years). Compared with medication, the placebo had the greatest response for those who were more educated (>12 years), to the point where the placebo almost outperformed medication.

Conclusions and directions for future research

This chapter discusses a conceptual model for understanding placebo responses in clinical trials for MDD and the empirical findings supporting the proposed model. Consistent with the proposed model, empirical findings support the potential to manipulate expectancy effects to maximize placebo responses in clinical practice and minimize it in clinical trials to allow a more valid testing of antidepressant drugs. The empirical literature suggests that some of the most promising approaches to manipulating placebo effects is manipulating expectancy and the therapeutic relationship.

Several methods have been suggested for manipulating the level of expectancy. One is to provide instructions to patients before the start of treatment regarding their chances of receiving the active drug. As both meta-analyses and RCTs have shown, this is a potent approach to manipulating expectancy.

In clinical practice, a similar approach can be implemented through psycho-education of the patients about findings showing the positive effects of the drugs prescribed to them. Another approach is to restore mechanisms under-pinning expectancy effects when these may be dysfunctional, for example, by enhancing processing speed in older adults with cerebrovascular lesions and executive dysfunction. We are aware of a current study to develop and test computerized cognitive training designed to increase processing speed and restore appropriate treatment expectancies, thereby enhancing antidepres-sant treatment response in older adults with MDD.

Several methods may be suggested to strengthen the therapeutic rela-tionship. One is to manipulate the number of contacts between the patients and clinicians. Based on meta-analyses conducted by our group and on our pilot study, which manipulated the number of visits provided, we recom-mend increasing visits in clinical practice and reducing them to the min-imum needed to ensure safety in clinical trials. The state of the art of clinical practice and research is based on exactly the opposite pattern. Currently, patients receive many more visits in clinical research than in clinical practice. Another approach is to personalize the number of visits and the techniques used by therapists to match patient characteristics (e.g., level of loneliness, social support). Empirical findings from the field of psychotherapy research identify specific techniques that are especially effective in strengthening the therapeutic alliance, such as alliance strengthening supportive work and rup-ture resolution strategies.[47] Additional research points to the ways in which such techniques can be matched to the patient's characteristics and needs to achieve maximum efficacy.[47–49]

Future studies on the factors contributing to placebo effects and their un-derlying mechanisms are crucial for manipulating the placebo effect. Such studies will be instrumental in establishing clear guidelines on how to min-imize placebo responses in clinical research and contribute to the accurate evaluation of new antidepressant medications. Studies crystalizing the factors contributing to placebo effects can also be instrumental in harnessing it in clinical practice to benefit patients.

References

1. Friedrich MJ. Depression is the leading cause of disability around the world. *JAMA.* 2017;317(15):1517–1517.
2. Hollon SD, Thase ME, Markowitz JC. Treatment and prevention of depression. *Psychological Science in the Public Interest.* 2002;3(2):39–77.

3. Kirsch I, Sapirstein G. Listening to Prozac but hearing placebo: A meta-analysis of anti-depressant medications. In: Kirsch I, ed. *How expectancies shape experience*. American Psychological Association; 1999:303–320. https://doi.org/10.1037/10332-012

4. Quitkin FM, Rabkin JG. Heterogeneity of clinical response during placebo treatment. *American Journal of Psychiatry*. 1991;148(2):193.

5. Nutt D, Goodwin G. ECNP summit on the future of CNS drug research in Europe 2011: Report prepared for ECNP by David Nutt and Guy Goodwin. *European Neuropsychopharmacology*. 2011;21(7):495–499.

6. Posternak MA, Zimmerman M. Is there a delay in the antidepressant effect? A meta-analysis. *Journal of Clinical Psychiatry*. 2005;66(2):9889.

7. Zilcha-Mano S, Roose SP, Brown PJ, Rutherford BR. Abrupt symptom improvements in antidepressant clinical trials: Transient placebo effects or therapeutic reality? *Journal of Clinical Psychiatry*. 2019;80:18m12353.

8. Zilcha-Mano S, Roose SP, Brown PJ, Rutherford BR. Early symptom trajectories as predictors of treatment outcome for citalopram versus placebo. *American Association for Geriatric Psychiatry*. 2017;25:654–661.

9. Weimer K, Colloca L, Enck P. Placebo effects in psychiatry-mediators and moderators. *Lancet Psychiatry*. 2015;2:246.

10. Petrie KJ, Rief W. Psychobiological mechanisms of placebo and nocebo effects: Pathways to improve treatments and reduce side effects. *Annual Review of Psychology*. 2019;70:599–625.

11. Wager TD, Rilling JK, Smith EE, et al. Placebo-induced changes in FMRI in the anticipation and experience of pain. *Science*. 2004;303(5661):1162–1167.

12. Wager TD, Scott DJ, Zubieta JK. Placebo effects on human μ-opioid activity during pain. *Proceedings of the National Academy of Sciences*. 2007;104(26):11056–11061.

13. Schafer SM, Geuter S, Wager TD. Mechanisms of placebo analgesia: A dual-process model informed by insights from cross-species comparisons. *Progress in Neurobiology*. 2018;160:101–122.

14. Stewart-Williams S, Podd J. The placebo effect: Dissolving the expectancy versus conditioning debate. *Psychological Bulletin*. 2004;130:324–340.

15. Wright AGC, Woods WC. Personalized models of psychopathology. *Annual Review of Clinical Psychology*. 2020;16:49–74.

16. Kisely S, Scott A, Denney J, Simon G. Duration of untreated symptoms in common mental disorders: Association with outcomes. *British Journal of Psychology*. 2006;189:79–80.

17. Rutherford BR, Mori S, Sneed JR, Pimontel MA, Roose SP. Contribution of spontaneous improvement to placebo response in depression: A meta-analytic review. *Journal of Psychiatric Research*. 2012;46:697–702.

18. Barnett AG, van der Pols JC, Dobson AJ. Regression to the mean: What it is and how to deal with it. *International Journal of Epidemiology*. 2005;34:215–220.

19. Marcus SM, Gorman JM, Tu X. Rater bias in a blinded randomized placebo-controlled psychiatry trial. *Stat Medical*. 2006; 25:2762–2770.

20. Furnham A. Response bias, social desirability and dissimulation. *Personality and Individual Differences*. 1986;7(3):385–400.

21. Rutherford BR, Sneed JR, Roose SP. Does study design affect outcome? The effects of placebo control and treatment duration in antidepressant trials. *Psychotherapy and Psychosomatics*. 2009;78:172–181.

22. Rutherford BR, Marcus SM, Wang P, et al. A randomized, prospective pilot study of patient expectancy and antidepressant outcome. *Psychological Medicine*. 2013;43(5):975–982.

23. Miller MD, Frank E, Reynolds CF. The art of clinical management in pharmacologic trials with depressed elderly patients. *American Journal of Geriatric Psychiatry*. 1999;7:228–234.

24. Rutherford BR, Wager TD, Roose SP. Expectancy effects in the treatment of depression: A review of experimental methodology, effects on patient outcome, and neural mechanisms. *Current Psychiatry Research and Reviews.* 2010;6:1–10.
25. Krell HV, Leuchter AF, Morgan M, Cook IA, Abrams M. Subject expectations of treatment effectiveness and outcome of treatment with an experimental antidepressant. *Journal of Clinical Psychiatry.* 2004;65(9):1174–1179.
26. Meyer B, Pilkonis PA, Krupnick JL, Egan MK, Simmens SJ, Sotsky SM. Treatment expectancies, patient alliance and outcome: Further analyses from the National Institute of Mental Health Treatment of Depression Collaborative Research Program. *Journal of Consulting and Clinical Psychology.* 2002;70(4):1051–1055.
27. Zilcha-Mano S, Brown PJ, Roose SP, Cappetta K, Rutherford BR. Optimizing patient expectancy in the pharmacologic treatment of major depressive disorder. *Psychological Medicine.* 2019;49:2414–2420.
28. Sneed JR, Rutherford BR, Rindskopf D, Lane DT, Sackeim HA, Roose SP. Design makes a difference: A meta-analysis of antidepressant response rates in placebo-controlled versus comparator trials in late-life depression. *American Journal of Geriatric Psychiatry.* 2008;16(1):65–73.
29. Rutherford BR, Sneed JR, Tandler JM, Rindskopf D, Peterson BS, Roose SP. Deconstructing pediatric depression trials: An analysis of the effects of expectancy and therapeutic contact. *Journal of the American Academy of Child & Adolescent Psychiatry.* 2011;50(8):782–795.
30. Rutherford BR, Wall MM, Glass A, Stewart JW. The role of patient expectancy in placebo and nocebo effects in antidepressant trials. *Journal of Clinical Psychiatry.* 2014;75(10):18710.
31. Kemeny ME, Rosenwasser LJ, Panettieri RA, Rose R., Berg-Smith SM, Kline JN. Placebo response in asthma: A robust and objective phenomenon. *Journal of Allergy and Clinical Immunology.* 2007;119(6):1375–1381.
32. Rutherford BR, Roose SP. A model of placebo response in antidepressant clinical trials. *American Journal of Psychiatry.* 2013;170:723–733.
33. Rutherford BR, Wall MM, Brown PJ, et al. Patient expectancy as a mediator of placebo effects in antidepressant clinical trials. *American Journal of Psychiatry.* 2017;174:135–142.
34. Zilcha-Mano S, Brown PJ, Roose SP, Cappetta K, Rutherford BR. Optimizing patient expectancy in the pharmacologic treatment of major depressive disorder. *Psychological Medicine.* 2019;49:2414–2420.
35. Peciña M, Bohnert AS, Sikora M, et al. Association between placebo-activated neural systems and antidepressant responses: Neurochemistry of placebo effects in major depression. *JAMA Psychiatry.* 2015;72(11):1087–1094.
36. O'Doherty JP, Deichmann R, Critchley HD, Dolan RJ. Neural responses during anticipation of a primary taste reward. *Neuron.* 2002;33:815–826.
37. Zilcha-Mano S, Wallace ML, Brown PJ, Sneed J, Roose SP, Rutherford BR. Who benefits most from expectancy effects? A combined neuroimaging and antidepressant trial in depressed older adults. *Translational Psychiatry.* 2021;11(1):1–5.
38. Rutherford BR, Pott E, Tandler JM, Wall MM, Roose SP, Lieberman JA. Placebo response in antipsychotic clinical trials: A meta-analysis. *JAMA Psychiatry.* 2014;71:1409–1421.
39. Rutherford BR, Bailey VS, Schneier FR, Pott E, Brown PJ, Roose SP. Influence of study design on treatment response in anxiety disorder clinical trials. *Depress Anxiety.* 2015;32:944–957.
40. Zilcha-Mano S, Roose SP, Brown PJ, Rutherford BR. Abrupt symptom improvements in antidepressant clinical trials: Transient placebo effects or therapeutic reality? *Journal of Clinical Psychiatry.* 2019;79(1):20250.
41. Bordin ES. The generalizability of the psychoanalytic concept of the working alliance. *Psychotherapy: Theory, Research & Practice.* 1979;16(3):252.

42. Rickels K, Downing RW, Winokur A. Antianxiety drugs: Clinical use in psychiatry. In: Iversen LL, Iversen SD, Snyder SH, eds. *Handbook of Psychopharmacology*. Springer, Boston, MA; 1978:395–430. https://doi.org/10.1007/978-1-4684-3189-6_7

43. Krupnick JL, Sotsky SM, Simmens S, et al. The role of the therapeutic alliance in psychotherapy and pharmacotherapy outcome: Findings in the NIMH Treatment of Depression Collaborative Research Program. *Journal of Consulting and Clinical Psychology*. 1996;64(3):532–539.

44. Zilcha-Mano S, Roose SP, Barber J, Rutherford BR. Therapeutic alliance in antidepressant trials: Cause or effect of symptomatic levels? *Psychotherapy and Psychosomatics*. 2015;84:177–182.

45. Fawcett JPSI., Epstein P, Fiester SJ, Elkin I, Autry JH. Clinical management: Imipramine/placebo administration manual. NIMH Treatment of Depression Collaborative Research Program. *Psychopharmacology Bulletin*. 1987;23:309–324.

46. Brown WA, Johnson MF, Chen MG. Clinical features of depressed patients who do and do not improve with placebo. *Psychiatry Research*. 1992;41:203–214.

47. Zilcha-Mano S, Fisher H. Distinct roles of state-like and trait-like patient-therapist alliance in psychotherapy. *Nature Reviews in Psychology*. 2022;1:194–210. https://doi.org/10.1038/s44159-022-00029-z

48. Zilcha-Mano S. Is the alliance really therapeutic? Revisiting this question in light of recent methodological advances. *American Psychologist*. 2017;72(4):311.

49. Zilcha-Mano S. Toward personalized psychotherapy: The importance of the trait-like/state-like distinction for understanding therapeutic change. *American Psychologist*. 2021;76(3):516.

4.2

Placebo and nocebo effects in depression

Implications for treatment and clinical trial designs

Winfried Rief, John M. Kelley, and Yvonne Nestoriuc

Introduction

In this chapter, we examine evidence for placebo and nocebo effects in depression, including their mechanisms of action, and then consider how these effects might be used clinically to benefit patients. Although meta-analyses of clinical trial data indicate that the efficacy of antidepressants is statistically greater than placebos, the effect sizes are small, which suggests that antidepressants provide only marginal clinical benefits over placebos. In addition, placebos appear to duplicate about 80% of the effects of antidepressants, and the available data from natural course controls suggests that regression toward the mean and natural history account for a relatively small fraction of placebo responses. Taken together, the negative side-effect profile of antidepressants and their small clinical benefit compared to placebo, along with the robust effect of placebos compared to natural course controls suggest that placebos could benefit patients nearly as much as antidepressants, but without the negative side effects that accompany pharmaceutical treatment. We discuss ways that this might be achieved, most prominently by the use of open-label placebos. In addition, we present evidence for the role of expectations as an important mechanism underlying placebo efficacy, the experience of nocebo effects, and the exacerbation of genuine negative side effects, as well as the augmentation of genuine drug effects. Finally, we discuss how expectations for treatment improvement, on the one hand, and expectations about side effects, on the other, might be manipulated to improve clinical outcomes and reduce the frequency and severity of side effects, as well as the implications that such expectancy manipulations might have for clinical trial design.

Placebo effects in antidepressant trials

Antidepressant medications are included in all evidence-based treatment guidelines for depression, and they are especially recommended as treatment for severe cases of the disorder. These treatment guidelines have relied upon decades of randomized controlled trials (RCTs) of the efficacy of antidepressants that have reported statistically significant effects, and they have led to widespread adoption of antidepressants as a first-line treatment for depression. Moreover, the introduction of the selective serotonin reuptake inhibitors (SSRIs) in the late 1980s, with their reported lower levels of side effects, led to enthusiastic single-case reports in the public media, and these reports, along with Peter Kramer's bestselling popular book, *Listening to Prozac*,[1] led to a tremendous increase in prescriptions for antidepressants, which has continued unabated until the present. For example, in 2017, about 13% of the US population took antidepressants within the past month. In addition, 20% of adults aged 60 years and older reported that they were currently being treated with antidepressants.[2]

Doubts about the effectiveness of antidepressants

However, over the past 2 decades, this enthusiastic endorsement of the efficacy of antidepressants has been increasingly challenged, leading some experts to even question whether antidepressants actually confer any clinically meaningful benefits at all as compared to placebos.[3] For example, after carefully reviewing previously published meta-analyses, Jakobsen and colleagues concluded that antidepressants seem to have minimal beneficial effects on depressive symptoms, and, problematically, they also increase the risk of *adverse events*, including serious ones (e.g., suicide attempt and/or ideation) albeit with a smaller absolute risk.[4] Importantly, the US Food and Drug Administration's focus on statistically significant effects, as opposed to clinically meaningful ones, as the standard for approval, has blurred the line between marginally beneficial treatments and treatments that provide robust benefits to patients.

Cipriani and colleagues have conducted perhaps the most comprehensive and highest quality meta-analysis of antidepressant drug trials to date.[5] Their network meta-analysis included 522 trials with 116,477 patients, and they calculated that the overall effect size for the benefit of antidepressants as compared to placebos was only a standardized mean difference (SMD) of .30. According to Cohen's widely-accepted conventions, an SMD = .30 is considered a small effect.[6] From a clinical perspective, an SMD = .30 can be converted to the number needed to treat to achieve a minimal therapeutic benefit, which in this case is 10. In other words, 10 persons would need to be treated with antidepressants in order for one to benefit, which means that 9 persons treated with antidepressants—who might, of course, also experience noxious side effects—would *not* show an advantage compared to placebo treatments. Similarly small effect sizes have been found for antidepressants in children with mental and behavioral disorders.[7]

The problem with such a small effect size is not only that it indicates a lack of robustness of the medication's effects, but it also raises the possibility that some other difference between the drug and placebo groups may account for the small difference in efficacy. For example, antidepressants often produce side effects that can reduce the effectiveness of patient and physician blinding and thus trigger more positive treatment expectations in the drug group.[8,9] Not surprisingly, the drug-specific effect of antidepressants can vanish if participants do not expect to receive the drug, suggesting that expectation is a major mediator of antidepressants' efficacy.[10,11] Indeed, when patients are led to believe that they are receiving an inert placebo, the effect of the SSRI escitalopram, for example, is reduced to a level that is not clinically meaningful.[11]

It has been increasingly recognized that the problem in demonstrating a benefit of antidepressants over placebos is mainly caused by strong effects in the placebo arms of clinical trials. Not infrequently, the placebo arms of antidepressant trials show improvements of more than 10 points on standard screening tools, such as the Hamilton Depression Scale.[12] Some authors report that the effect sizes of improvements in the placebo group have even increased over the last several decades,[13,14] although this conclusion has been questioned in a more recent publication.[3] These changes over time are likely caused in part by a steady reduction in the heterogeneity of clinical trials, which also reduces the generalizability of the results.[14] Further, the methodological quality of antidepressant studies has increased over time, which may have also contributed to smaller differences in efficacy between drugs and placebos.

Several meta-analyses have also shown that an advantage of antidepressants over placebos is only found if the study design limits the induction of placebo mechanisms. If patients are seen once a week, the improvements in the placebo group are much higher than in studies where patients are only seen every other week or less.[15] Social contact with study physicians or study nurses seems to have the potential to boost positive effects in placebo arms to the same effect size that was found in the drug arms.

A general question when considering these effects is the influence of statistical artifacts, instead of genuine clinical changes in the symptomatology of patients. One of these statistical effects is regression toward the mean, in which patients in the extreme areas of a distribution (e.g., very strong depressive symptoms) have a greater probability to move in the direction of average scores (e.g., moderate depression), while the probability of becoming even more depressed is much lower. In clinical trials, patients who are typically included have serious symptoms or are in a serious crisis. Therefore, the natural course (without treatment) is more likely to develop in the direction of lower depression scores rather than higher. These effects can only be investigated if the drug and placebo arms of clinical trials are compared to natural course groups. Unfortunately, however, this is rarely done. One of the few studies including an arm with patients who received only low intensity medical care confirmed that the substantial improvements found in the placebo arms of antidepressant trials are indeed much greater than any changes in the natural course group (see Figure 4.2.1).[16] Over the 10-week course of treatment, both the active drug group and the placebo group showed substantial improvements, whereas the supportive care group showed only minor changes. These results suggest that the strong effects in placebo arms of antidepressant trials are a real effect of placebo mechanisms, and not simply attributable to the effects of regression toward the mean and natural course.

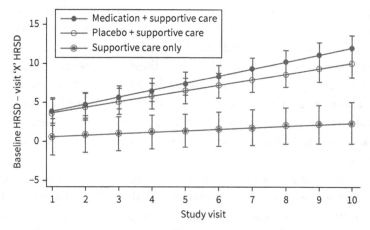

Figure 4.2.1 RCT on antidepressants including a supportive care–only arm. While improvements in pill taking arms were similar, they were higher than improvements in natural course.[16] This indicates that regression to the mean did not explain the improvements (e.g., in the placebo pill group).

The ascertainment strategy used to assess change can also contribute to larger improvements in outcome variables over time. In antidepressant trials, it has been shown that effect sizes are much higher when improvement is derived from expert ratings as compared to self-ratings.[14,17] One possible explanation for this finding is that many experts can correctly guess the group allocation of patients (i.e., drug vs. placebo) despite blinding, presumably because patients with more side effects are more likely to be taking an active drug.[18] Thus, the expectation of study physicians that a person with side effects is more likely allocated to the drug arm, and should also show more improvement, can contribute to larger drug-placebo differences when the effects are assessed by expert ratings.

To summarize, clinical trials investigating antidepressants suggest that strong placebo effects are involved, and they also indicate that expectations both on the part of the patients as well as the study personnel could contribute to treatment success. This is further supported by findings that the number of arms of the study design also affects improvement rates of placebo arms. If the study only uses two arms (i.e., drug vs. placebo), the likelihood of being in the placebo arm is 50%. If two or more active arms are compared to one placebo arm, the likelihood (and presumably the expectation) of being in the placebo arm is much lower. It has been shown that the response rate in the placebo arm is significantly lower in two-arm designs compared to three- or four-arm designs.[19] Again, this can be interpreted as meaning that a higher expectation on the part of both patient and physician that the patients may be in the placebo arm leads to lower response rates.

Experimental modulation of expectation in the affective system

The problem of the clinical trials cited above is that they are typically not designed to evaluate expectation effects, and therefore our conclusions come more from an indirect analysis of the results. Most clinical trials do not systematically modulate expectations, and, therefore, any conclusions about expectation effects are necessarily tentative. The conclusions would be much firmer if clinical trials used balanced-placebo designs and/or more trials also included natural course groups.

Although there is a paucity of high-quality, prospective clinical trial data on expectations, several experimental studies have systematically manipulated expectations and investigated the effects on affective outcomes. In one study, participants were exposed to movie clips designed to elicit sadness, but prior to viewing the clips, a placebo nasal spray was administered that participants were led to believe would either (a) protect them from experiencing sadness or (b) would exacerbate their feelings of sadness. Depending on the differing explanations of the expected effects of the "drug," the video clips either induced sadness, or the experience of sadness was substantially blocked.[20] While this effect was first shown in healthy volunteers, subsequent studies using similar designs have included patients who were diagnosed with major depression. These studies with depressed patients showed even stronger expectation effects.[21] The same research group was also able to demonstrate that these expectation modulations are not only effective in changing symptoms such as sadness, but they can also modulate other symptoms of depression such as rumination.[22] Finally, expectations can also influence the formation of intrusive memories.[23]

In other studies, the investigation of the role of expectations in depression was extended to examine not only outcome expectations for treatments, but also the processes and mechanisms that maintain depression in general.[24,25] Depression is characterized by expectations for social rejection and expectations for failure.[26,27] A depressed mood blocks the update of these negative expectations such that when positive experiences occur, the negative expectations are maintained.[28] This effect is crucially important for understanding why depressed patients remain depressed, even when positive events occur that contradict their negative view of themselves and their world. Further, many patients with depression use cognitive immunization strategies to prevent a positive update of negative expectations, which further explains the persistence of depression, especially in chronic depression. Given these findings, a prediction-processing perspective might offer new pathways to better understand the mechanisms that maintain depression, and to improve treatments for patients with depressive disorders.[24]

How to make use of these placebo mechanisms?

Given how strong placebo effects appear to be in clinical trials of antidepressants and given our increasing knowledge of the mechanisms that underlie these effects, the question arises whether we can make use of these insights to improve patient care for depressed patients. Deceptive administration of placebos is, of course, in conflict with medical ethics in most countries. However, administering placebos openly and without deception (i.e., open-label placebo (OLP)) could circumvent this problem. But given the fact that placebo effects seem to be driven, at least in part, by expectancies, could open administration of placebos be effective, even when a patient knows that she is receiving an inert treatment? Over the past decade, researchers have conducted clinical trials of open-label placebos that, importantly, were administered with a persuasive rationale for efficacy. A recent meta-analysis of 11 of these trials in a variety of disorders including low back pain, cancer-related fatigue, migraine headaches, depression, menopausal hot flashes, and irritable bowel syndrome found a significant overall effect favoring open-label placebo over treatment as usual (SMD = 0.72, p < 0.0001).[29] Regarding depression specifically, a pilot trial of open-label placebo administered in the context of a rationale for efficacy provided encouraging results, and suggested that OLP could be effective in alleviating major depression.[30] A larger trial investigating OLP in depression followed, which suggested that openly-administered placebos could be a treatment option, at least for some subgroups.[31] In particular, patients aged younger than 65 years seemed to respond better to OLP than patients aged 65 and older. It should be noted, however, that the sample size in this trial was small and the analysis was post hoc, so these findings regarding the moderating influence of age on OLP effects in depression should be considered tentative. To date, these are the only two clinical trials of OLP in depression; and in the absence of larger clinical trials, the evidence for the efficacy of OLP for the treatment of depression needs to be considered tentative.

Even if OLPs have positive effects in depression, there is some evidence that the effects of deceptive placebos are even larger.[32,33] Interestingly, this is also in accordance with a survey asking about the acceptability of the use of placebos that showed that double-blind placebo administration leads to more positive outcome expectations than OLP administration; and acceptability in the lay public for deceptive placebo applications is high.[34] These findings suggest that there is further potential to boost expectation effects to improve clinical outcomes, but the ethical issues associated with the use of deception in routine clinical practice would need to be carefully considered.

Another approach is to consider expectations in depression in a broader sense, with expectations being a core mechanism maintaining depressive states. Here, interventions can be further developed and improved that aim to counter dysfunctional expectations, while reducing the impact of cognitive immunization. Details can be found elsewhere.[25]

Nocebo effects in clinical trials of antidepressants

The influence of treatment expectations on antidepressant efficacy has been shown in numerous clinical trials and meta-analyses.[14] In particular, participants in placebo groups frequently report improvement of depressive symptoms that is comparable to the drug response (40% vs. 50% response rate, respectively).[5] At the same time, participants in the placebo arms of clinical trials often report debilitating side effects, known as nocebo effects.[35] Interestingly, these adverse events in the placebo groups often mimic the actual adverse events in the verum groups, suggesting that information about expected side effects that is provided to all patients creates negative expectations that in turn leads to placebo-treated patients then reporting those side effects.

A meta-analysis that included 143 antidepressant RCTs with over 12,000 patients documented nocebo rates that were two to six times higher in the placebo groups for trials of tricyclic antidepressants (TCAs) as compared to the placebo groups for trials of SSRIs, including adverse events such as blurred vision, fatigue, and constipation (see Table 4.2.1).[36] Since SSRIs have a well-known reputation for producing fewer side effects as compared to TCAs, these findings emphasize the importance of individual expectations for the efficacy and safety of antidepressants. Negative expectations regarding potential adverse effects of antidepressants might arise from treatment information provided to patients, through prior negative experiences with side effects to antidepressants, or by social observation of side effects experienced by friends or family.[37,38]

The fact that nocebo effects tend to mimic the actual side effects to the medication given in the verum arm has major consequences for the design and conduct of clinical trials. First, nocebo effects of placebo treatments are not a constant, but seem to be variable and specific to the active medication, and,

Table 4.2.1 Adverse events reported in the placebo arms of antidepressant trials of SSRIs versus TCAs

Adverse Events	TCA-Placebo	SSRI-Placebo	Odds Ratio
Blurred vision	7%	1%	OR = 6.1 (95%CI 2.6–14.5)
Fatigue	17%	6%	OR = 3.6 (95%CI 2.7–4.7)
Dry mouth	19%	6%	OR = 3.5 (95%CI 2.9–4.2)
Dizziness	14%	7%	OR = 2.7 (95%CI 2.2–3.4)
Constipation	11%	4%	OR = 2.7 (95%CI 2.1–3.6)
Sexual dysfunction	5%	2%	OR = 2.3 (95%CI 1.5–3.5)
Tremor	4%	2%	OR = 1.7 (95%CI 1.1–2.7)

Higher rates of nocebo effects resulted in the placebo arms of TCAs trials compared to the placebo arms of SSRIs trials.[36] This indicates that specific nocebo effects resulted depending on the side effects profile of the active drug, suggesting that treatment expectations and treatment information might play a role in explaining these nocebo effects.

thus, a single placebo control group does not suffice to control for different sources of nocebo effects in trials, in particular, if they compare different drugs. Separate placebo controls would be necessary to depict the nocebo effects of each single active arm. However, it remains unclear how practical this approach might be.

Second, the potential and highly likely interaction effects of placebo and verum groups need to be accounted for. Estimating the drug effect or the drug safety simply by subtracting adverse effects in the placebo arm from those in the verum arm, depends on the assumption that these effects are additive. The balanced-placebo design is a viable option to test these interaction effects while accounting for the potentially missing prerequisite of additivity.[39]

Third, including a placebo group in a clinical trial might influence participants' expectations per se. In a recent meta-analysis, adverse events rates were about 20% higher in antidepressant trials including a placebo group than in head-to head trials.[40] Thus, future studies should pay close attention to how participants' expectations are influenced by information about trial design. This can be done by documenting information procedures and assessing resulting treatment expectations.

Fourth and most obvious, adverse effects need to be systematically measured as patient-reported outcomes in order to analyze their occurrence and potential effect on positive treatment outcome. A systematic quantitative review documented that adverse event reporting was insufficient in RCTs of persistent depressive disorder, with some studies using unstructured assessment methods such as spontaneous recall.[41] This was also true for 46% of the included studies in the meta-analysis comparing nocebo effects in SSRI versus TCA trials.[36] Validated and structured tools to assess treatment side effects in clinical depression trials on pharmacological as well as psychological treatments such as the general assessment of side effects scale (GASE) are available.[42] Utilizing such structured tools to assess adverse events in randomized controlled depression trials enables researchers to compile risk-benefit information and thus use safety data to improve clinical decision-making and help patients optimally navigate the options available for treating depression.[43]

Modulating expectations to reduce side effects in antidepressant trials

Nocebo effects can significantly increase nonspecific symptoms and complaints in patient populations, resulting in psychological distress and reducing medication adherence. For example, over 30% of the patients who dropped out of the RCTs included in the meta-analysis on antidepressant nocebo effects actually came from the placebo groups.[36] Patient beliefs and expectations about medicines are some of the major mechanisms of nocebo effects, and they are shaped by personal and witnessed prior experiences, as well as by information provided by health care providers and the media. For example, headaches and other common side effects of antidepressants can result simply from the mention of headaches in the informed consent process as a potential side effect.[44]

Informed consent procedures have great potential to modify patients' treatment expectations in order to optimize treatment outcome by maximizing placebo effects and minimizing nocebo effects. However, today's informed consent processes are largely viewed as obligatory procedures to prevent litigation. In routine clinical practice, they are mainly focused on the potential risks and side effects of a given treatment, presented within a one-size-fits-all approach. The downsides of this approach have been critically discussed, particularly regarding the harm it may cause by shaping negative expectations and triggering nocebo-related side effects in routine clinical practice.[45]

On the positive side, treatment expectations can be influenced by short and economical psychological interventions.[46] Effective strategies to optimize treatment expectations within informed consent include framing of side effects information, either by emphasizing the probability of *being free from* adverse effects,[47] by elaborating on the anticipated positive effects and their mechanisms of action,[48] or by accompanying side-effect information with specific coping strategies.[46] Moreover, counteracting symptom misattribution by explicitly informing patients about the nocebo effect has been shown to be effective in reducing experimentally induced nocebo effects.[44]

A recent experimental study showed that a short patient-oriented interaction that provided information about the nocebo effect was effective in functionally adapting patient's informational needs regarding antidepressant medication.[49] This was the first empirical test of the feasibility and effectiveness of a contextualized informed consent procedure. Specifically, as compared to patients who were not informed about the nocebo effect, informed patients reported reduced needs for full information about possible side effects of antidepressants and stronger wishes to be informed about the desired effects and the mechanisms of action of antidepressants, including context and expectation effects.[49] This type of informational interaction might help healthcare practitioners optimize patient's treatment expectations via informed consent, while still respecting patient autonomy.

Taken together, contextualizing informed consent about antidepressants using framing strategies and information about the nocebo effect may help to functionally adapt patient's expectations and reduce nocebo-related adverse events.

Summary and conclusions

In this chapter on placebo and nocebo effects in depression, including their mechanisms of action, we reviewed clinical trial results, as well as data from laboratory experiments, and our conclusions can be summarized as follows:

(1) Although antidepressants show statistically greater efficacy compared to placebos, the effect sizes are small, and the specific effect of these drugs provides only a small clinical benefit to patients.

(2) Placebo responses in double-blind trials are about 80% as large as the response to antidepressants.

(3) Regression toward the mean and natural course account for only a small fraction of the antidepressant effect of placebos, which indicates that most of placebo responses are genuine placebo effects.

(4) Given these large placebo effects, and the small specific effect for antidepressants, as well as their negative side effects, efforts should be made toward harnessing placebo effects to benefit patients.

(5) OLPs show promise in treating depression, but larger studies of longer duration are needed.

(6) Nocebo effects are prevalent in antidepressant trials; they are detrimental to patient's quality of life and can motivate patients to stop taking the medication prematurely.

(7) Communication strategies such as contextualizing informed consent and framing treatment information are viable options to optimize treatment expectations and reduce nocebo-related adverse effects.

(8) Patient and physician expectations are an important mechanism underlying placebo and nocebo effects, and they likely also contribute to patient responses to genuine treatment, including both symptom improvement and the development of negative side effects. As such, expectations are an important target for future research aimed at improving our ability to reduce depressive symptoms, minimize the frequency and severity of negative side effects, and improve clinical trial design.

References

1. Kramer P. *Listening to Prozac: A Psychiatrist Explores Antidepressant Drugs and the Remaking of the Self.* Viking Press; 1993.
2. Winerman L. By the numbers: Antidepressant use on the rise. *Monitor on Psychology.* 2017;48(10). https://www.apa.org/monitor/2017/11/numbers
3. Kirsch I. Placebo effect in the treatment of depression and anxiety. *Frontiers in Psychiatry.* 2019;10:407. doi:10.3389/fpsyt.2019.00407
4. Jakobsen JC, Gluud C, Kirsch I. Should antidepressants be used for major depressive disorder? *BMJ Evidence-Based Medicine.* 2020;25(4):130–136.
5. Cipriani A, Furukawa TA, Salanti G, et al. Comparative efficacy and acceptability of 21 antidepressant drugs for the acute treatment of adults with major depressive disorder: A systematic review and network meta-analysis. *Lancet.* 2018; 391(10128):1357–1366. doi: 10.1016/S0140-6736(17)32802-7.
6. Cohen J. *Statistical Power Analysis for the Behavioral Sciences.* 2nd ed. Lawrence Erlbaum Associates; 1988.
7. Locher C, Koechlin H, Zion SR, et al. Efficacy and safety of selective serotonin reuptake inhibitors, serotonin-norepinephrine reuptake inhibitors, and placebo for common psychiatric disorders among children and adolescents a systematic review and meta-analysis. *JAMA Psychiatry.* 2017;74(10):1011–1020.
8. Rief W, Glombiewski JA. The hidden effects of blinded, placebo controlled randomized trials: An experimental investigation. *Pain.* 2012;153:2473–2477.
9. Berna C, Kirsch I, Zion SR, et al. Side effects can enhance treatment response through expectancy effects: An experimental analgesic randomized controlled trial. *Pain.* 2017;158(6):1014–1020.
10. Rutherford BR, Wall MM, Brown PJ, et al. Patient expectancy as a mediator of placebo effects in antidepressant clinical trials. *American Journal of Psychiatry.* 2017;174(2):135–142.
11. Faria V, Gingnell M, Hoppe JM, et al. Do you believe it? Verbal suggestions influence the clinical and neural effects of escitalopram in social anxiety disorder: A randomized trial. *Ebiomedicine.* 2017;24:179–188.
12. Stahl SM, Fava M, Trivedi MH, Caputo A, Shah A, Post A. Agomelatine in the treatment of major depressive disorder: An 8-week, multicenter, randomized, placebo-controlled trial. *Journal of Clinical Psychiatry.* 2010;71(5):616–626.
13. Walsh BT, Seidman SN, Sysko R, Gould M. Placebo response in studies of major depression: Variable, substantial, and growing. *Journal of the American Medical Association.* 2002;287:1840–1847.
14. Rief W, Nestoriuc Y, Weiss S, Welzel E, Barsky AJ, Hofmann SG. Meta-analysis of the placebo response in antidepressant trials. *Journal of Affective Disorders.* 2009;118(1–3):1–8.
15. Rutherford BR, Tandler J, Brown PJ, Sneed JR, Roose SP. Clinic visits in late-life depression trials: Effects on signal detection and therapeutic outcome. *American Journal of Geriatric Psychiatry.* 2014;22(12):1452–1461.
16. Leuchter AF, Hunter AM, Tartter M, Cook IA. Role of pill-taking, expectation and therapeutic alliance in the placebo response in clinical trials for major depression. *British Journal of Psychiatry.* 2014;205(6):443–449.
17. Cuijpers P, Li J, Hofmann SG, Andersson G. Self-reported versus clinician-rated symptoms of depression as outcome measures in psychotherapy research on depression: A meta-analysis. *Clinical Psychology Review.* 2010;30:768–778.
18. Margraf J, Ehlers A, Roth WT, et al. How blind a double blind study is. *Journal of Consulting and Clinical Psychology.* 1991;59:184–187.

19. Sinyor M, Levitt AJ, Cheung AH, et al. Does inclusion of a placebo arm influence response to active antidepressant treatment in randomized controlled trials? Results from pooled and meta-analyses. *Journal of Clinical Psychiatry*. 2010;71:270–279.

20. Glombiewski JA, Rheker J, Wittkowski J, Rebstock L, Rief W. Placebo mechanisms in depression: An experimental investigation of the impact of expectations on sadness in female participants. *Journal of Affective Disorders*. 2019;256:658–667.

21. Haas JW, Rief W, Glombiewski JA, Winkler A, Doering BK. Expectation-induced placebo effect on acute sadness in women with major depression: An experimental investigation. *Journal of Affective Disorders*. 2020;274:920–928.

22. Rebstock L, Schäfer LN, Kube T, Ehmke V, Rief W. Placebo prevents rumination: An experimental study. *Journal of Affective Disorders*. 2020;274:1152–1160.

23. Herzog P, Barth C, Rief W, Brakemeier EL, Kube T. How expectations shape the formation of intrusive memories: An experimental study using the trauma film paradigm. *Cognitive Therapy and Research*. 2022;46:809–826. https://doi.org/10.1007/s10608-022-10290-4

24. Kube T, Schwarting R, Rozenkrantz L, Glombiewski JA, Rief W. Distorted cognitive processes in major depression: A predictive processing perspective. *Biological Psychiatry*. 2020;87(5):388–398.

25. Rief W, Joormann J. Revisiting the cognitive model of depression: The role of expectations. *Clinical Psychology in Europe*. 2019;1(1):1–19. https://doi.org/10.32872/cpe.v1i1.32605

26. Kube T, D'Astolfo L, Glombiewski JA, Doering BK, Rief W. Focusing on situation-specific expectations in major depression as basis for behavioural experiments: Development of the Depressive Expectations Scale. *Psychology and Psychotherapy-Theory Research and Practice*. 2017;90(3):336–352.

27. Kirchner L, Schummer SE, Krug H, Kube T, Rief W. How social rejection expectations and depressive symptoms bi-directionally predict each other—A cross-lagged panel analysis. *Psychology and Psychotherapy-Theory Research and Practice*. 2022;95(2):477–492.

28. Kube T, Kirchner L, Gärtner T, Glombiewski JA. How negative mood hinders belief updating in depression: Results from two experimental studies. *Psychological Medicine*. 2023;53(4):1288–1301.

29. von Wernsdorff M, Loef M, Tuschen-Caffier B, Schmidt S. Effects of open-label placebos in clinical trials: A systematic review and meta-analysis. *Scientific Reports*. 2021;11(1):1–14.

30. Kelley JM, Kaptchuk TJ, Cusin C, Lipkin S, Fava M. Open-label placebo for major depressive disorder: A pilot randomized controlled trial. *Psychotherapy and Psychosomatics*. 2012;81(5):312–314.

31. Nitzan U, Carmeli G, Chalamish Y, et al. Open-Label placebo for the treatment of unipolar depression: Results from a randomized controlled trial. *Journal of Affective Disorders*. 2020;276:707–710.

32. Kube T, Rief W, Vivell MB, et al. Deceptive and nondeceptive placebos to reduce pain an experimental study in healthy individuals. *Clinical Journal of Pain*. 2020;36(2):68–79.

33. Gohler AC, Haas JW, Sperl MFJ, Hermann C, Winkler A. Placebo nasal spray protects female participants from experimentally induced sadness and concomitant changes in autonomic arousal. *Journal of Affective Disorders*. 2021;295:131–138.

34. Haas JW, Rief W, Doering BK. Open-label placebo treatment: Outcome expectations and general acceptance in the lay population. *International Journal of Behavioral Medicine*. 2021;28(4):444–454.

35. Meister R, Jansen A, Härter M, Nestoriuc Y, Kriston L. Placebo and nocebo reactions in randomized trials of pharmacological treatments for persistent depressive disorder: A meta-regression analysis. *Journal of Affective Disorders*. 2017;215:288–298.

36. Rief W, Nestoriuc Y, von Lilienfeld-Toal A, et al. Differences in adverse effect reporting in placebo groups in SSRI and tricyclic antidepressant trials: A systematic review and meta-analysis. *Drug Safety*. 2009;32(11):1041–1056.

37. Rheker J, Winkler A, Doering BK, Rief W. Learning to experience side effects after antidepressant intake—Results from a randomized, controlled, double-blind study. *Psychopharmacology*. 2017;234(3):329–338.

38. Zilcha-Mano S, Brown PJ, Roose SP, Cappetta K, Rutherford BR. Optimizing patient expectancy in the pharmacologic treatment of major depressive disorder. *Psychological Medicine*. 2019;49(14):2414–2420.

39. Enck P, Weimer K, Klosterhalfen S. Balanced placebo design, active placebos, and other design features for identifying, minimizing and characterizing the placebo response. In: Luana C, Magne Arve F, Karin M, eds. *Placebo and Pain: From Bench to Bedside*. Academic Press; 2013:159–173.

40. Cheung CP, Thiyagarajah MT, Abraha HY, et al. The association between placebo arm inclusion and adverse event rates in antidepressant randomized controlled trials: An examination of the nocebo effect. *Journal of Affective Disorders*. 2021;280:140–147.

41. Meister R, von Wolff A, Mohr H, et al. Adverse event methods were heterogeneous and insufficiently reported in randomized trials on persistent depressive disorder. *Journal of Clinical Epidemiology*. 2016;71:97–108.

42. Rief W, Barsky AJ, Glombiewski JA, Nestoriuc Y, Glaesmer H, Braehler E. Assessing general side effects in clinical trials: Reference data from the general population. *Pharmacoepidemiology and Drug Safety*. 2011;20(4):405–415.

43. Meister R, Lanio J, Fangmeier T, et al. Adverse events during a disorder-specific psychotherapy compared to a nonspecific psychotherapy in patients with chronic depression. *Journal of Clinical Psychology*. 2020;76(1):7–19.

44. Pan Y, Kinitz T, Stapic M, Nestoriuc Y. Minimizing drug adverse events by informing about the nocebo effect-an experimental study. *Frontiers in Psychiatry*. 2019;10:504.

45. Wells RE, Kaptchuk TJ. To tell the truth, the whole truth, may do patients harm: The problem of the nocebo effect for informed consent. *American Journal of Bioethics*. 2012;12(3):22–29.

46. Shedden-Mora M, Pan Y, Heisig S, et al. Optimizing expectations about endocrine treatment for breast cancer: Results of the randomized controlled PSY-BREAST Trial. *Clinical Psychology in Europe*. 2020;2(1):1–20.

47. Faasse K, Huynh A, Pearson S, Geers AL, Helfer SG, Colagiuri B. The influence of side effect information framing on nocebo effects. *Annals of Behavioral Medicine*. 2019;53(7):621–629.

48. Heisig SR, Shedden-Mora MC, Hidalgo P, Nestoriuc Y. Framing and personalizing informed consent to prevent negative expectations: An experimental pilot study. *Health Psychology*. 2015;34(10):1033–1037.

49. Nestoriuc Y, Pan Y, Kinitz T, Weik E, Shedden-Mora MC. Informing about the nocebo effect affects patients' need for information about antidepressants: An experimental online study. *Frontiers in Psychiatry*. 2021;12:587122.

4.3

Expectations and placebo effects in the context of cognitive training

Jocelyn Parong, Susanne Jaeggi, Aaron Seitz, and C. Shawn Green

Introduction

Basic cognitive skills such as attention or memory are important for most, if not all, of our daily activities, from remembering grocery lists, to keeping track of conversations, to carrying out specialized work-related or academic-related tasks. As such, there has been great interest in whether and how these basic cognitive skills can be improved through behavioral training. Over the past few decades, the proposition that by improving basic cognitive skills we could in turn produce significant real-world benefits has spurred dozens of experimental intervention studies aimed at improving a multitude of cognitive functions, including working memory (i.e., the active storage and manipulation of information),[1] selective attention (i.e., the ability to focus on particular inputs for further processing, while simultaneously ignoring irrelevant information),[2] and fluid intelligence (i.e., the ability to reason and problem solve).[3] Not only could enhancing such functions have a significant impact among populations who experience challenges in those domains, such as those with attention-deficit hyperactivity disorder or Alzheimer's disease or related dementias, but also could benefit typically developing individuals in everyday real-world situations.

Cognitive training is the superordinate category label that has been applied to all interventions designed with the purpose of enhancing cognitive skills, from music training to mindfulness meditation.[4] For the purposes of this chapter though, we will utilize the term *cognitive training* to specifically refer to the segment of the field that has employed various forms of computerized training, including commercial or custom video games or video game-like programs, as these strongly share the set of methodological considerations and areas of debate that we will examine here.[5-8] One major area of debate focuses on whether the observed changes in cognition produced by cognitive training are (1) of a large enough magnitude and (2) sufficiently broad to be practically meaningful.

Indeed, one of the more consistent findings across the learning sciences is that if individuals are given dedicated training on a particular task, they tend to improve on that very task. However, they do not then always show improvements in other tasks—even ones that seem to be quite like the one they trained on. This phenomenon has sometimes been referred to as the "curse of specificity"[9] because for training to produce real-world improvements, it is critical that the benefits extend not just beyond, but well beyond, the confines of the computerized training tasks. For example, imagine that a person receives dedicated training on the game Tetris, where players must mentally rotate and then organize 2D puzzle shapes as they descend the screen to form complete lines on the bottom. It is almost certainly the case that the individual will become better at playing Tetris as a result of this training. The bigger question is whether they would also then, for instance, show enhanced performance on mental rotation tasks in a laboratory setting, such as on the Shepard and Metzler 3D mental rotation tasks[10] and/or performance on real-world tasks that require the use of mental rotation, such as some math problems[11] or navigating in an unfamiliar environment.

The consensus in the field to date is that there is overwhelming evidence that computerized cognitive training improves performance on identical or nearly identical tasks (e.g., speed-of-processing training using a Useful Field of View training program increases performance on closely related laboratory measures of processing speed).[12] There is less, but still compelling evidence of improved performance on moderately similar tasks (e.g., working memory training improves performance on fluid intelligence tasks, or action video game training improves top-down attention).[2,13] And finally, there is much more uncertainty about whether computerized cognitive training consistently produces improved performance on vastly dissimilar tasks, especially real-world tasks.[7]

The very nature of cognitive training interventions makes placebo effects a possible concern

Though previous cognitive training studies have shown some promising outcomes for improving cognitive functions, the mechanisms of exactly how and when transfer from cognitive training occurs is still an ongoing research question. One popular critique of the field has posited that participants' expectations regarding outcomes play a major role in the positive outcomes that have been observed. In other words, it has been argued that perhaps participants are showing improvements in cognitive abilities following training not because of anything to do with the training itself, but instead they are showing improvements simply because they expected that the training would enhance their cognitive skills.

In considering this idea, it is worth briefly examining the basic premises and methods underlying cognitive training interventions (for a more extensive discussion, see Green et al.[5]). In most cognitive training studies, one group of participants is assigned to a treatment condition, which practices a computerized cognitive intervention (e.g., a video game or other computerized program) for a certain amount of time, while another group of participants is assigned to a control condition, which either completes no training at all (i.e., what is sometimes called a no-contact or waitlist control group) or more ideally, completes an activity assumed to lack the "active ingredient" that would induce changes in the targeted component of cognition in the same way the treatment intervention would. Posttreatment cognitive abilities, relative to baseline pretreatment cognitive abilities, are then compared between the treatment and control conditions. If the treatment group improves more than the control group, it can be concluded that the cognitive intervention (more specifically, its active ingredient, given an appropriate active control condition) was effective. However, ensuring that the active ingredient is the *only* element that differs between the treatment and control groups is particularly difficult in the case of cognitive training interventions. If a medical researcher is examining the efficacy of a particular drug compared to a placebo control, they can carefully match the appearance of the real pill and control pill (e.g., a sugar pill). If the research team and participants remain unaware of the condition to which participants have been assigned, any differences in outcomes between the experimental and control groups can be attributed solely to the active ingredient in the experimental drug. This is most often referred to as a double-blind design, in that neither the research team nor the participants can determine what condition participants have been assigned (although note that the use of the word *blind* in this context can be considered ableist and, thus, below we use alternative terms, such as *masking*).

To move in this methodological direction, researchers in the cognitive training domain have frequently attempted to use control conditions that are very similar to the true intervention, such as manipulating a custom racing game to include either multi-task or single-task requirements,[14] by comparing visual n-back training to auditory n-back training,[15] or by comparing easier and harder versions of the same task.[16] However, it remains the case that creating an outwardly identical active control activity that looks like the treatment intervention without the active ingredient is literally impossible; without the active ingredient, the mechanics of the game or program (e.g., content, challenges, and strategies) will *necessarily* change. Additionally, cognitive training interventions are designed to put at least some strain on certain cognitive systems, which may produce fatigue that participants can identify and make them aware of being in a certain cognitive training intervention.[17] It is interesting to note that a similar issue almost certainly exists in medical studies—even those that are referred to as double-blind (i.e., that participants form expectations or become aware based upon how they feel after taking their respective pills). Most active drugs will induce at least some side effects, which can in turn be used by participants to "guess" their condition.[18] Some researchers have argued that an ideal control pill should thus induce some side effects (if not identical side effects—e.g., rather than a sugar pill, or an antihistamine that would cause dry mouth) to ensure that participants cannot use the presence or absence of side effects to form intuitions about the condition to which they have been assigned.[19]

Given that differences in the look and feel of the true intervention and the active control cannot be fully eliminated in cognitive training designs, if these differences in look and feel in turn produce differences in expectations regarding the most likely outcome of the two forms of training, improvements in one condition over another may be due, at least in part, to differential placebo effects across conditions.[17] And indeed, there is reason to suspect that many people either carry positive expectations of cognitive training interventions before entering a study or quickly form expectations upon being exposed to the training tasks. For example, Rabipour and Davidson[20] asked participants to rate how successful they believe computerized cognitive training would be at improving their general cognitive function on a scale from 1 (completely unsuccessful) to 7 (completely successful). They found that 69% percent of respondents gave ratings of 5 or higher, suggesting that many people have existing positive expectations of cognitive training even before experiencing any training. They also found that these expectations can be manipulated by presenting evidence either advocating for or against brain training programs. Other studies have corroborated this finding, with most participants leaning toward positive views of cognitive training.[21-22]

Similarly, Boot and colleagues[23] asked participants to watch a video about either an action video game (Unreal Tournament; a game that has been used in the attempt to drive cognitive enhancements) or a game commonly used as a control game in cognitive training studies (Tetris or The Sims). They were then asked to read descriptions of a list of cognitive and perceptual laboratory tasks and indicate whether they thought the game they viewed would improve performance on each task. Participants expected that the action video game would lead to greater improvements in some tasks, such as tasks that measure visual spatial attention (the Multiple Object Tracking task, Useful Field of View), which generally aligned with the published results of cognitive training interventions (i.e., that action video games improve visual attention skills).[13] Another study found similar results, showing that participants who were trained on action video games generally expected greater improvements than those trained in a control game.[24]

All told, then, the available data do suggest that participants can and do form differential expectations about cognitive interventions. This in turn leads to the question: Do the expectations have practical consequences? In other words, Do they affect behavioral outcomes?

Are expectations related to behavioral outcomes in cognitive training?

To date, only a few studies have directly measured participants' expectations using self-report measures and compared those to actual outcomes and these studies have found somewhat mixed results. Baniqued and colleagues[25] found that participants' expectations did indeed differ between training and control conditions and that this at least partially related to differences in behavior. Participants were assigned to play either a gamified cognitive training program called Mind Frontiers or a group of control activities. Following training, the participants were then asked to rate their perceived improvements in various aspects of cognition. The results showed that the Mind Frontiers group not only improved on working memory, perceptual speed, and reaction time tasks to a great degree relative to the control group, but they also expected that they would show greater improvements on average.

However, expectations have not always been seen to be linked with actual behavioral outcomes. In some cases, participants have shown expectations of improvement, but no actual improvements in cognitive skill. For instance, Guye and von Bastian[26] compared a working memory training intervention to a visual search control group. Although participants in the working memory training group indicated higher posttraining expectations of improvement compared to the visual search group, there were no actual group differences on the transfer tests (see also Souders[27]). In other cases, improvements have been seen in cognitive skills, but have been unlinked to expectations. For example, in Zhang and colleagues,[24] participants were trained on either an action video game or a control video game. In aggregate, those individuals trained on an action video game showed both greater improvements in cognitive skill and higher expectations of improvement. However, when the data were examined at the individual level, there was no relation between the individuals' degree of expectation and behavioral outcomes.

In all then, the currently available data do not point to a strong link between expectations developed during cognitive training interventions and behavioral outcomes. Yet, studies that have examined the possible influence of expectations derived during true cognitive training interventions (i.e., where the methods are typically designed to minimize differences in expectations), cannot necessarily speak to the question of whether, under some conditions, such expectation-derived improvements can exist. For this, researchers must explicitly and deliberately attempt to produce such outcomes.

Can expectation effects be induced in cognitive training?

As discussed earlier, when measured through self-report, participants' expectations do not necessarily consistently match their behavioral outcomes in cognitive training studies. However, these inferences are limited by the fact that standard cognitive training paradigms are not meant to influence participants' expectations in the first place. This has sparked interest in whether these types of effects can be induced by explicitly manipulating participants' expectations in cognitive training. There have been a variety of methods used to induce placebo effects in cognitive training, and the results—like the other work reviewed thus far—have been somewhat mixed.

At a minimum, there is reason to think that participants' beliefs about their cognitive performance are related to their behavioral performance, and more importantly, that these beliefs can easily be manipulated. For example, Green and colleagues[28] gave participants a drink that contained either glucose or aspartame and either correctly or incorrectly labeled the drink, with the idea that participants would expect that glucose has a positive effect and aspartame has no effect on cognitive performance. The glucose drink improved performance on an attentional vigilance task when participants were told that they were ingesting glucose, suggesting that at least some of the improvement in cognition was due to the participants' expectancy. Similar results have been found in other studies related to food as well (e.g., whether or not a participant believes they are ingesting caffeine).[29-30]

More specifically in the context of cognitive training, some studies have shown that participant expectations can be manipulated and that these expectations are directly related to improvements in cognitive functions. In one example, Foroughi and colleagues[31] recruited participants into a cognitive training study using two different flyers. One flyer advertised the study as a brain training and cognitive enhancement study and stated that working memory training can increase fluid intelligence, while the other flyer stated that participating in research could earn class credits. All participants then completed a single session of dual n-back training (working memory). Those who joined the study through the brain training flyer showed improvements in a fluid intelligence measure comparable to a 5-to-10-point increase on a standard IQ test after the session, while those who responded to a nonsuggestive flyer showed no improvements. These results provide some evidence that participants' expectations can be manipulated, which affect subsequent cognitive outcomes. Contrary to these findings, in other studies, participants' expectations were manipulated, but were not related to any improvements in cognition. For example, Vodyanyk and colleagues[32] conducted a study in which they induced either positive or neutral expectations prior to a short session of cognitive training. They found no evidence for a placebo effect using various types of training (n-back, Tetris) in multiple domains (fluid intelligence, spatial skills).

While the aforementioned studies attempted to induce expectation-related changes in very short "training" studies (i.e., on the order of a few minutes to an hour or so), other work has examined the same question in longer cognitive training paradigms. In these studies, expectations have generally not been related to cognitive training outcomes. Using a similar flyer-recruitment method as used by Foroughi and colleagues,[31] Katz and colleagues[33] advertised a training experiment to participants that would either improve their intelligence or get paid for participating in the study. However, after completing either a dual n-back cognitive training intervention or a control knowledge-based task over the course of several weeks, the results showed no differences in improvements as a function of the expectation message. In another study, Tsai and colleagues[34] assigned participants to either a positive or negative expectation condition that received a narrated presentation about neuroscience-based "evidence" and then had them complete a week-long n-back training program or an active control activity. Overall, there were no differences in cognitive performance between the positive or negative expectation groups. Instead, the n-back group improved on an untrained working memory task while the control group showed no improvement, regardless of expectations in either training group. Similarly, Rabipour and colleagues[35] provided participants with either a positive message that cognitive training would improve their cognitive overall or a neutral message that it would not produce any benefits. They found that the expectation message had no effects on outcomes after a 5-week-long commercial cognitive training intervention called Activate.

Overall, placebo effects in the context of cognitive training seem to be nuanced, calling for further examination of the underlying mechanisms of placebo effects in cognitive training, such as when, how, and for whom they could occur.

Recommendations for future research

Now, research examining the influence of expectation effects in cognitive training interventions is limited and mixed. This is perhaps not surprising given that the research remains in its relative infancy, and, thus, there is simply not enough data to know what the central tendency in the field is, let alone how various possible mediators or moderators act in space. Available data do make several future needs quite clear.

First, there is at least sufficient evidence that expectation effects could be an issue to indicate that researchers should be as thoughtful as possible in their experimental methodology. Ideally, this should include an active control condition in addition to a passive one to match the levels of intent between conditions and to estimate possible effects in the active control.[5-6] Moreover, any active control group(s) should be closely matched to the treatment condition when possible. Compared to passive control conditions, active controls are thought to induce more similar expectations between the treatment and control participants, though they will rarely be identical expectations. In conjunction with an active control group, it would be important to get a sense of the participant's general expectations before, during, and/or after cognitive training. Questionnaires have been developed to measure exactly this purpose.[20] For example, asking participants to rate how effective they believe the cognitive training will be useful in later assessing whether expectations between conditions were similar, as well as controlling for these expectations as critical variables in statistical analyses. Yet open questions regarding such practices remain and will need careful consideration in future work (e.g., whether expectations that would not otherwise be present are created via the very act of making measurements).

Finally, while a great deal of the focus in cognitive training studies has been to minimize or eliminate expectation effects, from the perspective of real-world effects, if such effects can be induced, the opposite tactic may be preferable. For example, when examining whether cognitive skills can be improved, particularly in populations in need of cognitive improvement, rather than trying to minimize the possible effect of the participants' expectations, it may be more clinically valuable to induce and capitalize on optimistic expectations that can positively affect the outcomes of the intervention. The important outcome is seeing that cognitive skills can indeed be enhanced, whether through placebos or the intervention itself. Further, it may also be advantageous to identify which cognitive outcomes measures as well as which types of people are most susceptible to placebo effects in cognitive training. As there is evidence that cognitive training does not affect all aspects of cognition equally, there is reason to suspect placebo effects may also not be uniform across cognition. Additionally, some individual differences across participants, such as personality and motivation traits, may predict those who may be susceptible to placebo effects,[36] which in turn may be utilized to create more personalized training interventions.

In sum, it is important to understand, measure, and account for the role of participants' expectations in cognitive training. To date, there is mixed evidence whether they can account for the positive results seen from cognitive training interventions and further research is needed in this area to understand their effect sizes and how these are distributed across different types of outcome measures, differ across people, and differentially induced across manipulation types. Additionally further work would be beneficial in addressing how, in some cases, placebo effects may be of value in enhancing the real-world outcomes of cognitive training interventions.

References

1. Könen T, Strobach T, Karbach J. Working memory training. In: Strobach T, Karbach J, eds. *Cognitive Training*. Springer; 2021:155–167. http://doi:10.1007/978-3-030-39292-5_11
2. Bavelier D, Green CS. Enhancing attentional control: Lessons from action video games. *Neuron*. 2019;104(1):147–163. http://doi:10.1016/j.neuron.2019.09.031
3. Au J, Sheehan E, Tsai N, Duncan GJ, Buschkuehl M, Jaeggi SM. Improving fluid intelligence with training on working memory: A meta-analysis. *Psychonomic Bulletin & Review*. 2015;22(2):366–377. http://doi:10.3758/s13423-014-0699-x
4. Strobach T, Karbach J, eds. *Cognitive Training*. Springer; 2021. http://doi:10.1007/978-3-030-39292-5
5. Green CS, Bavelier D, Kramer AF, et al. Improving Methodological Standards in Behavioral Interventions for Cognitive Enhancement. *Journal of Cognitive Enhancement*. 2019; (3):2–29. http://doi:0.1007/s41465-018-0115-y
6. Au J, Gibson BC, Bunarjo K, Buschkuehl M, Jaeggi SM. Quantifying the difference between active and passive control groups in cognitive interventions using two meta-analytical approaches. *Journal of Cognitive Enhancement*. 2020;4(2):192–210. http://doi:10.1007/s41465-020-00164-6

7. Melby-Lervåg M, Redick TS, Hulme C. Working memory training does not improve performance on measures of intelligence or other measures of "far transfer": Evidence from a meta-analytic review. *Perspectives on Psychological Science.* 2016;11(4):512–534. http://doi:10.1177/1745691616635612

8. Simons DJ, Shoda Y, Lindsay DS. Constraints on generality (COG): A proposed addition to all empirical papers. *Perspectives on Psychological Science.* 2017;12(6):1123–1128. http://doi:10.1177/1745691617708630

9. Green CS, Bavelier D. Learning, attentional control, and action video games. *Current biology.* 2012;22(6):R197–R206. http://doi:10.1016/j.cub.2012.02.012

10. Sims VK, Mayer RE. Domain specificity of spatial expertise: The case of video game players. *Applied Cognitive Psychology.* 2002;16(1):97–115. http://doi:10.1002/acp.759

11. Hawes ZCK, Gilligan-Lee KA, Mix KS. Effects of spatial training on mathematics performance: A meta-analysis. *Developmental Psychology.* 2022;58(1):112–137. http://doi:10.1037/dev0001281

12. Ball K, Berch DB, Helmers KF, et al. Effects of cognitive training interventions with older adults: A randomized controlled trial. *JAMA: Journal of the American Medical Association.* 2002;288(18):2271–2281. http://doi:10.1001/jama.288.18.2271

13. Bediou B, Adams DM, Mayer RE, Tipton E, Green CS, Bavelier D. Meta-analysis of action video game impact on perceptual, attentional, and cognitive skills. *Psychological Bulletin.* 2018;144(1):77–110. http://doi:10.1037/bul0000130

14. Anguera JA, Boccanfuso J, Rintoul JL, et al. Video game training enhances cognitive control in older adults. *Nature.* 2013;501(7465):97–101. http://doi:10.1038/nature12486

15. Opitz B, Schneiders JA, Krick CM, Mecklinger A. Selective transfer of visual working memory training on Chinese character learning. *Neuropsychologia.* 2014;53:1–11. http://doi:10.1016/j.neuropsychologia.2013.10.017

16. Simon SS, Tusch ES, Feng NC, Håkansson K, Mohammed AH, Daffner KR. Is computerized working memory training effective in healthy older adults? Evidence from a multisite, randomized controlled trial. *Journal of Alzheimer's Disease.* 2018;65(3):931–949. http://doi:10.3233/JAD-180455

17. Denkinger S, Spano L, Bingel U, Witt CM, Bavelier D, Green CS. Assessing the impact of expectations in cognitive training and beyond. *Journal of Cognitive Enhancement.* 2021;5:502–518. http://doi:10.1007/s41465-021-00206-7

18. Hróbjartsson A, Forfang E, Haahr MT, Als-Nielsen B, Brorson S. Blinded trials taken to the test: An analysis of randomized clinical trials that report tests for the success of blinding, *International Journal of Epidemiology.* 2007;36(3):654–663. http://doi:10.1093/ije/dym020

19. Moscucci M, Byrne L, Weintraub M, Cox C. Blinding, unblinding, and the placebo effect: An analysis of patients' guesses of treatment assignment in a double-blind clinical trial. *Clinical Pharmacology and Therapeutics.* 1987;41(3):259–265. http://doi:10.1038/clpt.1987.26

20. Rabipour S, Davidson PSR. Do you believe in brain training? A questionnaire about expectations of computerised cognitive training. *Behavioural Brain Research.* 2015;295:64–70. http://doi:10.1016/j.bbr.2015.01.002

21. Hynes S. Internet, home-based cognitive and strategy training with older adults: A study to assess gains to daily life. *Aging Clinical & Experimental Research.* 2016;28(5):1003–1008. http://doi:10.1007/s40520-015-0496-z

22. Yeo SN, Lee TS, Sng WT, et al. Effectiveness of a personalized brain-computer interface system for cognitive training in healthy elderly: A randomized controlled trial. *Journal of Alzheimer's Disease.* 2018;66(1):127–138. http://doi:10.3233/JAD-180450

23. Boot WR, Simons DJ, Stothart C, Stutts C. The pervasive problem with placebos in psychology: Why active control groups are not sufficient to rule out placebo effects. *Perspectives on Psychological Science.* 2013;8(4):445–454. http://doi:10.1177/1745691613491271

24. Zhang R-Y, Chopin A, Shibata K, et al. Action video game play facilitates "learning to learn." *Communications Biology*. 2021;4(1):1154. http://doi:10.1038/s42003-021-02652-7

25. Baniqued PL, Allen CM, Kranz MB, et al. Working memory, reasoning, and task switching training: transfer effects, limitations, and great expectations? *PLoS ONE*. 2015;10(11):e0142169. http://doi:10.1371/journal.pone.0142169

26. Guye S, von Bastian CC. Working memory training in older adults: Bayesian evidence supporting the absence of transfer. *Psychology and Aging*. 2017;32(8):732–746. http://doi:10.1037/pag0000206

27. Souders DJ, Boot WR, Blocker K, Vitale T, Roque NA, Charness N. Evidence for narrow transfer after short-term cognitive training in older adults. *Frontiers in Aging Neuroscience*. 2017;9:41. http://doi:10.3389/fnagi.2017.00041

28. Green MW, Taylor MA, Elliman NA, Rhodes O. Placebo expectancy effects in the relationship between glucose and cognition. *British Journal of Nutrition*. 2001;86(2):173–179. http://doi:10.1079/bjn2001398

29. Fillmore MT, Mulvihill LE, Vogel-Sprott M. The expected drug and its expected effect interact to determine placebo responses to alcohol and caffeine. *Psychopharmacology*. 1994;115(3):383–388. http://doi:10.1007/BF02245081

30. Fillmore M, Vogel-Sprott M. Expected effect of caffeine on motor performance predicts the type of response to placebo. *Psychopharmacology*. 1992;106(2):209–214. http://doi:10.1007/BF02801974

31. Foroughi CK, Monfort SS, Paczynski M, McKnight PE, Greenwood PM. Placebo effects in cognitive training. *PNAS*. 2016;113(27):7470–7474. http://doi:10.1073/pnas.1601243113

32. Vodyanyk M, Cochrane A, Corriveau, A, Demko Z, Green CS. No evidence for expectation effects in cognitive training tasks. *Journal of Cognitive Enhancement*. 2021;5:296–310. http://doi:10.1007/s41465-021-00207-6

33. Katz B, Jaeggi SM, Buschkuehl M, Shah P, Jonides J. The effect of monetary compensation on cognitive training outcomes. *Learning and Motivation*. 2018;63:77–90. http://doi:10.1016/j.lmot.2017.12.002

34. Tsai N, Buschkuehl M, Kamarsu S, Shah P, Jonides J, Jaeggi SM. (Un)great expectations: The role of placebo effects in cognitive training. *Journal of Applied Research in Memory and Cognition*. 2018;7(4):564–573. http://doi:10.1037/h0101826

35. Rabipour S, Morrison C, Crompton J, et al. Few effects of a 5-week adaptive computerized cognitive training program in healthy older adults. *Journal of Cognitive Enhancement*. 2020;4:258–273. http://doi:10.1007/s41465-019-00147-2

36. Geers AL, Helfer SG, Kosbab K, Weiland PE, Landry SJ. Reconsidering the role of personality in placebo effects: Dispositional optimism, situational expectations, and the placebo response. *Journal of Psychosomatic Research*. 2005;58(2):121–127. http://doi:10.1016/j.jpsychores.2004.08.011

4.4

Why psychotherapy is an open-label placebo and open-label placebos are psychotherapy

Jens Gaab

Changeling placebos

Placebos come in all shapes and forms. There is the proverbial placebo pill in the context of psychopharmacological trials,[1] placebo nasal spray,[2] placebo oxygen,[3] placebo surgery,[4] placebo acupuncture needles,[5] there are placebo creams,[6] and as much as it possible to turn exercise,[7,8] wine,[9] violins,[10] and even real treatments[11,12] into placebo. Also, placebos not only have many appearances, but their effects have been found to surface in various forms, encompassing chronic and acute pain, sleep problems, disgust, the experience of music, itch, panic, high-altitude headache, performance in athletes, sexual dysfunction, mortality, self-esteem, depression, love sickness, obesity, symptoms of Parkinson's disease, posttraumatic stress disorder and even schizophrenia. As such, it seems harder to prove that a given treatment is not or does not contain any placebo effect than to show that a given treatment is or does contain any placebo effect, except for lethal poison or parachutes, in which case these would qualify as treatments (against life and free falling?).

With this multitude of forms and effects, the placebo is difficult to pin down into a straightforward definition. Therefore, the common definition of *placebo* being a pharmacological inert treatment used for its nonspecific, psychological, or psychophysiological effect is both unhelpful as well as illogical. Placebos can have specific physiological effects; active treatments can be used as placebo; and a placebo can still be a placebo even though it has no effect. However, would either turn any nonpharmacological treatment (e.g., psychotherapy) as much as any treatment having psychological effects (e.g., again, psychotherapy) directly into a placebo? Consequently, Kirsch identified both practical and conceptual problems "to extend the placebo concept from the medical setting to the psychotherapeutic setting" and aptly stated, "practically, it cannot be done; conceptually, it makes no sense to try"[13] (p. 796). This a well-founded and sensible claim as psychotherapy "placebo" control conditions are ripe with methodological biases and as it has been concluded that "whether a given psychotherapeutic intervention is to be considered a specific treatment or not is influenced by the operationalization of the placebo control condition" it is compared against[14] (summary).

Is psychotherapy *placebo* spelled backward?

Still, there are several strands of reasoning that preclude an exceptional status of psychotherapy about placebo or, to put it positively, to search for a placebo definition that also allows for psychological interventions (i.e., allows the definition of nonpharmacological placebos). First, the history as much as the present of psychotherapy is paved with placebo references, both justified as well as unjustified. This not only includes the shrouded ancestry of Freud's psychoanalysis in Mesmer's Animal Magnetism and de Puységur's Magnetic Sleep,[15] but also lists Eysenck's infamous claims in 1952 that "the general tenor of the evidence produced in recent years seems to be that the conclusion [. . .] is still valid: psychotherapy works, as far as it does, by means of non-specific or placebo effects"[16] (p. 16; see also[17]). This is echoed in valid concerns that "insight-oriented psychotherapies are highly susceptible to generating placebo insights, that is, illusions, deceptions, and adaptive self-misunderstandings that convincingly mimic veridical insight but have no genuine explanatory power"[18] and the position that "medicine today is disturbed by the placebo effect in a way psychotherapy is not. [. . .] It is because psychotherapy is less burdened by doubts about the placebo effect that it was able to come to its aid when it was orphaned by medicine."[19]

Even though "Eysenck was probably wrong,"[20] as various psychotherapies for depression fare significantly better than control conditions, including placebo control conditions, the observed specific effect is small and only marginally above the cutoff for minimal significant difference in the treatment of depression when adjusting for known sources of bias.[20] This sobering empirical perspective is supplemented by meta-analyses showing that psychotherapies for depression were only significantly better than "nondirective supportive" control groups when researchers' allegiance was uncontrolled for[21] and direct comparisons between psychotherapy and either pill or psychotherapy placebos, showing a significant effect above placebo, but which again is below the proposed cut-offs for clinical significance.[22,23] Besides the empirical (near-) equivalence between pill or control placebo conditions and psychotherapy, there are also examples of assumed or indented placebo psychotherapies. This encompasses of course "the extremely controversial subject"[24] of Eye Movement Desensitization Reprocessing (EMDR), which has been shown to be efficacious, but which has been labeled as a pseudoscientific therapeutic technique[25] and downright equaled with Mesmer's Animal Magnetism,[26,27] the first scientifically exposed placebo.[28] Further, at least two psychotherapies—interpersonal therapy and present-centered therapy—set out as control conditions in pharmacological or nonpharmacological clinical trials, but subsequently turned into empirically supported therapies.[29,30]

Besides this empirical and theoretical proximity between placebos and psychotherapy, the underlying mechanisms of these two psychological interventions appear to have more in common than readily accepted. While the importance of expectancy—either induced by verbal instructions or through conditioning—and the therapeutic alliance has repeatedly been shown as the main drivers of a placebo response,[31,32] the therapeutic factors underlying psychotherapy's often-substantial effects are subject to a long-standing and often-heated debate.[33] However, even if the invitation to the "dance of specificity"[13] is rejected, the therapeutic alliance—either its components or as a whole—as well as patient's expectations, are shown to be powerful, if not the most powerful, ingredients of psychotherapy.[33] This similarity in mechanisms between placebo and psychotherapy might best be exemplified by both interventions being described as "meaning" interventions.[34,35] Unsurprisingly, proximity between these two psychological interventions was noticed: "The old debate about whether or not psychotherapy and placebos have similar mechanisms consists of ascertaining whether psychotherapy is nothing but a placebo effect, and thus whether a placebo procedure is a very simple form of psychotherapy"[36] (pp. 141–143).

An ethical definition of *placebo*

As shown above, it is both pragmatically as well conceptually unwarranted to subordinate psychotherapy to a placebo definition derived from Medicine as much as it is not reasonable to assume that psychotherapy is fully immune to placebos. Thus, neither is psychotherapy a placebo by nature nor is it acceptable that psychotherapists can tell their patients anything as long as it works—informed consent and the respect of patient's autonomy are practical and moral obligations for psychotherapists as much as they are for surgeons, primary care doctors, and emergency physicians or in fact any other health care provider.[37,38,39] For this, an applicable definition of *placebo* would best not rely on the physical property of the placebo nor on the existence of its effects, but rather approach this phenomenon from a theoretical perspective. Here, the definition provided by Adolf Grünbaum[40,41] is considered "by far the best proposal" (see for review and revision[42]) as it on the one hand bases the definition of so-called characteristic and incidental treatment constituents relative to a given treatment theory, while on the other hand ethically defines *placebo* as the deceptive administration of a treatment solely consisting of incidental treatment constituents. With this definition, it is possible to define an active treatment as a placebo (when a given treatment theory does not define it as characteristic for the condition at hand) as much as a *psychotherapy* can be defined as a placebo, when it contains nothing more than incidental treatment constituents, again relative to a given treatment theory. Thus, this definition could best be considered as an ethical definition as the moment of deception is decisive, whereas the property of the treatment and its effects (or their absence) are not definitive criteria.

Interestingly and following this definition, a placebo openly described as placebo would not be a placebo anymore, but rather an example of verum as the treatment provider would not deceive the treatment recipient about the nature (i.e., characteristic) (e.g., expectancy/conditioning/meaning and therapeutic relationship) and incidental constituents (e.g., form, ingrediencies, and administration) of the treatment. In fact, it could be reasoned that an openly administered placebo might even be the purest form of a nonplacebo/verum treatment because there is nothing the patient cannot know (and thus be deceived about), and everything that works is anything the patient makes of it. It has been said of placebos that "Nothing works better," so it might be fitting to say that openly administered placebos are "Anything you want them to be."

Placebos show the way

Returning to the issue of the relationship between placebos and psychotherapy, Grünbaum's definition of *placebo* provides firm ground to expand the placebo concept without turning psychotherapy automatically into placebo nor automatically excluding the possibility of placebo in psychotherapy. Importantly, the fact that both interventions share and employ characteristic psychological and interpersonal constituents, such as expectancy, conditioning, meaning, and therapeutic alliance, is not of relevance for the definition of a psychotherapy being a placebo, but rather whether these constituents are openly administered (i.e., whether the client or patient is fully informed and gives consent to be treated by this treatment with these characteristic psychological and interpersonal constituents). From an empirical perspective, the open communication of psychotherapy's therapeutic factors (i.e., the therapeutic alliance, the personality, and interpersonal skills of the therapist as much as the expectancy of clients/patients; see for comprehensive review[33]), would not only be well-founded but also easy to communicate, as these constructs are assumingly understood even by nonpsychologists.

While this appears straightforward on paper or in theory, respectively, there seems to be reluctance to "go open."[43] For example, Leder[44] criticized this approach as "(1) the information about common factors is not necessary for informed consent and (2) clarity about specific mechanisms of change in therapy is consistent with 'many theory-specific forms of psychotherapy.'"[45] While there are epistemological arguments against this position,[45] this might also be answered empirically by considering what happens when the therapeutic factors of psychotherapy are disclosed. Based on evidence from psychotherapy-naïve participants, the content of disclosure had the expected effects (i.e., participants informed about these therapeutic factors rated them to be more important than participants informed about (assumingly) treatment-specific effects).[46] Interestingly, a similar survey in psychotherapy trainees indicated a lack of ethical, conceptual, and procedural knowledge in future psychotherapists, which "raises important questions about the preparedness of psychotherapy students to fulfill their ethical obligations."[47] This preliminary evidence suggests that, on the one hand, openly informing patients about psychotherapies' therapeutic factors does not confuse but rather empower patients, while, on the other hand, psychotherapists are lacking the needed ethical footing. This is ever so striking as there is little reservation to use just that what should be disclosed. For example, even though different therapeutic schools use different models and methods, they share their aim to promote a plausible narrative for the therapy at hand (see for a review[48]). Further, the (nondisclosed!) use of placebo mechanisms to increase the response expectancy in a psychological intervention is seen to use "placebo mechanisms (to) increase a proven psychological intervention's efficacy for healthy participants [. . .] if offered combined with a positive communication style."[49] While this is without doubt an interesting result of a carefully conducted scientific study, its transfer into clinical reality is ethically problematic (see[38]).

Interestingly, placebo is not only the problem here, but it also provides an excellent solution. Contrary to intuition, common lore, and scientific belief, openly administered placebos work,[50] and they work as good as the deceptive placebos.[6] Interestingly, open-label placebos (OLPs) are not only effective but also well accepted. In an online case vignette study, 63% of participants thought OLPs to be acceptable for the exemplary complaint of insomnia, and 48% indicated willingness to take an OLP.[51] Further, the administration of OLPs in patients with irritable bowel syndrome showed that "OLP participants reflected more on their treatment, often involving noticeable cognitive and emotional processes of self-reflection."[52]

Regarding psychotherapy, a recent survey among psychotherapists in Switzerland indicates that informed consent is seen as a constant process and both as a challenge as well as a resource.[53] Interestingly, therapists were mostly concerned with providing information to patients to allow making self-determined decisions, whereas providing information on the mode of action of the given therapy was seen as a challenge by about 50% of therapists.[53] The discussion and empirical test of what and how is to be disclosed to patients needs to advanced, encompassing not only the usual suspects (i.e., confidentiality, frequency of meetings, treatment goals, and empirical effectiveness),[53] but also include the mode of action (i.e., the characteristic and incidental treatment constituents of psychotherapy).[38]

Open-label placebos are psychotherapy and psychotherapy should be an open-label placebo

In the light of the above, OLPs can be seen as psychotherapy as its best (i.e., the open and fully transparent application of proven psychological principles with sound empirical evidence). With regard to the latter, it needs to be noted that placebos might be the most-tested intervention of all as they are used in all placebo-controlled clinical trials. Further, considering that placebo conditions are usually not treated fairly,[54] the often-substantial effects could be considered as conservative estimates of its potential. Contrariwise, psychotherapy might not be a placebo per se, but psychotherapy clearly can be a placebo as much as any other intervention can be turned into a placebo. To avoid the problem for psychotherapy to become placebo (i.e., to deceive patients about its characteristic and incidental treatment constituents), it would be best to follow the principles of OLP and to go open[43]—there is little to lose and much to gain.

References

1. Locher C, Koechlin H, Zion SR, et al. Efficacy and safety of selective serotonin reuptake inhibitors, serotonin-norepinephrine reuptake inhibitors, and placebo for common

psychiatric disorders among children and adolescents: A systematic review and meta-analysis. *JAMA Psychiatry.* 2017;74(10):1011–1020. http://doi:10.1001/jamapsychia try.2017.2432

2. Darragh M, Yow B, Kieser A, Booth RJ, Kydd RR, Consedine NS. A take-home placebo treatment can reduce stress, anxiety and symptoms of depression in a non-patient population. *Australian and New Zealand Journal of Psychiatry.* 2016;50(9):858–865. http:// doi:10.1177/0004867415621390

3. Benedetti F, Durando J, Giudetti L, Pampallona A, Vighetti S. High-altitude headache: The effects of real vs sham oxygen administration. *Pain.* 2015;156(11):2326–2336. http:// doi:10.1097/j.pain.0000000000000288

4. Jonas WB, Crawford C, Colloca L, et al. To what extent are surgery and invasive procedures effective beyond a placebo response? A systematic review with meta-analysis of randomised, sham controlled trials. *BMJ Open.* 2015;5(12):e009655. http://doi:10.1136/ bmjopen-2015-009655

5. Takakura N, Takayama M, Kawase A, Kaptchuk TJ, Yajima H. Double blinding with a new placebo needle: a further validation study. *Acupuncture in Medicine.* 2010;28(3):144–148. http://doi:10.1136/aim.2009.001230

6. Locher C, Frey Nascimento A, Kirsch I, Kossowsky J, Meyer A, Gaab J. Is the rationale more important than deception? A randomized controlled trial of open-label placebo analgesia. *Pain.* 2017;158(12):2320–2328. http://doi:10.1097/j.pain.0000000000001012

7. Desharnais R, Jobin J, Côté C, Lévesque L, Godin G. Aerobic exercise and the placebo effect: A controlled study. *Psychosomatic Medicine.* 1993;55:149–154. http://dx.doi.org/ 10.1097/00006842-199303000-00003

8. Crum AJ, Langer EJ. Mind-set matters: Exercise and the placebo effect. *Psychological Science.* 2007;18(2):165–171. http://doi:10.1111/j.1467-9280.2007.01867.x

9. Fritz C, Curtin J, Poitevineau J, Morrel-Samuels P, Tao FC. Player preferences among new and old violins. *Proceedings of the National Academy of Sciences U S A.* 2012;109(3):760–763. http://doi:10.1073/pnas.1114999109

10. Werner C, Birkhäuer B, Locher C, et al. Price information influences the subjective experience of wine: A framed field experiment. *Food Quality and Preference.* 2021;92:104223. https://doi.org/10.1016/j.foodqual.2021.104223

11. Colloca L, Lopiano L, Lanotte M, Benedetti F. Overt versus covert treatment for pain, anxiety, and Parkinson's disease. *Lancet Neurology.* 2004;3(11):679–684. http://doi:10.1016/ S1474-4422(04)00908-1

12. Tondorf T, Kaufmann LK, Degel A, et al. Employing open/hidden administration in psychotherapy research: A randomized-controlled trial of expressive writing. *PLoS ONE.* 2017;12(11):e0187400. http://doi:10.1371/journal.pone.0187400

13. Kirsch I. Placebo psychotherapy: Synonym or oxymoron? *Journal of Clinical Psychology.* 2005;61(7):791–803. http://doi:10.1002/jclp.20126

14. Locher C, Hasler S, Gaab J. When do psychotherapeutic placebos work? A critical review on the example of systematic desensitization. *Verhaltenstherapie.* 2016;26:9–20. http:// doi:10.1159/000443464

15. Crabtree A. *From Mesmer to Freud: Magnetic Sleep and the Roots of Psychological Healing (New).* Yale University Press; 1994.

16. Eysenck HJ. The outcome problem in psychotherapy: What have we learned? *Behaviour Research and Therapy.* 1994;32(5):477–495. http://doi:doi:10.1016/0005-7967(94)90135-x

17. Eysenck HJ. The effects of psychotherapy: An evaluation. *Journal of Consulting Psychology.* 1992 [1952];16:319–324.

18. Jopling DA. Placebo insight: The rationality of insight-oriented psychotherapy. *Journal of Clinical Psychology.* 2001;57:19–36. http://dx.doi.org/ 10.1002/1097-4679

19. Justman S. From medicine to psychotherapy: The placebo effect. *History of the Human Sciences*. 2011;24:95–107. http://dx.doi.org/10.1177/0952695110386655

20. Cuijpers P, Karyotaki E, Reijnders M, Ebert DD. Was Eysenck right after all? A reassessment of the effects of psychotherapy for adult depression. *Epidemiology and Psychiatric Sciences*. 2019;28(1):21–30. http://doi:10.1017/S2045796018000057

21. Cuijpers P, Driessen E, Hollon SD, van Oppen P, Barth J, Andersson G. The efficacy of non-directive supportive therapy for adult depression: A meta-analysis. *Clinical Psychology Review*. 2012;32(4):280–291. http://doi:doi:10.1016/j.cpr.2012.01.003

22. Cuijpers P, Turner EH, Mohr DC, et al. Comparison of psychotherapies for adult depression to pill placebo control groups: A meta-analysis. *Psychological Medicine*. 2014;44(4):685–695. http://doi:doi:10.1017/S0033291713000457

23. Baskin TW, Tierney SC, Minami T, Wampold BE. Establishing specificity in psychotherapy: A meta-analysis of structural equivalence of placebo controls. *Journal of Consulting and Clinical Psychology*. 2003;71:973–979. http://dx.doi.org/10.1037/0022-006X.71.6.973

24. American Psychological Association, Society of Clinical Psychology. *Research-Supported Psychological Treatments*. n.d. Retrieved March 15, 2014. http://www.div12.org/Psychological Treatments/disorders/ptsd_main.php

25. Herbert JD, Lilienfeld SO, Lohr JM, et al. Science and pseudoscience in the development of eye movement desensitization and reprocessing: Implications for clinical psychology. *Clinical Psychology Review*. 2000;20:945–971.

26. McNally, R. J. EMDR and Mesmerism: A comparative historical analysis. *Journal of Anxiety Disorders*. 1999;13:225–236. http://dx.doi.org/10.1016/S0887-6185(98)00049-8

27. Justman, S. The power of rhetoric: Two healing movements. *Yale Journal of Biology and Medicine*. 2011;84:15–25.

28. Franklin B, Majault L, Sallin B, et al. Report of the commissioners charged by the King with the examination of animal magnetism. *International Journal of Clinical and Experimental Hypnosis*. 2002;50:332–363. http://dx.doi.org/10.1080/00207140208410109

29. Weissman MM. A brief history of interpersonal psychotherapy. *Psychiatric Annals*. 2006;36(8):553–557.

30. Frost ND, Laska KM, Wampold BE. The evidence for present-centered therapy as a treatment for posttraumatic stress disorder. *Journal of Traumatic Stress*. 2014;27:1–8.

31. Kaptchuk TJ, Kelley JM, Conboy LA, et al. Components of placebo effect: Randomised controlled trial in patients with irritable bowel syndrome. *British Medical Journal*. 2008;336:999–1003. http://dx.doi.org/10.1136/bmj.39524.439618.25

32. Gaab J, Kossowsky J, Ehlert U, Locher C. Effects and components of placebos with a psychological treatment rationale—Three randomized-controlled studies. *Scientific Reports*. 2019;9(1):1421. http://doi:doi:10.1038/s41598-018-37945-1

33. Wampold BE, Imel ZE. *The Great Psychotherapy Debate: Models, Methods, and Findings*. 2nd ed. Routledge; 2015.

34. Frank JD. Psychotherapy—The transformation of meanings: Discussion paper. *Journal of the Royal Society of Medicine*. 1986;79:341–346.

35. Moerman DE, Jonas WB. Deconstructing the placebo effect and finding the meaning response. *Annals of Internal Medicine*. 2002;136:471–476. http://dx.doi.org/10.7326/0003-4819-136-6-200203190-00011

36. Benedetti F. *Placebo Effects: Understanding the Mechanisms in Health and Disease*. Oxford University Press; 2009.

37. Blease CR, Lilienfeld SO, Kelley JM. Evidence-based practice and psychological treatments: the imperatives of informed consent. *Frontiers in Psychology*. 2016;7:1170. http://doi:10.3389/fpsyg.2016.01170

38. Trachsel M, Gaab J. Disclosure of incidental constituents of psychotherapy as a moral obligation for psychiatrists and psychotherapists. *Journal of Medical Ethics*. 2016;(8):493–495. doi:10.1136/medethics-2015-102986.

39. Trachsel M, Gaab J, Biller-Andorno N, Tekin S, Sadler J. *The Oxford Handbook of Psychotherapy Ethics*. Oxford University Press; 2021. http://doi:10.1093/oxfordhb/978019 8817338.001.0001

40. Grünbaum A. The placebo concept. *Behaviour Research and Therapy*. 1981;19(2):157–167

41. Grünbaum A. The placebo concept in medicine and psychiatry. *Psychological Medicine*. 1986;16(1):19–38.

42. Howick J. The relativity of "placebos": Defending a modified version of Grünbaum's definition. *Synthese*. 2016;194(4):1363–1396.

43. Gaab J, Blease C, Locher C, Gerger H. Go open—A plea for transparency in psychotherapy. *Psychology of Consciousness: Theory, Research, and Practice, American Psychological Association*. 2016;3(2):175–198. http://dx.doi.org/10.1037/cns0000063

44. Leder G. Psychotherapy, placebos, and informed consent. *Journal of Medical Ethics*. 2020;47(7):444–7. doi:10.1136/medethics-2020-106453.

45. Blease C. Psychotherapy is still failing patients: Revisiting informed consent-a response to Garson Leder. *Journal of Medical Ethics*. 2020:medethics-2020-106865. doi:10.1136/medethics-2020-106865.

46. Blease CR, Kelley JM. Does disclosure about the common factors affect laypersons' opinions about how cognitive behavioral psychotherapy works? *Frontiers in Psychology*. 2018; 9:2635. http:// doi:10.3389/fpsyg.2018.02635

47. Blease CR, Arnott T, Kelley JM, et al. Attitudes about informed consent: An exploratory qualitative analysis of UK psychotherapy trainees. *Frontiers in Psychiatry*. 2020;11:183. http://doi:10.3389/fpsyt.2020.00183

48. Locher C, Meier S, Gaab J. Psychotherapy: A world of meanings. *Frontiers in Psychology*. 2019; 10:460. http://doi:10.3389/fpsyg.2019.0046

49. Salzmann S, Wilhelm M, Schindler S, Rief W, Euteneuer F. Optimising the efficacy of a stress-reducing psychological intervention using placebo mechanisms: A randomized controlled trial. *Stress Health*. 2022;38(4):722–735. doi:10.1002/smi.3128.

50. von Wernsdorff M, Loef M, Tuschen-Caffier B, et al. Effects of open-label placebos in clinical trials: A systematic review and meta-analysis. *Science Reports*. 2021;11:3855. https://doi.org/10.1038/s41598-021-83148-6

51. Haas JW, Rief W, Doering BK. Open-label placebo treatment: Outcome expectations and general acceptance in the lay population. *International Journal of Behavioral Medicine*. 2021;28(4):444–454. http://doi:10.1007/s12529-020-09933-1

52. Haas JW, Ongaro G, Jacobson E, et al. Patients' experiences treated with open-label placebo versus double-blind placebo: a mixed methods qualitative study. *BMC Psychology*. 2022;10(1):20. doi:10.1186/s40359-022-00731-w.

53. Eberle K, Grosse Holtforth M, Inderbinen M, Gaab J, Nestoriuc Y, Trachsel M. Informed consent in psychotherapy: A survey on attitudes among psychotherapists in Switzerland. *BMC Medical Ethics*. 2021;22(1):150. http://doi:10.1186/s12910-021-00718-z

54. Blease CR, Bishop FL, Kaptchuk TJ. Informed consent and clinical trials: Where is the placebo effect? *British Medical Journal*. 2017;356:j463. http://doi:10.1136/bmj.j463

5

PUTTING PLACEBOS INTO PRACTICE

This section provides practical insights and guidance for implementing placebo effects in clinical practice. By understanding the mechanisms, ethical considerations, and contextual factors, healthcare professionals can optimize treatment outcomes and enhance patient care.

The first chapter explores the correlation between consciousness, subjective experiences of wellness or illness, and the pathways that influence physiological processes. Relevant processes are overviewed, emphasizing an evidence-based approach to utilizing placebo responses in specific clinical scenarios while preserving the moral integrity of the clinical encounter. Chapter two highlights the debates surrounding their utility and ethical implications in clinical practice. The emergence of placebo-controlled trials and landmark meta-analyses is explored, leading to a call for a paradigm shift in placebo research. The chapter advocates for the increased implementation of existing research findings for the benefit of patients and emphasizes the need for clinically applicable research.

Recognizing the influence of contextual factors on treatment outcomes, the third chapter emphasizes the significance of managing cognitive, relational, and environmental contextual factors. The role of beliefs, expectations, and mindsets in shaping a person's experience is considered, along with the importance of establishing an empathic therapeutic relationship.

The fourth chapter addresses the challenges in determining treatment effectiveness, emphasizing the need for person-centered perspectives in research designs using placebo control groups, going beyond regulatory considerations. The implications of placebo responses (and placebo effects) for interpreting results from randomized placebo-controlled clinical trials are analyzed, along with discussions on identifying "good evidence" of therapeutic effects that can be applied in clinical practice.

5.1

Placebo responses and effects

Processes, potential, and ethical considerations in clinical care

Nikola Boris Kohls, Monica A. Leyva, and James Giordano

Placebo (responses and effects) in context

When addressing mechanisms by which consciousness, and the subjective experiences of "wellness," or "illness" and suffering evoked by injury or disease are correlated, it becomes apparent that all engage pathways that can affect a variety of physiological, salutogenic, and/or maladogenic processes.[1] Indeed, external events—whether environmental, ritual, or interpersonal—engage one or more sensory systems, activate the peripheral and central nervous system, evoke cognitive substrates involved in different types of memory and emotion, and generate a change in the somatic state.[2] This instigates both directed actions/behaviors and the phenomenon of the bodily response and external provocation that are perceived as a "mind state." This is what Damasio has called the "feeling of what happens" and this is intrinsic to sentient experience.[3]

Neural systems are characteristically nonlinear, adaptive, and responsive to the internal and external milieu, and they can be environmentally and circumstantially conditioned.[4] While such responses are common, if not universal (not only to humans, but perhaps many mammalian species), the extent to which these systems are responsive, and the fortitude and pattern of responses, appear to be individually variant. Individual responses are determined by genetic predisposition and epigenetic-phenotypic interactions with various environmental factors throughout the lifespan.

Wachholtz and Pargament have shown that ritual experiences and practices can decrease anxiety, and can reduce negative, cognitive and behavioral features associated with pain and distress.[5] If we accept physician/philosopher Leon Kass's definition of *health* as an integrated "wholeness,"[6] then a role of certain environmental and interpersonal experiences and practices may facilitate salutogenic effects in the strictest sense: by preserving or enhancing the sense and, perhaps, the functional basis of "integration" that is "health," and by decreasing the dis-integration incurred by injury, disease, and illness.

The growing recognition that such experiences and the effects they generate are relevant to the clinical encounter should not be wholly surprising, as the use of ritual to enhance susceptibility and promote readiness to healing experiences has been characteristic of shamanic practices throughout history.[7] Creating a sense of expectation that a healing would occur thereby established the reciprocity of the encounter. In the Asclepian tradition, it was believed that the attendance of the graces (notably Hygieia and Panacea) established and maintained the durable healing power of the Asclepian "cure."[8] To be sure, the notion of a ritual evoked by the physician's demeanor and actions was critical to Hippocratic Medicine.[9]

The focus of the clinical encounter is the good of the patient, for it is the patient who seeks the physician's professed skills to enable healing. The satisfactory outcome of the clinical encounter may not entail cure but must involve care. To paraphrase Hippocrates, the regard for the patient is the art, and such positive regard is therefore instrumental to the ends of Medicine to render a right and good healing.[10,11] Is it not rational to assume that the supposedly "mystical" nature of shamanic healing—when interpreted in light of our contemporary understanding of neural mechanisms of expectation and belief—may, in fact, still be an important element of the modern clinical encounter? Simply, if the patient seeks the physician with some expectation (i.e., "hope") of healing that is based upon the physician's profession (i.e., literal declaration of knowledge intent and skills), then it is clear that the moral obligation of the physician is to prudently act within reason to attempt to realize that which has been professed—by maximizing the good for, and of, the patient.[12] In this sense, the tenor of the clinical encounter should "please" the patient by meeting the expectation for a positive interaction with the physician (that, at very least, does not harm).

It is in this light that we propose re-examination of the concept of the placebo. Literally translated from the Latin, *placebo* means "*I shall please.*" Given the aforementioned premises of the clinical encounter, is that not essential to the act of Medicine, at least in the context of care, hope and expectation arising from, and within, the physician-patient interaction? The notion of placebo as an "inert agent"—while relatively viable in the research literature to refer to a sham treatment—should be reconsidered, both in terms of the apparently nonspecific effects that such "inert" treatments produce, and the relevance of such "placebo effects" to clinical practice. Taken in accordance with the literal definition of *placebo*, "to please," it is important not to misinterpret placebo as mere placation. This is etymologically incorrect, conceptually inaccurate, and ethically unacceptable. Rather, placebo effects are those processes—or events that engage resultant processes—that are facilitative to healing.[12]

In this way, placebo effects might be better considered as patient-specific biopsychosocial effects. Unfortunately, however, the ambiguous terms *placebo* and *placebo effect*—retaining a considerable burden of "folk" meaning and reflecting a connotation of sham treatment—still persist. It is this folk interpretation that has led to definitional ambiguity and ethical consternation regarding the use of the placebo effect in medical practice. Not unlike the notion of "spirituality" (as confused with religion or religiosity), such definitional ambiguity can sustain both philosophical and pragmatic problems.[13] Also, like spirituality, a mechanistic understanding may be critical to increasing the relevance and resonance of such processes to Medicine.

Placebo effects can be regarded as physiological and psychological responses that can mitigate signs and symptoms of several types of conditions and disorders, and somewhat more generally, induce salutary effects. As noted elsewhere in this volume, placebo responses and effects have been somewhat enigmatic to both research and medical practices, at least in part because of ambiguous and/or insufficient theoretical orientations to the nature of these effects and responses. In many ways, this reflects the mechanistic conundrum common to much of Western Science and Medicine: namely, the reticence to accept that something can or may be effective unless there is demonstration of a viable mechanism for such effects. Indubitably, mechanistic understanding is important to define substrates involved, the potential for these substrates to be elicited in particular individuals, and if and how such processes might incur various beneficial, desirable, or deleterious effects.

Relevant putative mechanisms of placebos

Several neural loci and networks are likely involved in and by placebo responses. However, here we believe it important to discuss neural substrates as contributory to an understanding both of the placebo (response and effect) phenomena, and its utility and relevance to clinical intervention(s). Brain stem systems engage sensory input from a range of stimuli from external and internal environments to attend to feature orientation and processing. Differential activation of reticulothalamic neuraxes involved in attention, emotion, and directed consciousness (i.e., consciousness of a circumstance and the attendant emotional valance) can create a basal emotional state that, when taken together with activation of networks involving the amygdala, insula, and regions of the associative, cingulate, temporal, and parietal cortices evoke a sense of intentionality. Concomitant and/or subsequent engagement of hippocampal, and parahippocampal cortical neuraxes conjoin working and declarative memory to frame experience within past and current circumstance. Networks of the right and/or left prefrontal and orbitofrontal cortices participate, at least to some extent, in higher order expectation or anticipatory cognitions involved in situational experience, and relating such experience to prior, current, or potential future consequences (see Chapter 2.1).

Frontal and prefrontal cortical networks, which contribute to processing of expectation, decrease activity of the anterior insula, specific nuclei of the thalamus, anterior cingulate gyrus, and activate midbrain periaqueductal and periventricular gray regions to evoke direct sensory—rather than perceptual—modulation of physiological input. Later stage mechanisms involve reduced activity of the anterior and medial cingulate gyrus and amygdala, and support progressive relatively durable, conditionable placebo responses.

The role of neurocognitive processes in placebo *effects* has led to specific disciplinary foci that are dedicated to elucidating these substrates, and the possible bases and utility of these experiences. To be sure, several neurochemical systems play a role in placebo effects, and studies have provided evidence for training effects derived from placebo-induced stimuli.[14] These dimensions involve multifactorial cognitive domains and functions and, therefore, are unlikely to be subserved by, or relegated to, a single neural network, region, site, or neurotransmitter system. Rather, it seems that placebo *effects* are complex phenomena that, although facilitated by neurophysiological processes, are largely dependent upon personal and cultural contexts and, thus, are reliant upon multiple types and extents of biopsychosocial variables and effects.

Our prior work has posited that placebo effects might be regarded as complementary "mind-body" phenomena that involve "bottom-up" (i.e., bodily input to brain) and "top-down" (i.e., brain output to bodily functions) neurological substrates.[15] There is a growing body of literature, and increasing interest, to further elucidate how such mechanisms could deepen insights to the proverbial "mind-body problem," and perhaps open promising venues for various forms of care and healing. Yet, while certain nodes and networks of the brain appear to mediate aspects of placebo experiences and responses, it is important to avoid what Bennett and Hacker refer to as the "mereological fallacy," namely, the error of ascribing the function of the system as a whole to its particular component parts, when addressing putative roles of neural substrates and mechanisms.[16] In this case, it appears that there is not a specific brain site or network that mediates placebo effects, but rather the differential spatial and temporal activation of a number of networks.

Moreover, caution is warranted when addressing putative neural substrates in reference to cognitions, emotions, and behaviors. While we may discuss neural mechanisms involved in these processes, the experiences themselves are higher order phenomenon of the organism in which the nervous system is embodied and the reciprocally interactive effects of the environment in which the embodied organism is embedded. The embedded nature of organisms within social-cultural environments reflects "hierarchical levels of brain function, from acquisition of purely sense data, to the more extrapolated cognitive events of linking emotions and memories to expectation and/or contextual objectification."[2] This may suggest reciprocity and predisposition of these functions and effects; and the role, and importance of belief, expectation, and environmental conditioning in eliciting these psychobiological events and their manifestations.

Clinical potential

Clinical studies have identified three importance components for healing and coping processes; (1) hope in the face of illness, (2) receiving and giving a sense of acceptance, and (3) meaning and purpose (as focal to a particular point and/or context of the lived experience). Medical sociologist Aaron Antonovsky has attempted to determine why and how some individuals are able to adapt and overcome distress and remain healthy, while others more easily and/or rapidly succumb to such events.[17,18] The core concept of Antonovsky's theory is the "sense of coherence" that entails three subcomponents representing, first, a global orientation that expresses the extent to which one has a pervasive, enduring, dynamic feeling of confidence that the stimuli deriving from one's internal and external environments in the course of living are structured predictably and explicitly (i.e., comprehensibility); second, that these resources are available to meet the demands posed by stimuli and challenges (i.e., manageability); and third, that these demands and challenges are worthy of investment and engagement (i.e., meaningfulness). Per Antonovsky, individuals may be able to develop such coherence if able to perceive their environment(s) as comprehensible, manageable, and their life situation as meaningful.

In this context, it is interesting to compare salutogenic theory (which is often defined as a *sense of coherence*) with clinical observations associated with placebo responses. There have been suggestions that at least two encompassing psychological processes appear to be relevant for eliciting health-related placebo phenomenon: (1) a feeling of security and support, emanating from the encouragement from others, described by the authors as "feeling cared for, being helped, or receiving treatment," thereby suggesting that this process may be related to the manageability component of a sense of coherence; and (2) "a sense of empowerment," and "achieving health, taking care of one's self," that may be related to the meaningfulness—and perhaps comprehensibility—component(s) of the sense of coherence.[19]

These processes can be seen as healing attempts, which are driven by endogenous or exogenous interpersonal, and/or socioenvironmental factors. The components of meaningfulness can incur health effects rising from internal resource management, which influence perception, expectancy, motivation, and external resource management, inclusive of establishing relationships, and engaging with significant symbols and rituals. This is reflected in eight actions that, according to Barrett and coworkers, clinicians may perform to facilitate induction of placebo responses, these are: (1) speak positively about treatments, (2) provide encouragement, (3) develop trust, (4) provide reassurance, (5) support the clinical relationship, (6) respect individuality and uniquity, (7) explore values, and (8) create ceremony.[19]

To this last point, on a psychological level, the use of a placebo may be valuable for fostering perception and increasing meaningfulness of the clinical encounter. On a behavioral level, the use of a placebo may allow an individual to express such meaningfulness, and engagement. Functionally, placebo-inductive stimuli and practices may activate corresponding neural networks that are involved in eliciting health effects by the activation of physiologic (neuroendocrinologic and immunologic) processes.

Based upon extent evidence, we opine that it is at least plausible, if not likely, that there are complex interplays of inter- and intrapersonal factors that are necessary for placebo effects and responses. In this light, the placebo phenomenon may be regarded as "therapeutic meaning response," a definition that may infer (and perhaps afford better understanding of) body, brain, mind, and culture interacting in healing effects.[20] As studies have suggested, defining the placebo effects as a "positive healing action," resulting from the use of interventions mediated, at least to some extent, by the effect(s) that meanings have upon the patient, is to both mainstream as well as more integrative and complementary approaches (e.g., chiropractic, therapeutic touch, and homeopathy).[20–22]

Such a definition seems to be in accordance with cultural anthropologic findings demonstrating that symbolic interventions and shamanic treatments have been used within the context of Medicine throughout history for pleasing, encouraging and fortifying—rather than curing—patients.[23] Hence, we posit that an extended concept of the "meaning response" may also be useful to explain how and why experience can be conjoined with personal value, so as to allow or elicit potential placebo (or nocebo) mechanisms.

To date, two important models for explaining underlying cognitive and behavioral mechanisms of the placebo effect have been proposed: expectancy theory and classical conditioning.[24] While expectancy theory assumes that implicit or explicit expectancies can influence placebo-type organic processes (viz., of health/wellness; disease, injury, and illness), conditioning theory suggests that placebo effects can be regarded as a type of classical (Pavlovian), or mixed classical-operant (quasi-Skinnerian) conditioning. Studies examining if and how placebo effects might be due to expectancy or conditioning have suggested that both processes are involved and cannot be mechanistically disentangled.[25]

Therefore, meaningfulness might be regarded as an overarching concept or process, describing the effects of both expectancy and conditioning models, and insight to neurocognitive and behavioral mechanisms of meaningfulness may be viable and, therefore, of value to explain health-related effects of placebos. Personal values may contribute to expectancies (e.g., anticipations about the nature and extent of disease and illness, treatment, and/or trust in the clinician) that can influence or engage top-down networks operative in brain-mind-body responses to affect health and health-related dispositions. Such anticipations and expectancies could be environmentally and circumstantially paired, patterned, and reinforced, and, therefore, conditioning theory may also explain some of the placebo responses and effects incurred on individual and group (i.e., cohort) levels.

Ethical issues and considerations

Given the personal and individually unique nature of these experiences, we have argued that "acknowledgement of patients' needs . . . desire for resources permit the clinician to assume an accepting stance and . . . may fortify the clinician-patient relationship as a fundamental domain of healing."[2] This latter dimension (i.e., a positive clinician-patient relationship) is essential to (1) generating trust, (2) creating an environment in which the patient feels safe and secure, and (3) enabling the clinician to operate within this environment to evaluate whether certain beliefs or practices may exert salutary or negative influences relevant to patients' health and care.[1]

Understanding biopsychosocial processes is important when attempting to meet the clinical adage of "the right treatment for the right diagnosis." Thus, ongoing research will be crucial to determining what works (and what doesn't); in whom, when, and under what conditions; and what mechanisms are involved. Such studies can be useful to define how psychophysiological (and physio-psychological) variables mediate patient responses and therapeutic outcomes as influential and applicable, albeit with caveats, to the conduct of the clinical encounter.

The key elements of the clinical encounter are determination of what is wrong with the patient; what can be done (given knowledge of and about the disorder, and the range of potential interventions that target its pathologic mechanisms and effects); and from these factors, what should be done.[26] But "should" implies, if not explicates, some underlying system of values and judgments about what is "right" and "good."[27] Thus, it is necessary to recognize the multidimensional nature of "good" relative to what is biomedically sound, and how the application or engagement of biomedical factors can affect an individual patient's predicament of illness, circumstances, values, and choices. For disorders that have been shown to involve neural substrates that have been demonstrated to be affected in and by placebo effects, evoking placebo may, therefore, be aptly considered as alignment of the treatment with the disorder. Apropos this consideration, we (and others in this volume) urge re-examination of the concept, and perhaps use of placebos.

To wit, the definition of *placebo* as used in the research literature, to refer to a sham treatment, should be redefined. Considering the placebo to be processes that induce neuropsychological effects that are facilitative to healing can, and should, be more validly considered for potential therapeutic utility in light of current neuroscientific information and understanding. But such consideration should not be cavalier; to the contrary, adherence to resolving clinical equipoise dictates that like any potential therapeutic approach, the use of the placebo (effects and responses) must be weighed against other possible and viable interventions in light of available evidence, particulars of the case, and the relative balancing of benefits, burdens, risks, and harms.[28] Simply, knowing that a particular treatment *can* evoke mechanisms to produce positive outcomes does not explicitly compel or sustain that it *should* be used.

While placebo responses and effects may be viewed as valid means to mitigate signs and symptoms of certain types of disorders, we believe, pro philosopher Sissela Bok, that achieving these means by blatant deception incurs ethical harms through (1) intentional misleading of the patient, (2) undermining the veracity that establishes and maintains trust within the clinical encounter and relationship, (3) denying patients information necessary for valid informed consent, and (4) impugning patients' autonomy (in this sense, the negative right to refuse particular treatments).[29]

This speaks to the viability and ethical probity of utilizing "open placebo" (viz., an intervention employed to evoke a placebo response that is explicitly defined as such). Disclosing that a certain interventions may induce placebo responses does not necessarily reduce the potential for its effect, particularly if and when circumstances in which this information is provided afford sufficiently positive reinforcement for patients' expectations.[30] A clinician could assert that a particular intervention may engage mechanisms that in some ways can reduce feelings of subjective illness (i.e., "placemo" responses and effects) and perhaps evoke physiological processes that are recuperative, and that the actual mechanisms of these effects are not fully known. Indeed, despite myriad advances in bioscience and technology, in many ways, Medicine remains a relatively uncertain practice. Communicating this uncertainty to patients with a sense of optimism allows for veracity and intellectual honesty, while still fostering trust and hope.

Ethico-legal questions also center on the cost of interventions that may be used to evoke placebo responses. Namely, should these interventions be billable? One line of rationalization might be that if a technique is revealed to produce positive outcomes (even in the absence of demonstrated, specific underlying mechanism's effect) then it is billable (what might be called the *valued ends justification*). Another is that if (even a putative) is shown (as in the case at least in part for the placebo) then this supports the "reality" of the technique as scientifically valid and thus, a billable intervention (i.e., the *mechanistic justification*). Lastly, the mere fact that a clinician must devote some particular amount of time to rendering said interventions may be used to justify incurring costs (the *professional services justification*).

Each may be sustainable on some level, and, as historically shown, there have been ample instances of techniques being rendered, and patients billed, without (partial, complete, and/or correct) understanding of underlying mechanisms (e.g., aspirin, lithium, and cyclic antidepressants), or even definitive therapeutic benefit (e.g., frontal lobotomy). Therefore, if it is determined that placebos may be employed as a "formal" treatment modality, it will then become necessary to establish not only particular indications for placebo inducing methods, but also billing requirements and codifications for these uses in practice.

The fundamental ethical issue is how placebo effects might be elicited and engaged in patient care. While there is certainly "discretionary space" that the clinician must carefully establish to afford some latitude in how much information should be provided to a particular patient, as noted above, outright deception is contrary to the veracity that establishes trust within the clinician-patient relationship.[31,32] The asymmetry of knowledge and power between clinician and patient reinforces the fact that the clinician, as steward of knowledge, must utilize both objective knowledge of fact and subjective knowledge of the patient to best provide care that is right and good.[33] Beneficent actions must be grounded by prudent selection and use of such knowledge. The moral obligation is to provide therapeutically competent care that focuses upon the patient's best interest. Further, the therapeutic obligation must adhere to the moral ends of Medicine as humanitarian practice, and so moral and therapeutic intentions and actions are reciprocal and remain somewhat inseparable. Understanding that there are endogenous mechanisms that can facilitate pain modulation, healing responses, and enhance medical intervention(s) to improve therapeutic outcomes affords considerable insight into if, and perhaps how, such responses may be elicited in clinical practice.[22] Toward such ends, employing placebos could be justifiable in accordance with the principle of double effect, if (and only if): (1) the intervention is not intrinsically wrong (thus, sustaining the necessity of ongoing research to support evidence and mechanisms of placebo responses as salutogenic), (2) the use of a placebo has inherent benefit and is not simply a (dubious) means to a desired end, and (3) that any such interventions are consented to by the patient (see, e.g., the above discussion of "open placebo").[22] To this latter point, we concur with Jonsen and colleagues, who have argued that placebos should only be considered as a last resort in those situations when patients explicitly request (and/or require) some form of "active" care.[34] Application of any knowledge lies not in its potential, but in the prudent decisions and acts that allow its use as a tool that is both consistent with, and pursuant to, the primacy of the patient's best interest(s), as fundamental to the morally sound ends of Medicine.

Conclusions

How then can, and should, placebos and placebo effects be utilized within clinical care? Toward such ends we advocate a refocus upon the placebo not merely as an inert agent that induces some positive effect(s), but upon the actions of the clinician as *an agent* to evoke (placebo) responses and effects that are contributory to more positive therapeutic outcomes. Without doubt, there are times when diagnosis and/or effective treatment will remain enigmatic and elusive, and when the patient may frustrate the expert knowledge of the clinician. That is the nature of Medicine, and understanding this is fundamental to the realities of exercising practical clinical care. It is in this context that we have described previously placebo as ". . . not a sham intervention . . . but as a consequence of the clinical encounter itself."[28]

Understanding the patient is just as important as understanding the processes of illness and suffering, for such processes ultimately produce subjective effects within the life-world and objective body of the person who has become the patient. Determining the right treatment often requires pairing objective knowledge (of pathologic mechanisms and differing therapeutics) to the subjective context of a particular patient. And while the right treatment may require trial and error within an empirical approach, it is often the "good" of the treatment—the communication of intention, nonabandonment, and hope—that sustains the trust necessary to meet a patient's expectations within continued care. The placebo effect does not involve deceiving patients about inactive treatments. Instead, we argue that placebo effects can be gained by the clinician's active affirmation of her/his role in upholding patient's hope: by both the use of the most modern skills, techniques, and technologies and by the preservation of the durable interpersonal dimensions of clinical care as a humanitarian art.

References

1. Giordano J. Chronic pain and spirituality. *Practical Pain Management.* 2007;7(3):64–68.
2. Giordano J, Engebretson J. Neural and cognitive basis of spiritual experience: Biopsychosocial and ethical implications for clinical medicine. *Explore.* 2006;2:216–225.
3. Damasio A. *The Feeling of What Happens, Body and Emotion in the Making of Consciousness.* Harcourt; 1999.
4. Maricich Y, Giordano J. Pain, suffering and the ethics of pain medicine: Is a deontic foundation sufficient? *American Journal of Pain Management.* 2007;17:130–138.
5. Wachholtz A, Pergament K. Is spirituality a critical ingredient in medication? Comparing the effect of spiritual meditation, secular meditation and relaxation on spiritual, psychological, cardiac and pain outcomes. *Journal of Behavioral Medicine.* 2005;28(4):369–384.
6. Kass L. *Beyond Therapy: Biotechnology and the Pursuit of Happiness.* President's Council on Bioethics; 2003.
7. Winkleman M. Shamanism as the original neurotheology. *Zygon.* 2004;39(1):193–218.
8. Grmek MD. *Diseases in the Ancient Greek World.* Johns Hopkins University Press; 1989.
9. Smith WD. *The Hippocratic Tradition.* Cornell University Press; 1979.
10. Hippocrates *Works Volume Two.* Jones WHS, Withington ET, Potter P, Smith WD, eds. and trans. Loeb Classical Library; 1923.
11. Pellegrino ED. Medical ethics: Entering the post Hippocratic era. *American Board of Family Medicine.* 1988;1:120–137.
12. Giordano J. Pain, the patient and the physician: Philosophy and virtue ethics in pain medicine. In: Schatman ME, ed. *Ethical Issues in Chronic Pain Management.* Informa; 2006:1–18.
13. Benedetti F, Mayberg HS, Wager TD, Stohler CS, Zubieta JK. Neurobiologic mechanisms of the placebo effect. *Journal of Neuroscience.* 2005;25(45):10390–10402.

14. Amanzio M, Benedetti F. Neuropharmacological dissection of placebo analgesia: Expectation-activated opioid systems versus conditioning-activated specific subsystems. *Journal of Neuroscience.* 1999;19:484–494.

15. Kohls N, Sauer S, Offenbächer M, Giordano J. Spirituality: An overlooked predictor of placebo effects? *Philosophical Transactions of the Royal Society B: Biological Sciences.* 2011;366:1938–1948.

16. Bennett M, Hacker PMS. *The Philosophical Basis of Neuroscience.* Blackwell Publishing; 2003.

17. Antonovsky A. *Health, Stress, Coping: New Perspectives on Mental and Physical Wellbeing.* Jossey-Bass; 1979.

18. Antonovksy A. *Unraveling the Mystery of Health. How People Manage Stress and Stay Well.* Jossey-Bass; 1987.

19. Barrett B. Muller D, Rakel D, Rabago D, Marchand L, Scheder J. Placebo, meaning and health. *Perspectives in Biology and Medicine.* 2006;49(2):178–198.

20. Moerman DE, Jonas WB. Deconstructing the placebo effect and finding the meaning response. *Annals of Internal Medicine.* 2002;136:471–476.

21. Spiro HM. *Doctors, Patients and Placebos.* Yale University Press; 1986.

22. Giordano J, Boswell MV. Pain, placebo, and nocebo: Epistemic, ethical and practical issues. *Pain Physician.* 2005:8:331–333.

23. Giordano, J, Jonas WB. Asclepius and hygieia in dialectic: Philosophical, ethical and educational basis of an integrative medicine. *Integrative Medicine Insights.* 2007;23(3):89–101.

24. Voudouris NJ, Peck CL, Coleman J. The role of conditioning and verbal expectancy in the placebo response. *Pain.* 1990;43:121–128.

25. Stuart-William S, Podd J. The placebo effect: Dissolving the expectancy versus conditioning debate. *Psychological Bulletin.* 2004;130(2):324–340.

26. Pellegrino ED. The healing relationship: Architectonics of clinical medicine. In: Shelp EE, ed. *The Clinical Encounter: The Moral Fabric of the Patient-Physician Relationship.* Riedel; 1983:153–172.

27. MacIntyre A. *What Justice, Which Rationality?* University of Notre Dame Press; 1988.

28. Giordano J. Placebo and placebo effect: Practical considerations, ethical concerns. *American Family Physician.* 2008;77(9):1212–1214.

29. Bok S. The ethics of giving placebos. *Scientific American.* 1974;231:17–23.

30. Colloca L, Benedetti F. Placebos and painkillers: Is mind as real as matter? *Nature Reviews Neuroscience.* 2005;6(7):545–552.

31. Petrovic P, Dietrich T, Fransson P, Andersson J, Carlsson K, Ingvar N. Placebo in emotional processing-induced expectations of anxiety relief activate a generalized modulatory network. *Neuron.* 2005;46:957–969.

32. Phan KL, Fitzgerald DA, Nathan PJ, Moore GJ, Uhde TW, Tancer ME. Neural substrates for voluntary suppression of negative affect: A functional magnetic resonance imaging study. *Biological Psychiatry.* 2005;57:210–219.

33. Bloche MG. Fidelity and deceit at the bedside. *JAMA.* 2000;283:1881–1884.

34. Jonsen AR, Siegler M, Winslade WJ. *Clinical Ethics.* 2nd ed. Macmillan; 1986.

5.2

Putting placebos into practice

From mechanisms to making patients better

Damien G. Finniss, Jeremy Howick, and Przemyslaw Babel

Introduction: the growth of the Placebo field

Placebos have been part of the medical lexicon for over 200 years. Over these 2 centuries, there has been discussion about the use of placebos in clinical practice with various interpretations (positive and negative) from utility and ethical perspectives.[1] The advent of the placebo-controlled trial in the 1950s, coupled with Beecher's seminal meta-analysis in 1955,[2] raised the profile of the topic area and arguably marked a new phase in research on placebos and placebo effects.

The remainder of the twentieth century saw relatively modest growth and development in the field of Placebo Research (when compared to that of the twenty-first century). There was further investigation into responses to placebo in clinical trials, and a new focus on understanding the mechanisms of placebo effects. The latter originated in animal studies[3] and progressed to humans including early work in clinical populations (e.g., Levine and colleagues in 1978).[4]

Many of these studies have used more traditional placebos such as sugar tablets or inert tablets. What is often inadequately explained in publications from these studies is that the placebo pills are administered in the psychosocial context of a therapeutic ritual designed to simulate a specific treatment in a particular context (and thus the nature of the placebo is not as important as what it is intended to do).[5] When one administers a traditional placebo, it is intended to assess the effect of the psychosocial context on the patients' brain and body.[6] It is the context that engages the placebo mechanisms, resulting in genuine psychobiological phenomena and health improvements. Importantly, in the setting of a negative context, nocebo effects can occur and can either detract from proven treatments or cause negative health outcomes.

Alongside the research into placebo mechanisms, there has been a substantial number of epidemiological studies. This includes a host of narrative reviews (e.g., Houston 1938) [7] and clinical trials (e.g., Egbert 1964)[8] where there is no specific mention of placebo effects nor administration of traditional placebos, yet conceptually the authors have been referring to and experimenting with specific contextual interventions to improve clinical outcomes. For example, in Egbert et al.'s study (1964), a "special care" group, where patient expectations and doctor-patient interactions were optimized, resulted in significant opioid reduction post major abdominal surgery.

This bourgeoning research has provided important support for work in clinical populations. For example, in the field of Pain and Analgesia, there has been dedicated work in experimental and clinical pain assessing various psychological and biological mechanisms of placebo analgesia and nocebo hyperalgesia (Section 2 of the book). Further, there have been some novel clinical trials, such as that conducted by Kaptchuk and colleagues in 2008, that blended the use of a traditional placebo (sham acupuncture) with very specific contextual interventions focused on the patient-doctor interaction. This trial demonstrated a "dose-response" effect to sham (placebo) acupuncture when adding specific elements to a therapeutic context intervention, such as empathy, thoughtful listening, and targeted symptom inquiry.[9] Further, there have been some novel clinical trials assessing "open-label" placebo prescription.[10] In these trials, the traditional placebo is given in a nondeceptive manner, but this administration is coupled with very controlled information and reinforcement of expected outcomes delivered in a therapeutic context (the setting of meeting a physician in a trial). Taken together there has been a synergy between the work with traditional placebos and that of broader research on therapeutic context,[11] supported by a growing amount of basic science and experimental research.

The call for a shift

The rich field of Placebo Studies has shown how placebo treatments produce their effects and that they benefit patients. We therefore believe that Placebo Studies now must focus on implementation for patient benefit. Such meaningful translation of placebo science to clinical practice requires at least three key elements. First, there needs to be an acknowledgment of a formal field that is genuinely multidisciplinary in nature and facilitates interaction between a wide range of scientists, clinicians, and leaders. Second, there needs to be more translational research from the laboratory to the clinic with the goal of exploring clinically meaningful effects (specifically with respect to duration and not only magnitude). Third, the research needs to be implemented vigorously.

Acknowledging the need for placebo research that directly benefits patients

The first of these elements has arguably been achieved. It has been over 25 years since the Harvard University interdisciplinary exploration of placebo effects. This initiative involved a select few academics from broad backgrounds working together to promote understanding and progress toward further understanding placebo effects.[12] At a similar time (late 1990s), the International Association for the Study of Pain developed an interest group on placebos, which culminated in a broad membership base and several academic meetings, namely in Copenhagen in 2008, which saw over 100 clinicians and academic researchers meet.

Further evidence of the progression of this specialty field comes in the form of *The Journal of Interdisciplinary Placebo Studies* (JIPS) database, which was developed in 2004.[13] It has served as an important central database for placebo research and is actively updated, disseminating new research findings on placebo to its members. JIPS is affiliated with the Society for Interdisciplinary Placebo Studies, an initiative founded in 2014, which has become a key organization with global representation from placebo researchers, clinicians, and academics from a broad range of disciplines. Of note, this organization has facilitated key meetings and publications addressing conceptual, definitional, and clinical application aspects of placebo research.[14,15] Taken together these ongoing initiatives are evidence of the formalization of a genuine multidisciplinary specialty, and one which can promote ongoing translational research.

There has been an exponential rise in research on placebo effects.[16] Further, a more recent analysis of the JIPS database revealed that while the absolute number of studies with patients has increased, there has been a relative reduction when compared to the entire literature growth, resulting in less than one in four papers including patients (a clinical population).[13] The true number of trials with direct clinical extrapolation (e.g., the Egbert (1964) or Kaptchuk (2008)) mentioned above would be much lower.

Taken together, there is a very strong foundation for a time-period shift. There is recognition of a dedicated field with core organizations, a critical number and breadth of constituents, and an impressive body of mechanism research to provide foundation for translational work. The exponential growth in publications now needs to be matched with parallel initiatives promoting translational research, medical and health education, policy development, and broader philosophy.

More translational research from bench to bedside

Learning mechanisms serve as a model for translational research, showcasing the growth of placebo research and its remarkable potential to be applied in patient care. Placebo effects have long been recognized as learning phenomena, with classical conditioning identified as a fundamental mechanism. More recently, observational learning and operant conditioning have been proposed as additional learning mechanisms in the context of placebo effects.

Learning mechanisms as a model for translational research

Learning mechanisms are a demonstration of the growth of placebo research and the wonderful potential to translate this work to patient care. Placebo effects have been learning phenomena since the 1950s, when classical conditioning was suggested as their underlying mechanism.[17-19] In 2002, observational learning was proposed as a second learning process,[20] and very recently, operant conditioning as an additional learning mechanism.[21]

There is growing evidence that classical conditioning induces placebo and nocebo effects, and that they are not necessarily mediated by expectancy.[22-25] Further, there is evidence that placebo effects can be induced without conscious awareness.[26,27] In keeping with the principles of classical conditioning, it has been shown that the magnitude of the conditioned placebo effects depend on the strength of the unconditioned response[28] and that placebo effects undergo a generalization process.[29,30] The phenomenon of extension has also been demonstrated; although, a higher number of trials and partial schedule of unconditioned stimuli prevent the extinction.[31,32]

Research shows that observational learning is another potent learning mechanism of placebo effects.[33] It induces placebo effects regardless of the type of modeling,[34] type of placebo intervention,[35] and characteristics of the model.[36,37] However, the characteristics of the model are related to the magnitude of placebo effects induced by observational learning. It has been found that male models [38] of higher social status,[37] who demonstrate more self-confident behaviors,[39] induce stronger placebo effects. Interestingly in one case of verbal modeling, which involves presentations of pain ratings rather than observation of a person experiencing benefit (a placebo effect), individual reported pain ratings were found to be more effective than those coming from a group of people.[40] Further, there is some evidence that the magnitude of placebo effects induced by observational learning may be related to the empathy levels of the observers.[38,41]

There is some promising initial research supporting the role of operant conditioning.[21] It seems that reinforcement of responding to a placebo together with the punishment of reacting in the opposite direction may induce the placebo effect.[42] There is also evidence for placebo-like effects induced by operant conditioning.[43,44] This may represent an important area of focus and opportunity, particularly in Pain and Analgesia, given the well-established role of operant conditioning in that field.[45]

Significant progress has been made in recent years with respect to understanding the psychological determinants of placebo effects. The discussion has progressed from a "expectation vs conditioning" debate [46] to understanding the potential contribution of multiple learning processes with that of verbal suggestion and expectancies. For example, stronger placebo and nocebo effects have been demonstrated when learning processes were accompanied by verbal suggestions that were congruent with classical conditioning principles.[47,48] Equally, there is recent evidence demonstrating that a stronger placebo effect is observed when the suggestion of the improvement preceded rather than followed classical conditioning.[49] Interestingly, these findings have not been replicated for nocebo effects,[50] where classical conditioning may not contribute to the verbally induced nocebo effect.[51] Of note are the findings that verbal suggestions can completely abolish the effect of conditioning[52] and classical conditioning can reverse or nullify the effect of suggestions.[29,53]

The results of the studies on the learning mechanisms of placebo effects provide important clinical implications on how to harness learning mechanisms to induce and boost placebo effects and prevent, diminish, or nullify nocebo effects. Firstly, from the perspective of classical conditioning, a history of previous positive therapeutic context(s) should be sought, and attempts made to replicate as much of the previous positive contexts as possible into the planned intervention. Equally, a focused assessment should be made of any negative contextual elements that may potentiate nocebo effects. These may be addressed through altering the clinical context (e.g., a change in environment) or through targeted cognitive intervention. In the setting of concurrent placebo use with treatments (e.g., use of placebos with analgesics to optimize analgesia and reduce analgesic side effect), caution should be given to adequately alternate the pairing of active analgesic with a placebo to potentiate long-lasting placebo effects.

Secondly, from the observational learning viewpoint, consideration should be given to observing improvement in other patients in a similar context. This may include group therapy or the use of technology to permit patients to see and hear from others who had responded well to treatment. For example, in one clinical trial, an information package included a video of a news interview in which patients in a similar trial reported excellent benefits.[54] Of course, observing negative results in others should be avoided as best possible. Further research is needed with respect to understanding and applying specific modeling characteristics, and equally the modulation of empathy in observational learning is also worthy of consideration.

Thirdly, clinicians should help patients recognize the positive effects of placebo and active interventions and then reinforce those effects, particularly the notion that routine therapies engage placebo mechanisms even if a traditional placebo is not given. Clinicians should also help patients interpret nocebo effects and side effects of active interventions as signals that they are providing efficacy. This reconceptualization or reframing coupled with reinforcement of treatment progress represents an application of fundamental cognitive and behavioral therapy coupled with contemporary placebo and nocebo science.

Finally, learning mechanisms should be seen in the broader context of multiple placebo mechanisms. Therefore, verbal suggestions congruent with previous experience should be provided to patients to boost learning processes. When positive effects of placebo and active interventions are observed, they should still be boosted by providing a further positive experience and verbal suggestions of improvement. However, when adverse effects of placebo and active interventions are observed, positive experience and verbal suggestions should be provided to nullify and reverse them.

Taken together, learning mechanisms demonstrate the rapid progression in knowledge about placebo and nocebo effects. Placebo and nocebo effects are learning phenomena—they can be learned and unlearned. This is of relevance in the translation to clinical practice, where over the continuum of a health care encounter, there is opportunity to assess, modify, and both reinforce learning processes and integrate them with other cognitive mechanisms to optimize the harnessing of placebo effects. One way to facilitate clinical translation is to embed these concepts into a framework that is clinically applicable across healthcare and already adopts some of the broader psychological and environmental principles that are fundamental to placebo and nocebo science.

A broader sociopsychobiological framework for implementation of placebo and nocebo research

As previously discussed, the growth of the field of Placebo Research has come both from research using traditional placebos and broader research around therapeutic context. There is clinically relevant evidence to support combined learning processes as key mechanisms of placebo effects, and that these processes encompass both cognitive and behavioral elements. Further, the role of the broader context (environment) is emphasized when considering multiple learning processes. Taken together, it is reasonable to suggest that the clinical application of placebo effects involves consideration of biological, psychological (including cognitive and behavioral elements) and overarching social or environmental contributors. This is the model originally presented by Engel in 1977 to challenge Biomedicine,[55] which has been further developed in the field of Pain Management, as an example,[56] and advocated by leading global health[57] and professional organizations.[58]

The Placebo field has provided compelling evidence that therapeutic ritual (or the psychosocial context around the patient) medicates multiple, specific placebo effects, and these effects can be clinically significant.[48] The open-hidden paradigm is a powerful demonstration of the power of the psychosocial context on clinical outcomes, underscoring the concept that placebo mechanisms can be harnessed *without* the use of a traditional placebo.[6,59] In this model, a drug is given in full view of the patient (through an intravenous drip) in one condition, and in the other, the drug is infused silently with minimal clinical interaction. The pharmacology of the drug is identical; however, the context is dramatically varied. Many drugs, such as morphine, are up to 50% less effective when most of the contextual element of the therapeutic ritual is removed, underscoring the role of context mediated endogenous analgesic mechanisms (the placebo component of routine care) in the overall outcome to a drug treatment. Therefore, from the perspective of the Placebo field, one could not only argue for routine incorporation of a biopsychosocial framework to application of placebo science at the bedside but argue for a sociopsychobiological framework that places context front and center. In fact, this has been suggested recently in the field of Pain and Analgesia.[60]

A sociopsychobiological framework permits longitudinal assessment of patients. This is useful in understanding factors that affect response to treatment both acutely and longer term. There is a strong body of evidence demonstrating that psychological and environmental factors are associated with variance in treatment outcomes after injury[61] or surgery[62,63] and that targeted psychosocial interventions can have meaningful longer term outcomes (e.g.,[64]). In addition to the previously mentioned trial by Egbert in 1964, a recent targeted perioperative trial using a contextual intervention (specifically a special care group with an expectancy modulating intervention) was able to show clinically meaningful effects on pain, physiological stress response and outcome at 6 months.[65] Importantly, both of these trials clearly emphasize the role of psychosocial interventions in a *longitudinal* manner over a time period of up to several weeks. This is undoubtedly of importance when planning for clinically meaningful harnessing of placebo mechanisms in practice and is underscored by the nature of our understanding of learning mechanisms and the importance of verbal, social, and behavioral reinforcement over time.

Vigorous implementation of the research

The evidence-based medicine movement has demonstrated that research, including research that benefits patients, sometimes is not implemented.[66] It follows that open acknowledgment that placebo research needs to take a practical turn, bolstered by more translational research, and will not benefit patients unless the knowledge is implemented. Implementing research (or indeed ideas in general) requires different skills from doing research. Hence, getting useful research to patients may require that the Placebo Research community develop new skills or outsource the implementation. One possibility of translating the science of placebos to clinical practice is to incorporate what constitutes good evidence with patient engagement. Partnership among researchers, stakeholder partners, and patients will help implement research into clinical practice. These parties should work together to identify patients' needs and values and bring these elements into the design, implementation, and dissemination of the science, ensuring an optimal translation that gets useful research to patients (see Chapter 5.4 for an in-depth discussion of this concept).

Conclusions

Placebo researchers have successfully provided evidence explaining how placebo effects arise, and that they can benefit patients. They have organized themselves into a large interdisciplinary, international, and influential group. More recently, they have provided a model—the biopsychosocial model—which has shown promise for implementing research to improve human health. Here we have shown that the time is ripe for a shift toward implementation so that real patients can benefit from the success of placebo researchers.

References

1. Finniss DG. Placebo effects: Historical and modern evaluation. *International Review of Neurobiology*. 2018;139:1–27.
2. Beecher HK. The powerful placebo. *JAMA*. 1955;159:1602–1606.
3. Herrnstein R. Placebo effect in the rat. *Science*. 1962;138:677–678.
4. Levine JD, Gordon NC, Fields HL. The mechanism of placebo analgesia. *Lancet*. 1978;2(8091):654–657.
5. Price DD, Finniss DG, Benedetti F. A comprehensive review of the placebo effect: Recent advances and current thought. *Annual Review of Psychology*. 2008;59:565–590.
6. Finniss DG, Kaptchuk TJ, Miller FG, Benedetti F. Biological, clinical, and ethical advances of placebo effects. *Lancet*. 2010;375(9715):686–695.
7. Houston WR. The doctor himself as a therapeutic agent. *Annals of Internal Medicine*. 1938;11(8):1416–1425.
8. Egbert LD, Battit GE, Welch CE, Bartlett MK. Reduction in postoperative pain by encouragement and instruction of patients—A study of doctor-patient rapport. *New England Journal of Medicine*. 1964;270(16):825–827.
9. Kaptchuk TJ, Kelley JM, Conboy LA, et al. Components of placebo effect: Randomised controlled trial in patients with irritable bowel syndrome. *British Medical Journal*. 2008;336(7651):999–1003.
10. Kaptchuk TJ, Miller FG. Open label placebo: Can honestly prescribed placebos evoke meaningful therapeutic benefits? *British Medical Journal*. 2018;363:k3889. doi:10.1136/bmj.k3889.
11. Howick J, Moscrop A, Mebius A, et al. Effects of empathic and positive communication in healthcare consultations: A systematic review and meta-analysis. *Journal of the Royal Society of Medicine*. 2018;111(7):240–252.
12. Harrington A. Introduction. In: Harrington A, ed. *The Placebo Effect—An Interdisciplinary Exploration*. Harvard University Press; 1997:1–11.
13. Enck P, Horing B, Broelz E, Weimer K. Knowledge gaps in placebo research: With special reference to neurobiology. *International Review of Neurobiology*. 2018;139:85–106.
14. Evers AWM, Colloca L, Blease C, et al. Implications of placebo and nocebo effects for clinical practice: Expert consensus. *Psychotherapy and Psychosomatics*. 2018;87(4):204–210.
15. Evers AWM, Colloca L, Blease C, et al. What should clinicians tell patients about placebo and nocebo effects? Practical considerations based on expert consensus. *Psychotherapy and Psychosomatics*. 2021;90(1):49–56.
16. Weimer K, Colloca L, Enck P. Age and sex as moderators of the placebo response—An evaluation of systematic reviews and meta-analyses across medicine. *Gerontology*. 2015;61(2):97–108.
17. Kurland AA. The drug placebo–its psychodynamic and conditional reflex action. *Behavioral Science*. 1957;2(2):101–110.
18. Wolf S. Effects of suggestion and conditioning on the action of chemical agents in human subjects—The pharmacology of placebos. *Journal of Clinical Investigation*. 1950;29(1):100–109.
19. Gliedman LH GW, Teitelbaum HA. Some implications of conditional reflex studies for placebo research. *American Journal of Psychiatry*. 1957;113:1103–1107.

20. Bootzin RR, Caspi O. Explanatory mechanisms for placebo effects: Cognition, personality and social learning. In: Guess HAKA, Kusek JW, Engel LW, eds. *The Science of the Placebo: Toward an Interdisciplinary Research Agenda*: BMJ Books; 2002:108–132.

21. Babel P. Operant conditioning as a new mechanism of placebo effects. *European Journal of Pain*. 2020;24(5):902–908.

22. Babel P. Classical conditioning as a distinct mechanism of placebo effects. *Frontiers in Psychiatry*. 2019;10:449. doi: 10.3389/fpsyt.2019.00449.

23. Bąbel P, Bajcar EA, Adamczyk W, et al. Classical conditioning without verbal suggestions elicits placebo analgesia and nocebo hyperalgesia. *PLoS ONE*. 2017;12(7):e0181856.

24. Bajcar EA, Adamczyk WM, Wiercioch-Kuzianik K, Bąbel P. Nocebo hyperalgesia can be induced by classical conditioning without involvement of expectancy. *PLoS ONE*. 2020;15(5):e0232108.

25. Babel P, Adamczyk W, Swider K, Bajcar EA, Kicman P, Lisinska N. How classical conditioning shapes placebo analgesia: Hidden versus open conditioning. *Pain Medicine (Malden, Mass)*. 2018;19(6):1156–1169.

26. Egorova N, Park J, Orr SP, Kirsch I, Gollub RL, Kong J. Not seeing or feeling is still believing: Conscious and non-conscious pain modulation after direct and observational learning. *Scientific Reports*. 2015;5:16809.

27. Jensen KB, Kaptchuk TJ, Kirsch I, et al. Nonconscious activation of placebo and nocebo pain responses. *Proceedings of the National Academy of Sciences USA*. 2012;109(39):15959–15964.

28. Price DD, Milling LS, Kirsch I, Duff A, Montgomery GH, Nicholls SS. An analysis of factors that contribute to the magnitude of placebo analgesia in an experimental paradigm. *Pain*. 1999;83(2):147–156.

29. Voudouris NJ, Peck CL, Coleman G. Conditioned response models of placebo phenomena: Further support. *Pain*. 1989;38:109–116.

30. Weng L, Peerdeman KJ, Della Porta D, van Laarhoven AIM, Evers AWM. Can placebo and nocebo effects generalize within pain modalities and across somatosensory sensations? *Pain*. 2022;163(3):548–559.

31. Colloca L, Petrovic P, Wager TD, Ingvar M, Benedetti F. How the number of learning trials affects placebo and nocebo responses. *Pain*. 2010;151(2):430–439.

32. Yeung STA, Colagiuri B, Lovibond PF, Colloca L. Partial reinforcement, extinction, and placebo analgesia. *Pain*. 2014;155(6):1110–1117.

33. Bajcar EA, Bąbel P. How Does Observational Learning Produce Placebo Effects? A Model Integrating Research Findings. *Frontiers in Psychology*. 2018;9:2041. doi:10.3389/fpsyg.2018.02041.

34. Hunter T, Siess F, Colloca L. Socially induced placebo analgesia: A comparison of a prerecorded versus live face-to-face observation. *European Journal of Pain (London, England)*. 2014;18(7):914–922.

35. Świder K, Bąbel P. The effect of the type and colour of placebo stimuli on placebo effects induced by observational learning. *PLoS ONE*. 2016;11(6):e0158363.

36. Bajcar EA, Wiercioch-Kuzianik K, Farley D, Adamczyk WM, Buglewicz E, Bąbel P. One of us or one of them? The effects of the model's and observer's characteristics on placebo analgesia induced by observational learning. *PLoS ONE*. 2020;15(12):e0243996.

37. Bieniek H, Bąbel P. The effect of the model's social status on placebo analgesia induced by social observational learning. *Pain Medicine (Malden, Mass)*. 2022;23(1):81–88.

38. Swider K, Bąbel P. The effect of the sex of a model on nocebo hyperalgesia induced by social observational learning. *Pain*. 2013;154(8):1312–1317.

39. Brączyk J, Bąbel P. The role of the observers' perception of a model's self-confidence in observationally induced placebo analgesia. *Journal of Pain*. 2021;22(12):1672–1680.

40. Bajcar EA, Wiercioch-Kuzianik K, Brączyk J, Farley D, Bieniek H, Bąbel P. When one suffers less, all suffer less: Individual pain ratings are more effective than group ratings in producing placebo hypoalgesia. *European Journal of Pain.* 2021;26(1):207–218.
41. Colloca L, Benedetti F. Placebo analgesia induced by social observational learning. *Pain.* 2009;144(1-2):28–34.
42. Adamczyk WM, Wiercioch-Kuzianik K, Bajcar EA, Bąbel P. Rewarded placebo analgesia: A new mechanism of placebo effects based on operant conditioning. *European Journal of Pain (London, England).* 2019;23(5):923–935.
43. Janssens T, Meulders A, Cuyvers B, Colloca L, Vlaeyen JWS. Placebo and nocebo effects and operant pain-related avoidance learning. *Pain Reports.* 2019;4(3):e748.
44. Jung WM, Lee YS, Wallraven C, Chae Y. Bayesian prediction of placebo analgesia in an instrumental learning model. *PLoS ONE.* 2017;12(2):e0172609.
45. Fordyce WE. *Behavioural science and chronic pain.* Postgraduate Medical Journal. 1984;60:865–868.
46. Stewart-Williams S, Podd J. The placebo effect: Dissolving the expectancy versus conditioning debate. *Psychological Bulletin.* 2004;130(2):324–340.
47. Petersen GL, Finnerup NB, Colloca L, et al. The magnitude of nocebo effects in pain: A meta-analysis. *Pain.* 2014;155(8):1426–1434.
48. Vase L, Riley JL 3rd, Price DD. A comparison of placebo effects in clinical analgesic trials versus studies of placebo analgesia. *Pain.* 2002;99(3):443–452.
49. Colloca L, Benedetti F. How prior experience shapes placebo analgesia. *Pain.* 2006;124(1-2):126–133.
50. Bajcar EA, Wiercioch-Kuzianik K, Farley D, Buglewicz E, Paulewicz B, Bąbel P. Order does matter: The combined effects of classical conditioning and verbal suggestions on placebo hypoalgesia and nocebo hyperalgesia. *Pain.* 2021;162(8):2237–2245.
51. Colloca L, Sigaudo M, Benedetti F. The role of learning in nocebo and placebo effects. *Pain.* 2008;136(1-2):211–218.
52. Benedetti F, Pollo A, Lopiano L, Lanotte M, Vighetti S, Rainero I. Conscious expectation and unconscious conditioning in analgesic, motor, and hormonal placebo/nocebo responses. *Journal of Neuroscience.* 2003;23(10):4315–4323.
53. Bajcar EA, Wiercioch-Kuzianik K, Adamczyk WM, Bąbel P. To experience or to be informed? Classical conditioning induces nocebo hyperalgesia even when placebo analgesia is verbally suggested-results of a preliminary study. *Pain Medicine (Malden, Mass).* 2020;21(3):548–560.
54. Carvalho C, Caetano JM, Cunha L, Rebouta P, Kaptchuk T, Kirsch I. Open-label placebo treatment in chronic low back pain: A randomized controlled trial. *Pain.* 2016;157(12):2766–2772.
55. Engel GL. The need for a new medical model: A challenge for biomedicine. *Science.* 1977;196(4286):129–136.
56. Gatchel RJ, Peng YB, Peters ML, Fuchs PN, Turk DC. The biopsychosocial approach to chronic pain: Scientific advances and future directions. *Psychological Bulletin.* 2007;133(4):581–624.
57. World Health Organization. *Guidelines on the Management of Chronic Pain in Children.* 2020. https://www.who.int/publications/i/item/9789240017870.
58. UK FoPM. *Faculty of Pain Medicine Statement on National Institute for Health and Care Excellence Guideline on Chronic pain (primary and secondary) in Over 16s: Assessment of All Chronic Pain and Management of Chronic Primary Pain.* 2021. https://fpm.ac.uk/sites/fpm/files/documents/2021-04/FPM%20Statement%20on%20NICE%20Chronic%20Pain%20Guidelines%202021-04-07.pdf.
59. Colloca L, Lopiano L, Lanotte M, Benedetti F. Overt versus covert treatment for pain, anxiety, and Parkinson's disease. *Lancet Neurology.* 2004;3:679–684.

60. Mardian AS, Hanson ER, Villarroel L, et al. Flipping the pain care model: A sociopsychobiological approach to high-value chronic pain care. *Pain Medicine.* 2020;21(6):1168–1180.

61. Nicholas MK, Linton SJ, Watson PJ, Main CJ; Group tDotFW. Early identification and management of psychological risk factors ("yellow flags") in patients with low back pain: A reappraisal. *Physical Therapy.* 2011;91(5):737–753.

62. Yang MMH, Hartley RL, Leung AA, et al. Preoperative predictors of poor acute postoperative pain control: A systematic review and meta-analysis. *BMJ Open.* 2019;9(4):e025091.

63. Harris I, Mulford J, Solomon M. Association between compensation status and outcome after surgery a meta-analysis. *JAMA.* 2005;293(13):1644–1652.

64. Nicholas MK, Costa DSJ, Linton SJ, et al. Implementation of early intervention protocol in Australia for 'high risk' injured workers is associated with fewer lost work days over 2 years than usual (stepped) care. *Journal of Occupational Rehabilitation.* 2020;30(1):93–104.

65. Rief W, Shedden-Mora MC, Laferton JA, et al. Preoperative optimization of patient expectations improves long-term outcome in heart surgery patients: Results of the randomized controlled PSY-HEART trial. *BMC Medicine.* 2017;15(1):4.

66. Howick J. *The Philosophy of Evidence-Based Medicine.* Wiley-Blackwell, BMJ Books; 2011.

5.3

Management of contextual factors to enhance placebo and minimize nocebo effects in clinical practice

Marco Testa, Giacomo Rossettini, Diletta Barbiani, and Maxi Miciak

Enhancing the "how to do" in clinical practice

As clinicians, we are focused on looking for new and more specific techniques, exercises, and drugs that match and improve a patient's structural or functional disorder. We look for one particular manipulation to precisely address a spinal segment facet joint, an exercise that can train a specific portion of a muscle, and a specific drug to target pain. This attitude is considered the "what to do" part of therapeutic interventions. Though professionally correct, it is only a part of our work. Another component of our intervention is at least as important as the "what to do," and it is the "how to do." Clinical conditions often present multiple features in complex ways. Physical features such as pain, fatigue, resistance, force, and precision of movement can be influenced by interactions between individual perception and cognitive and emotional processes. Moreover, internal and external contextual factors can easily influence how all of these features respond.

As a result, the clinical outcomes are determined by both the appropriateness of the specific therapy adopted ("what to do") and by the contextual factors around it ("how to do"). Several studies[1-4] on pain conditions such as low back pain, fibromyalgia, and osteoarthritis, have clearly shown that from 60%–80% of the positive therapy outcome is attributable to the nonspecific, contextual components of the treatment. This point invites us to reconsider the weight of the specific element of the therapy and the critical role that contextual factors could have in the therapeutic encounter. Alongside the evidence-based intervention components, we should carefully manage the nonspecific components of the therapy that are capable of producing placebo effects. Clinically, these effects are configured as physiological (e.g., pain, muscle tone) and behavioral (i.e., motor performance, disability) changes.

Classical conditioning and conscious expectation are the two most relevant mechanisms behind the placebo effects. The first is unconscious and based on sensory and precognitive association. The second depends on a conceptual process, a conscious construction of the situation, position, and role of the «self» into the context, contributing to the determination of the expectation.

The process leading to a placebo or nocebo effect is then considered a learning process where both conscious and unconscious mechanisms are deeply integrated and result in a physiological or behavioral output. In 2011, Colloca and Miller[5] proposed a model of observational social learning to interpret placebo effects. Their model combines the unconscious mechanisms of conditioning with conscious learning in a dynamic process that forms the «Self-in-context» construct by integrating all the information coming from a meaningful context of healing. This process has been shown to affect pain perception and induce immune, autonomic, and motor system responses.

The ventromedial prefrontal cortex area of the brain is dedicated to forming the representation of the «self-in-context», the basis for creating event expectation and anticipation.[6] This cerebral area integrates information from many other areas, including memories, beliefs, emotions, and associations, allowing the formation of "priors" organized in a predictor model.[7] This model is continuously and dynamically modified by current sensory and environmental information to form the posteriors, the ongoing condition of the «self-in-context».

The sound psychological and neurobiological mechanisms behind placebo effects invite us to know how to manage contextual factors in our professional practice. A model to guide the translation of such principles into practice was proposed in 2001 by Di Blasi[8] and reclaimed in 2016 by Testa and Rossettini.[9] It classifies the contextual factors that belong to the therapeutic context into five categories: (1) clinician characteristics, (2) patient characteristics, (3) relationship between clinician and patient, (4) treatment characteristics, and (5) healthcare setting. The clinician can use this conceptual framework to assess specific, modifiable contextual factors to tailor them to specific interventions.

By doing so, the clinician can create conditions to favor the patients' learning process, helping them recognize positive and meaningful healing scenarios and tuning their sensory and perceptual experiences.

The pre-eminent contextual factors is the relationship between clinician and patient. Communication is the most powerful agent in changing a patient's mindset.[10] Mindsets result from people's conceptual frames and interpretative lenses through which individuals shape their expectations. Patients are very attentive to our verbal and nonverbal messages. They will use them to construct predictions about the healing context and expectations toward the treatment. However, we should not forget that patients also use their body language to respond to our explicit and implicit messages. Therefore, continuously interpreting the patient's nonverbal reactions is critical to understand and to manage the communicative context effectively.

It is evident that "what" we use as a specific intervention (the evidence-based therapy) and "how" we provide it (the control of contextual factors) may also be relevant to the clinical, patient-based outcome. Therefore, we should stay focused on the healing context to potentially bolster our therapeutic intervention's power. While management of contextual factors might be erroneously interpreted as deceptive behavior toward patients, this perplexity is avoided by transparent and open communication, explaining the mechanisms behind placebo effects. A recent study reported results of a survey conducted in a population of people with musculoskeletal pain, and found the patients perceived the providers' adoption of contextual factors, when associated with evidence-based therapy, in clinical practice was indeed ethical.[11]

The following sections will present a more comprehensive view of the role of contextual factors in clinical practice. They will provide detailed descriptions of the mechanisms of action of mindsets and the multifaceted aspects of the therapeutic relationship between patient and clinician.

Improving musculoskeletal pain: patients' subjective outcomes by positively managing contextual factors—a clinical guide

In care settings, clinicians frequently deal with unexpected positive and negative changes in patients' symptoms that challenge their clinical reasoning and decision-making patterns. Under these circumstances, clinicians may have asked themselves questions such as "why do patients sometimes get worse even though evidence-based guidelines are followed?" Or "why do patients sometimes improve more than others although both receive the same, specific therapy?" These questions find an answer in the contextual factors and their effects. In the following paragraphs, the reader will be guided in understanding the value of contextual factors through a review of their: (a) defining characteristics, (b) mechanisms of action, and (c) clinical relevance.

As proposed by Balint in *The Lancet* in 1955, the context represents "the whole atmosphere around the therapy."[12] It is characterized by five psychosocial elements or dimensions (reported above) present during all clinical encounters between the patients and clinicians, identified and defined as "contextual factors."[8,13,14] To better understand contextual factors, we can consider a clinical scenario in which patients seek help from clinicians for osteoarthritic knee pain. After a thorough history-taking and physical exam, clinicians decide which specific evidence-based therapies (e.g., joint injections, therapeutic exercise, and drugs) to administer to reduce the patient's symptoms. Throughout the clinical encounter, from reception to completion, patients are continually influenced by five contextual factors represented by the features of:[9,15]

1. The healthcare professionals (HCPs) (e.g., appearance, attire, and professional reputation).
2. The patients (e.g., expectations, beliefs, mindset, and previous experiences).
3. The relationship between HCPs and patients (e.g., verbal and nonverbal elements of communication).
4. The treatment (e.g., rituality, invasiveness, and brand).
5. The healthcare settings (e.g., environment, architecture, and interior design).

Depending on how they are used, contextual factors directly influence the patient's perception and symptoms by positively or negatively shaping their experience.[16] Accordingly, contextual factors can trigger two effects: placebo and nocebo effects. Placebo effects occur when clinicians adopt appropriate contextual factors (e.g., empathetic approach); alternately, nocebo effects occur with inappropriate contextual factors (e.g., underestimating the patient's expectations).[16] In the following paragraphs, the mechanisms of action of contextual factors will be reviewed.

To understand the mechanisms of action of contextual factors, we will use an example of how the therapy is administered, using a patient with osteoarthritic knee pain as an example.

When patients receive pain relief therapies (e.g., joint injections, drugs), their five sensory systems are influenced by the treatment and the five types of contextual factors.[6] For example, the taste is stimulated by the flavor of the tablet (e.g., bitter), and the sense of smell is activated by the aroma of the sanitary disinfectant (e.g., intense). Sight is provoked by healthcare devices (e.g., the ultrasound machine); touch is provoked by the healthcare procedure (e.g., the needle penetrating the knee); and hearing is stimulated by the clinician's words (e.g., "This therapy will reduce your knee pain").

All contextual factors offer stimuli encoded by patients' brains, which interpret them and evaluate their meaning based on patients' mindsets (e.g., expectations and previous positive or negative experiences). Accordingly, if the contextual factors are interpreted as positive, the placebo effects are triggered, and if interpreted as negative, nocebo effects are stimulated[17] (see Figure 5.3.1). These positive or negative effects are sustained by a cascade of psycho-neuro-immuno-endocrinological events capable of influencing patients' nervous systems at multiple levels to release neurotransmitters and activate brain areas.[18,19]

For example, positive contextual factors influence patients' brain chemistry by increasing the release of endogenous opioids, endocannabinoids, and dopamine.[18,19] Conversely, negative contextual factors increase cholecystokinin and cyclooxygenase-prostaglandins systems while reducing the activation of the dopaminergic and opioid pathways.[18,19] Further, contextual factors can influence the activity of the dorsolateral prefrontal cortex, anterior cingulate

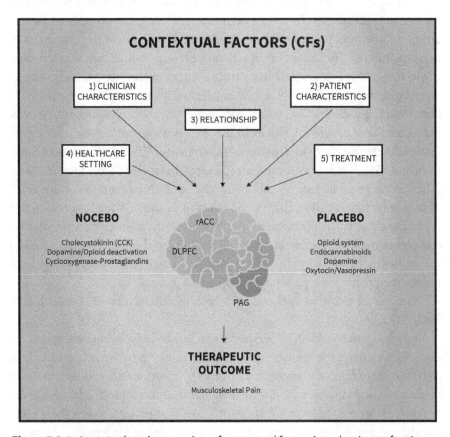

Figure 5.3.1 A comprehensive overview of contextual factors' mechanisms of action.
Reprinted with permission from Rossettini G, Carlino E, Testa M. Psycho-neurobiological mechanism of contextual factors (modified from Rossettini et al.[20]).

cortex, periaqueductal gray, and the dorsal horn of the spine. Altogether, they represent the network mainly involved in context-induced analgesia and hyperalgesia.[18,19]

Finally, contextual factors translate their actions into changes in the patient's outcomes at the clinical level. Using pain as an example, if contextual factors offered are positive, patients will perceive a relief of symptoms. In contrast, if the contextual factors proposed are negative, the patients will experience an aggravation of symptoms.

Contextual factors: clinical relevance

Although patients often unconsciously value the contextual factors around the therapies as relevant,[11] clinicians are not trained to manage them in clinical settings.[21-23] This attitude represents a missed opportunity to improve treatment under three different circumstances. First, the contextual factors are an adjunct component of the therapy that adds value to the specificity of each treatment.[24] Because they are always present in the clinical encounter, clinicians should understand "how to use" them to stimulate placebo effects and avoid nocebo effects. Second, contextual factors influence subjective outcomes (e.g., satisfaction, pain) that patients consider meaningful, to evaluate their care process.[25] For example, in knee osteoarthritis,[1] contextual factors determine changes in patients' outcomes for 75% of pain, 71% of function, and 83% of stiffness, representing useful therapeutic tools for clinicians. Third, contextual factors are ethically and morally acceptable strategies.[26] Thus, contextual factors enhance the effect of evidence-based therapies, not replacing them with approaches without a scientific basis (e.g., homeopathy, complementary, and alternative medicine). Accordingly, clinicians should use contextual factors in clinical settings to increase their effectiveness and reduce the potential for patients to drop out of treatment.

Examples of positive application of contextual factors are presented in Table 5.3.1.

Therefore, from a clinical perspective, it is not only "what" clinicians do that matters (e.g., the specificity of the therapy); "how" clinicians apply it also has value (e.g., the contextual factors). Clinicians should use the best evidence-based therapies within their clinical reasoning and decision-making. However, they should also not forget that patients assess their therapeutic outcomes, considering if the contextual factors offered to them are favorable or unfavorable.

Table 5.3.1 Examples of positive application of contextual factors in clinical care

Features of the HCPs	• Pay attention to habitus, wearing the medical coat or uniform • Be aware of beliefs and behaviors that can influence patients' mindsets
Features of the patients	• Use previous positive experiences to guide the clinical reasoning and the decision-making process • Boost positive expectations and beliefs during the caring process
Features of the therapeutic relationship	• Adopt positive messages associated with treatment for pain relief (e.g., "the therapy will improve the symptoms") • Use eye contact, affirmative head nodding, and an open body posture during the communication
Features of the treatment	• Adopt the therapeutic touch to assist, prepare and treat patients • Adopt an "open treatment," showing and telling the patient that therapy is applied
Features of the healthcare settings	• Combine positive distractors such as light, music, temperature, and aromas • Decorate the therapeutic environment with artworks and ornaments

However, there are still various open challenges in research that need to be tackled: choosing (a) which contextual factors to adopt, (b) when to integrate them into the care process, and (c) how to use them with their patients.

Mindsets matter: using contextual factors to shape mindsets and enhance treatment outcome

Mindsets are lenses or frames of mind that guide individuals toward a particular set of expectations and are a critical yet still underappreciated variable that can influence physical and mental health. Mindsets may be shaped by contextual factors, such as culture, religion, and social influences, and can alter objective reality through behavioral, psychological, and physiological mechanisms. In healthcare, mindsets may be shaped through positive patient-physician interaction, promoting therapeutic advantage. Given the malleability of mindsets, physicians' words and behavior become central—not superfluous—aspects of medical care, which may help to induce more adaptive mindsets that help patients cope with their illness better.

Mindsets are frames of mind that guide an individual toward a particular set of associations and expectations.[27] Mindsets are similar to beliefs, as they steer motivation and attention in a way that shapes behavior and physiology. They may facilitate adaptation, allowing one to make decisions under uncertainty and to refine problem-solving strategies through mental shortcuts.[28] Mindsets represent a simplified and stereotypical picture of one's reality. Examples of these include considering what is right or wrong, good or bad, inevitable or possible (e.g., "being skinny is a token of value," "stress is debilitating," "men are more intelligent than women," and "this side effect is as a sign that the treatment is working"). Individuals unknowingly depend upon their mindsets to make sense of and downsize the overwhelming complexity of reality.[28] While natural and inevitable, the effects of mindsets may leave indelible marks on individuals' health and well-being.[10] However, these mindsets are not fixed since they may be molded by contextual factors, such as culture, media, religion, and social networks. In healthcare, mindsets about illness and treatment are particularly relevant as they may positively or negatively guide the therapeutic process.

Mindsets share common ground with placebo effects. Placebo effects do not lie in the sham treatment itself; instead, they are fueled by the psychosocial forces and environmental cues that are part of the whole atmosphere around the therapy. Conscious expectations are considered among the candidate mechanisms of placebo effects.[17] Expectations are also central to mindsets.[10] For example, the mindset that "being skinny is a token of value" may be associated with many different expectations. Examples are "this food is bad because it will make me fat" or "I will not be able to cope if I know that I am gaining weight." However, these expectations go beyond the more specific expectations on the effectiveness of treatment and are broader and more pervasive. In the clinical context, patients may hold the specific expectation that a treatment will relieve their suffering. However, this expectation may stem from the broader mindset that illness is manageable.[10] These mindsets and the expectations they generate activate specific pathways and regions in the brain that are associated with reward, pain, and anxiety.[29,30] Further, diet, stress, and exercise studies have shown that mindsets affect psychological variables and objective markers of physical health, such as weight loss, blood pressure, cortisol response, and hormone secretion.[27,31,32] Mindsets may modify individuals' motivational and attentional processes, shaping behavior accordingly. However, their effects may bypass a behavior change and directly affect health outcomes. For example, hotel attendants were taught that their work provided a generous amount of daily physical activity and showed improvement in vital measures, though without a corresponding behavior change.[31] This suggests that mindsets may act via self-fulfilling processes without necessarily involving explicit expectations and awareness.

Although patients may hold their pre-existing mindsets in the healthcare setting, the fact that these mindsets are not fixed but malleable leaves space for HCPs to act on them positively. For example, helping patients internalize the mindset that illness is manageable and something that one can deal with (as opposed to a "doom") may change patients' expectations about their illness progression, the efficacy of treatments, and the nature of their symptoms.[9] Differently from placebo manipulations, in which patients are deceptively informed that a drug will ease specific symptoms,[33] mindset interventions do not necessarily entail deception. They may consist of simple attitude and communication changes. Words and actions of healing elicit patients' expectations and trust, which, in turn, may induce changes in how symptoms are perceived and how an illness progresses.[17] Although in some cases, patients may be particularly "receptive" to changing dysfunctional mindsets, in others, overthrowing a deeply ingrained mindset may require a more complex combination of information and emotional care. For example, one study found that the effect of a placebo cream on allergic reactions was of greater magnitude when the patient perceived the physician to be not just competent ("the doctor gets it") but also warm and empathic ("the doctor gets me").[34] This suggests that doctors have the power to craft patients' mindsets.

In summary, physicians have the exceptional opportunity to influence patient mindsets about health and healing. Instilling the mindset that the body is capable, and illness is manageable may be as simple as emphasizing certain information or making subtle changes in how that information is framed.[10] Thus, physicians should be aware of each patient's tendencies and personality traits, focusing on addressing the origin of their deeply ingrained and maladaptive mindsets to mobilize more adaptive ones.

Therapeutic relationship and safety: being present and receptive in the clinical interaction

Humans seek relationships that help us feel secure and allow us to be ourselves. In this regard, therapeutic relationships are no different than any other relationship. The term *therapeutic relationship* encompasses the intentions and attitudes people bring to the clinical encounter, the established professional and personal connections, and the affective bond formed.[35] The therapeutic relationship is a key contextual factor[20] and a pillar of person-centered care.[36] Although better quality relationships can positively influence satisfaction, adherence, and clinical outcomes,[37,38] the question of *how* this occurs in the messy reality of clinical encounters is not as clear given that relating is an "... emergent, self-regulating process...."[39]

Understanding the therapeutic relationship in healthcare encounters has evolved from a rather limited characterization as clinician-patient "rapport" to include the concept of "safety." *Safety* can be generically defined as the "freedom from the occurrence or risk of injury, danger, or loss."[40] Within the therapeutic relationship, safety can be described as implicit or explicit. *Implicit safety*, the unconscious sense of feeling at ease, is hardwired into our nervous system.[41-43] Porges coined this ability to assess our environment for nonverbal social cues of threat or safety "neuroception."[41] When we neuroceptively detect a threat, we autonomically respond by fighting, fleeing, or freezing.[41-43] *Explicit safety* is related to our psychological and social development and inherent rights to be seen, express ourselves, be heard, and be acknowledged and respected as individuals[44] (p. 216). When we convey our acceptance of others, we are more likely to foster an environment where others feel at ease and can socially engage. Although implicit safety and explicit safety are not mutually exclusive, distinguishing them is helpful when identifying actions for creating safety. Further, nurturing safety in our clinical relationships allows us to activate placebo effects.[20] A safe context stimulates autonomic nervous system regulation and placebo effects, while a dangerous context elicits dysregulation and nocebo effects. The neurobiological consequences of safety are apparent and round out the support for a therapeutic relationship as a cornerstone of effective clinical encounters.

Miciak et al.[45] have outlined the necessary conditions for developing therapeutic relationships. The status and intentions that clinicians and patients bring to the clinical encounter shape patients' attitudes, influencing how they relate to their conditions. These attitudes of engagement—presence, receptivity, genuineness, and commitment—form a safe therapeutic container (see Figure 5.3.2). Of the four conditions, being present and being receptive are considered foundational for creating implicit and explicit safety. These two conditions, forming the bottom and the walls of the container, respectively, are described below.

Being present is the intention and ability to remain in the moment of the clinical encounter and be a grounded, calming presence.[45] People who are present are focused[46] and embodied (e.g., aware of their thoughts, emotions, and sensations),[45] and aware of time and their physical environment.[45,46] The opposite of being present is being distracted.[46] Cultivating presence requires clinicians to draw attention to their personal state in order to regulate their nervous system and park professional and personal distractions. Clinicians can foster their ability to be present by developing personal practices (e.g., keywords, breathwork) that can be used prior to and during clinical encounters.

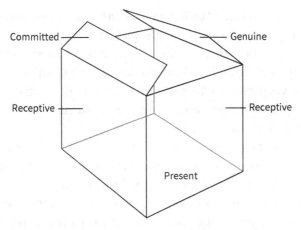

Figure 5.3.2 The safe therapeutic container formed by the conditions of engagement.
Reproduced from Miciak et al.[12] under Creative Commons Attribution 4.0 International License (http://creativecommons.org/licenses/by/4.0/).

BOX 5.3.1 Examples of clinician nonverbal behaviors that foster patient presence

---

- Making soft eye contact
- Welcoming and congruent facial expressions
- Prosody (tone, volume, and speed of vocalization)
- Adjusting proximity to patient
- Pacing the interaction
- Matching the patient (e.g., postures)

Being present has various positive consequences. As clinicians, we can intentionally regulate our stress levels, making ourselves "implicitly safe" to patients, which can reflexively affect patients' neurobiology through "coregulation."[42,43] Being present also allows us to be responsive in the dynamic social process, invoking a greater ability to be person-centered. For example, when present, we can more intentionally and authentically use nonverbal behaviors to translate presence to patients (see Box 5.3.1).[41,43,47]

Receptivity is the ability to be attentive and attuned to patients.[45] Receptivity can take two forms: focused receptivity and open attitude.[45] *Focused receptivity* is being attentive in order to become aware of patients' salient states, issues, needs, and wants.[45] Having an *open attitude* means suspending judgment and being willing to work with the patient.[45]

Receptivity can be cultivated in various ways. Focused receptivity can be enacted by *tracking* and *making contact* with what patients say and do.[44] *Tracking* involves gently attuning to the patient to notice verbal and nonverbal cues.[44] Examples of various verbal and nonverbal cues that can be tracked (and contacted) are found in Table 5.3.2.

Clinicians can *make contact*, or acknowledge patient cues, nonverbally (e.g., head nods, look of concern, and affirming vocalizations) or verbally.[44] Examples of verbal contact statements are found in Box 5.3.2.

Clinicians can manifest an open attitude by being willing to *make room for the patient's story*.[45] Inviting and allowing the patient to tell their story is acknowledging and transferring power to the patient. It is important to suspend judgment and not discuss patients' experiences while contacting parts of the story. Clinicians can also demonstrate an open attitude by *collaborating and negotiating* [45] with patients. For example, clinicians can solicit and acknowledge patients' feedback and adjust the treatment plan with them.

Table 5.3.2 Examples of patient verbal and nonverbal cues that can be tracked and contacted

Body	Postures, tensions, twitches, relaxation
Speech	Tone, speed, volume
Feelings	Sadness, happiness, frustration
Comments/'the story'	People, places, circumstances, poignant phrases
Resources	Resilience, strengths

BOX 5.3.2 Examples of verbal contact statements

"Sounds like you're afraid you'll hurt yourself."

"Your breath seems more relaxed."

"You are moving much better."

"That sounds like a special kind of happy."

"Frustrating, huh?"

"Your shoulders tighten talking about the accident."

"That must have been a very difficult" situation."

"This seems really important to you."

Conclusions

Clinicians should deliberately develop therapeutic relationships. To do so, we need to manifest safety by being a calming, stable presence in the relationship. We can then be receptive to patients' states and needs and meaningfully engage them (and ourselves) as partners in the care process.

References

1. Zou K, Wong J, Abdullah N, et al. Examination of overall treatment effect and the proportion attributable to contextual effect in osteoarthritis: Meta-analysis of randomised controlled trials. *Annals of the Rheumatic Diseases.* 2016;75(11):1964–1970. http://doi:10.1136/ANNRHEUMDIS-2015-208387
2. Puhl AA, Reinhart CJ, Rok ER, Injeyan HS. An examination of the observed placebo effect associated with the treatment of low back pain: A systematic review. *Pain Research and Management.* 2011;16(1):45–52. http://doi:10.1155/2011/625315
3. Menke JM. Do manual therapies help low back pain? A comparative effectiveness meta-analysis. *Spine (Phila Pa 1976).* 2014;39(7) E463–472. doi:10.1097/BRS.0000000000000230.
4. Whiteside N, Sarmanova A, Chen X, et al. Proportion of contextual effects in the treatment of fibromyalgia—A meta-analysis of randomised controlled trials. *Clinical Rheumatology.* 2018;37(5):1375. http://doi:10.1007/S10067-017-3948-3
5. Colloca L, Miller FG. How placebo responses are formed: A learning perspective. *Philosophical Transactions of the Royal Society B: Biological Sciences.* 2011;366(1572):1859. http://doi:10.1098/RSTB.2010.0398
6. Wager TD, Atlas LY. The neuroscience of placebo effects: Connecting context, learning and health. *Nature Reviews Neuroscience.* 2015;16(7):403–418. http://doi:10.1038/NRN3976
7. Geuter S, Koban L, Wager TD. The cognitive neuroscience of placebo effects: Concepts, predictions, and physiology. *Annual Review of Neuroscience.* 2017;40:167–188. http://doi:10.1146/ANNUREV-NEURO-072116-031132
8. di Blasi Z, Harkness E, Ernst E, Georgiou A, Kleijnen J. Influence of context effects on health outcomes: A systematic review. *Lancet.* 2001;357(9258):757–762. http://doi:10.1016/S0140-6736(00)04169-6
9. Testa M, Rossettini G. Enhance placebo, avoid nocebo: How contextual factors affect physiotherapy outcomes. *Metropolitan Area Network.* 2016; 24:65–74. doi:10.1016/j.math.2016.04.006.
10. Zion SR, Crum AJ. Mindsets matter: A new framework for harnessing the placebo effect in modern medicine. *International Review of Neurobiology.* 2018;138:137–160. http://doi:10.1016/BS.IRN.2018.02.002
11. Rossettini G, Palese A, Geri T, Mirandola M, Tortella F, Testa M. The knowledge of contextual factors as triggers of placebo and nocebo effects in patients with musculoskeletal pain: Findings from a national survey. *Frontiers in Psychiatry.* 2019 Jul 4;10:478. doi:10.3389/fpsyt.2019.00478.
12. Balint M. The doctor, his patient, and the illness. *Lancet.* 1955;268(6866):683–688. http://doi:10.1016/S0140-6736(55)91061-8

13. Miller FG, Kaptchuk TJ. The power of context: reconceptualizing the placebo effect. *Journal of the Royal Society of Medicine*. 2008;101(5):222–225. http://doi:10.1258/jrsm.2008.070466

14. Miciak M, Gross DP, Joyce A. A review of the psychotherapeutic "common factors" model and its application in physical therapy: The need to consider general effects in physical therapy practice. *Scandinavian Journal of Caring Sciences*. 2012;26(2):394–403. http://doi:10.1111/J.1471-6712.2011.00923.X

15. Palese A, Rossettini G, Colloca L, Testa M. The impact of contextual factors on nursing outcomes and the role of placebo/nocebo effects: A discussion paper. *Pain Reports*. 2019;4(3):e716. doi:10.1097/PR9.0000000000000716.

16. Rossettini G, Camerone EM, Carlino E, Benedetti F, Testa M. Context matters: The psychoneurobiological determinants of placebo, nocebo and context-related effects in physiotherapy. *Archives of Physiotherapy*. 2020;10(1):1–12. http://doi:10.1186/S40945-020-00082-Y

17. Benedetti F. Placebo and the new physiology of the doctor-patient relationship. *Physiological Reviews*. 2013;93(3):1207–1246. http://doi:10.1152/PHYSREV.00043.2012

18. Carlino E, Benedetti F. Different contexts, different pains, different experiences. *Neuroscience*. 2016;338:19–26. http://doi:10.1016/J.NEUROSCIENCE.2016.01.053

19. Carlino E, Frisaldi E, Benedetti F. Pain and the context. *Nature Reviews Rheumatology*. 2014;10(6):348–355. http://doi:10.1038/NRRHEUM.2014.17

20. Rossettini G, Carlino E, Testa M. Clinical relevance of contextual factors as triggers of placebo and nocebo effects in musculoskeletal pain. *BMC Musculoskeletal Disorders*. 2018;19(1):1–15. http://doi:10.1186/S12891-018-1943-8

21. Palese A, Cadorin L, Testa M, Geri T, Colloca L, Rossettini G. Contextual factors triggering placebo and nocebo effects in nursing practice: Findings from a national cross-sectional study. *Journal of Clinical Nursing*. 2019;28(9–10):1966–1978. http://doi:10.1111/JOCN.14809

22. Rossettini G, Geri T, Palese A, et al. What physiotherapists specialized in orthopedic manual therapy know about nocebo-related effects and contextual factors: Findings from a national survey. *Frontiers in Psychology*. 2020 Oct 20;11:582174. doi:10.3389/fpsyg.2020.582174.

23. Rossettini G, Palese A, Geri T, Fiorio M, Colloca L, Testa M. Physical therapists' perspectives on using contextual factors in clinical practice: Findings from an Italian national survey. *PLoS ONE*. 2018;13(11):e0208159. http://doi:10.1371/JOURNAL.PONE.0208159

24. Rossettini G, Testa M. Manual therapy RCTs: Should we control placebo in placebo control? *European Journal of Physical and Rehabilitation Medicine*. 2018;54(3):500–501. http://doi:10.23736/S1973-9087.17.05024-9

25. Rossettini G, Latini TM, Palese A, et al. Determinants of patient satisfaction in outpatient musculoskeletal physiotherapy: A systematic, qualitative meta-summary, and meta-synthesis. *Disability and Rehabilitation*. 2020;42(4):460–472. http://doi:10.1080/09638288.2018.1501102

26. Thomson OP, Rossettini G. "Don't focus on the finger, look at the moon"—The importance of contextual factors for clinical practice and research. *International Journal of Osteopathic Medicine*. 2021;40:1–3. http://doi:10.1016/J.IJOSM.2021.06.001

27. Crum AJ, Salovey P, Achor S. Rethinking stress: The role of mindsets in determining the stress response. *Journal of Personality and Social Psychology*. 2013;104(4):716–733. http://doi:10.1037/A0031201

28. Crum A, Zuckerman B. Changing mindsets to enhance treatment effectiveness. *JAMA*. 2017;317(20):2063–2064. http://doi:10.1001/JAMA.2017.4545

29. Benedetti F, Carlino E, Pollo A. How placebos change the patient's brain. *Neuropsychopharmacology.* 2011;36(1):339. http://doi:10.1038/NPP.2010.81

30. Bingel U, Wanigasekera V, Wiech K, Ni Mhuircheartaigh R, Lee MC, Ploner M, Tracey I. The effect of treatment expectation on drug efficacy: Imaging the analgesic benefit of the opioid remifentanil. *Science Translational Medicine.* 2011;3(70):70ra14. doi:10.1126/scitranslmed.3001244.

31. Crum AJ, Langer EJ. Mindset matters: Exercise and the placebo effect. *Psychological Science.* 2007;18(2):165–171. http://doi:10.1111/J.1467-9280.2007.01867.X

32. Crum AJ, Corbin WR, Brownell KD, Salovey P. Mind over milkshakes: Mindsets, not just nutrients, determine ghrelin response. *Health Psychology.* 2011;30(4):424–429. http://doi:10.1037/A0023467

33. de la Fuente-Fernández R, Ruth TJ, Sossi V, Schulzer M, Calne DB, Stoessl AJ. Expectation and dopamine release: mechanism of the placebo effect in Parkinson's disease. *Science.* 2001;293(5532):1164–1166. http://doi:10.1126/SCIENCE.1060937

34. Howe LC, Goyer JP, Crum AJ. Harnessing the placebo effect: Exploring the influence of physician characteristics on placebo response. *Health Psychology.* 2017;36(11):1074–1082. http://doi:10.1037/HEA0000499

35. McCabe E, Miciak M, Roduta Roberts M, Sun H, Gross DP. Measuring therapeutic relationship in physiotherapy: Conceptual foundations. *Physiotherapy Theory and Practice.* 2022;38(13):2339–2351. doi:10.1080/09593985.2021.1987604.

36. Constand MK, MacDermid JC, Dal Bello-Haas V, Law M. Scoping review of patient-centered care approaches in healthcare. *BMC Health Services Research.* 2014;14(1):1–9. http://doi:10.1186/1472-6963-14-271/COMMENTS

37. Kelley JM, Kraft-Todd G, Schapira L, Kossowsky J, Riess H. The influence of the patient-clinician relationship on healthcare outcomes: A systematic review and meta-analysis of randomised controlled trials. *PLoS ONE.* 2014;9(4):e94207. doi:10.1371/journal.pone.0094207. Erratum in: PLoS One. 2014;9(6):e101191.

38. Hall AM, Ferreira PH, Maher CG, Latimer J, Ferreira ML. The influence of the therapist-patient relationship on treatment outcome in physical rehabilitation: A systematic review. *Physical Therapy.* 2010;90(8):1099–1110. http://doi:10.2522/PTJ.20090245

39. Adler HM. Toward a biopsychosocial understanding of the patient–physician relationship: An emerging dialogue. *Journal of General Internal Medicine.* 2007;22(2):280. http://doi:10.1007/S11606-006-0037-8

40. Safety Definition & Meaning | Dictionary.com. Accessed March 28, 2022. https://www.dictionary.com/browse/safety

41. Porges SW. The polyvagal theory: New insights into adaptive reactions of the autonomic nervous system. *Cleveland Clinic Journal of Medicine.* 2009;76(Suppl 2):S86. http://doi:10.3949/CCJM.76.S2.17

42. Porges SW, Dana D. *Clinical Applications of the Polyvagal Theory.* W. W. Norton &Company; 2018. https://wwnorton.com/books/Clinical-Applications-of-the-Polyvagal-Theory/

43. Geller SM. Therapeutic presence and polyvagal theory: Principles and practices for cultivating effective therapeutic relationships. In: Porges SW, Dana D, eds. *Clinical Applications of the Polyvagal Theory: The Emergence of Polyvagal-Informed Therapies.* W.W. Norton & Company; 2018:106–126. https://psycnet.apa.org/record/2018-26629-007

44. Kurtz R. Body-centered psychotherapy: The Hakomi method. The integrated use of mindfulness, nonviolence, and the body. 1990; Mendocino, CA: LifeRhythm.

45. Miciak M, Mayan M, Brown C, Joyce AS, Gross DP. The necessary conditions of engagement for the therapeutic relationship in physiotherapy: An interpretive description study. *Archives of Physiotherapy.* 2018;8:3. doi:10.1186/s40945-018-0044-1.

46. Brown-Johnson C, Schwartz R, Maitra A, et al. What is clinician presence? A qualitative interview study comparing physician and non-physician insights about practices of human connection. *BMJ Open.* 2019;9(11):e030831. http://doi:10.1136/BMJOPEN-2019-030831

47. Geller SM, Porges SW. Therapeutic presence: Neurophysiological mechanisms mediating feeling safe in therapeutic relationships. *Journal of Psychotherapy Integration.* 2014;24(3):178–192. http://doi:10.1037/A0037511

5.4

Placebo effects and research quality

What is good evidence?

*Wayne B. Jonas, David Goldman, Salim Muhammed,
C. Daniel Mullins, and Luana Colloca*

Introduction

Currently, randomized controlled trials (RCTs) are critical to assessing the efficacy of pharmacological, nonpharmacological, and surgical treatments and interventions. In phase III RCTs, the experimental treatment group(s) is compared with a placebo group. In contrast, an untreated control group (no-treatment group) is indicated only when no standard treatments exist for the disease under consideration. Many RCTs compare the new treatment with a standard treatment with established efficacy (the active control group). *Placebo effects* refer to a beneficial effect produced by a placebo drug or treatment or a manipulation of the participant's belief, which cannot be attributed to the properties of the placebo or manipulation itself, and is, therefore, due to the cascade of neurobiological changes related to expectancy, prior therapeutic experiences, observation of benefits in others, contextual and treatment cues, and interpersonal interactions.[1] We argue that a no-treatment control group is necessary to dissociate placebo effects from the placebo responses. Thus, clinical trials that only include the new-treatment group, the active control group, and a placebo group, but not a no-treatment group, capture various nonspecific effects driven by the natural history, regression to the mean, false positive and negative errors, and biases that can confound findings.[2]

Methodological considerations and confounding variables

Natural history refers to spontaneous fluctuations in symptoms attributable to relapses and remissions.[2] When placebo treatments are taken, patients can experience a symptom reduction, and they may attribute the benefit to the placebo. Therefore, spontaneous remission can lead to an erroneous interpretation of cause-effect relationships. To prove the presence of placebo effects, it is necessary to show a difference between the natural history no-treatment group and the placebo group.

All measurements are subject to random error.[2] *Regression to the mean* refers to the tendency of results that are extreme by chance on first measurement (much higher or lower than average) to move closer to the mean after repeated measurements. Therefore, subsequent measurements of an extreme initial outcome can be lower or higher because of regression to the mean, rather than biologically mediated placebo effects.[3] Regression to the mean can coexist with placebo effects in RCTs, making it difficult to separate placebo effects from placebo responses. A reliable way to document that the observed improvement is attributable to placebo effects, is to compare the group receiving a placebo with the no-treatment group.

Another source of experimental confusion is bias, or false positive or negative errors by clinicians, researchers, patients, or both. *Bias* is a flaw in the study design or the method of collecting or interpreting information. Biases can lead to incorrect conclusions about the results of a given study or clinical trial. Bias in research results in deviation from the "truth."[4] It includes selection bias, information bias, and other types of biases. *Selection bias* refers to the absence of comparability among groups being investigated. *Information bias* is related to incorrect exposure and/or outcome determination. When information is gathered differently among groups, bias is triggered.

In this regard, biases in the form of false positive or false negative errors have been often described under the framework of signal detection theory, a model for the detection of ambiguous signals.[5] The ambiguity of signals leads to bias and a patient and/or a clinician can report and detect that a treatment is effective by mistake (i.e., false positive error) or not identifying that the treatment is effective (false negative error). In RCTs, the reported "success rate" may be due to one or more of the above-mentioned factors—natural history, regression to the mean, bias, and false positive or false negative errors—as well as unidentified cointerventions that can induce clinical benefits.[2] Another factor is that a patient, once included in a trial, can experience therapeutic benefits (i.e., Hawthorne effect[6,7]).

Placebo-related designs

Different clinical trial designs have been suggested to identify placebo responses.[8,9] Most RCTs use the placebo-controlled design. However, other designs, such as the balanced placebo design,[10] the double-blind versus deceptive design,[11] the open-hidden treatment administration (also called overt-covert treatment administration),[12,13,14] open-label placebo design,[15,16] sequential parallel comparison,[17] enriched enrollment with randomized withdrawal design,[18] among others, have been devised to identify placebo responses.

The balanced placebo design formulated by Ross (1962),[10] is an orthogonal manipulation of verbal suggestion (told drug versus told placebo) and drug administration (received drug versus received placebo). This design has been primarily used in clinical studies in participants who use alcohol,[19,20] nicotine,[21] and amphetamine,[22] as well as with participants who have psychiatric disorders.[23] This design determines the influences of verbally induced expectancies in therapeutic outcome related to both the placebo and the active groups. For example, the aerosolized, bronchoconstrictor (carbachol) administered to asthmatic subjects produced more airway resistance and dyspnea when patients were instructed that they were given *bronchoconstrictor* as compared to patients who were instructed that they were given a *bronchodilator*.[24] However, this design is difficult to adapt to conventional clinical trials because it requires deception. The recently proposed authorized deception[25] in consenting prospective patients allows implementation of this design in randomized placebo-controlled studies.

The double-blind versus deceptive design includes the administration of an active drug with a comparator group that receives deceptive administration of the same drug. Deception thus limits the use of designs, which compare the therapeutic outcomes of a double-blind administration of an active drug with a deceptive administration of the same drug despite this approach not requiring the administration of placebo as controls. But this design has not been applied outside experimental clinical settings. An example that should be replicated is a study with clinically used opioid drugs.[26] Patients in the postoperative setting received opioids under distinct verbal instructions: "It can be either a placebo or a painkiller, and, therefore, we are not certain that the pain will subside," versus "It is a potent painkiller, and, therefore, we expect the pain will subside soon." The latter statement led to a significant reduction of postoperative opioid administration.[26] Therefore, manipulating verbally induced expectations can modulate treatment outcomes.

Another procedure that can be used to separate active treatment from psychosocial effects related to placebo effects is the overt-covert treatment[12] administration procedure, also known as the open-hidden procedure.[13,14] This procedure refers to a doctor-initiated versus machine-initiated administration of a treatment. A therapeutic outcome is the result of the specific treatment effects and the placebo component. A hidden administration entails that the patient is unaware of the treatment administration (i.e., pre-programmed computer-controlled infusion pump). An open administration entails that the patient is aware of the treatment being administrated at a given time. This procedure has proven to be reliable in studying placebo effects in the fields of pain, anxiety, and Parkinson's disease.[12] This design has the advantage of not using placebos. The deception is also minimized. For the hidden arm, the onset of the treatment delivery is covered (e.g., patients do not know the exact time of the treatment administration), but patients know that they are going to be treated with standard treatment.[27]

Open-label placebo designs refer to the use of adjuvant placebos given along with the standard treatment. First introduced by Park and Covi (1965)[28] in psychiatric patients suffering from anxiety symptoms, the design has been revamped in 2010 by Ted Kaptchuk and his team[16] with the largest number of studies being published using this design. Despite the notion that placebo treatments or interventions work because people think that they may have received an active treatment or intervention, recent studies showed that open-label placebos (i.e., Zeebo pills) may also improve clinical outcomes related to irritable bowel syndrome in adults[16,29] and children,[30] chronic low back pain,[31,32] depression,[33] rhinitis,[34] cancer-related fatigue,[35] and menopausal hot flashes.[36] However, criticisms have been raised about the clinical implications and the weaknesses of current evidence because of lack of control for recruitment biases, blinding, and randomization.[37-39]

Other designs that have been suggested for reducing placebo responses (and sample size) are the sequential parallel comparison[17] and enriched enrollment with randomized withdrawal design.[18] The sequential parallel comparison involves parallel comparisons of one or more treatments with placebo.[17] Criticisms have been raised about the enriched enrollment with randomized withdrawal design and the open-label run-in phase.[18] While the latter can unblind study participants and investigators, using drug allocation concealment as a pretest to remove potential unblinded study participants does not seem to control for placebo responses.[40]

Once designs, control conditions, and confounding factors have been scrutinized, the goal is to demonstrate that a treatment or intervention is effective. The gold standard to prove efficacy often assumes additivity—the effect of a treatment is the result of subtraction of the effect observed in the placebo group from the effect observed in the active treatment group.[41] The *additivity* has been extensively discussed in placebo analgesia,[42] and additive effects have been also documented.[43] Using a 2 × 2 factorial placebo design, Schenk et al.[44] showed that lidocaine or prilocaine effects on pain ratings are associated with neural responses in anterior insular cortex, rostral anterior cingulate cortex, and ventral striatum. However, clinical findings suggest that placebo and drug effects are not merely additive.[12] The additive versus interactive effect may depend on the mechanisms of action of each specific treatment. Positron Emission Tomography studies with radiotracers can help address the issue of additivity from a mechanistic perspective, yet it is difficult to make inferences about additivity in RCTs.

In summary, ruling out placebo responses requires an adequate study design.[45,46] Additionally, placebo effects can be controlled by introducing proxies of expectations[47] (also see Chapter 1.2). Distinct scales for measuring expectations[48] have been proposed including sets of validated questions or visual analogue scales.[49] It is possible to measure anticipated outcomes, desire of benefits, allocation guess, and perception of benefits and patients' direct experiences. Other aspects to be taken into consideration are assay's sensitivity, outcome perception (e.g., teens and parents value different outcomes), and outcome choice (e.g., use of pain disability versus pain intensity).[8]

The current evidence quality model

The current model for judging evidence in research is the "evidence hierarchy," at the top of which is the randomized, placebo-controlled design (Box 5.4.1). However, this design is based on several assumptions about the placebo effects and its components that are challenged by results from many studies.[8,45,46] First, it assumes that a simple two-group design with a single placebo comparison group is sufficient to capture placebo effects and their interactions with the "active" treatment and, therefore, is sufficient to determine that the active treatment's effect is real. We now know that placebo effects consist of multiple dissociable mechanisms.[1] For example, the effects of the cultural variation of placebo responses and effects (also see Chapter 1.4) need to be considered in any model that purports to determine good evidence. Indeed, Moerman and colleagues showed large variability in the placebo groups of randomized placebo-controlled trials of drug treatment for ulcers, hypertension, and other conditions, based on the country in which the studies were done.[50] This variability often ranges from 0 to 100% treatment effect.[50]

BOX 5.4.1   Definitions

Placebo effects: "A beneficial effect produced by a placebo drug or treatment or a manipulation of the participant's belief, which cannot be attributed to the properties of the placebo/manipulation itself, and is therefore due to the cascade of neurobiological changes related to expectancy, prior therapeutic experiences, observation of benefits in others, contextual and treatment cues, and interpersonal interactions."[1]

Placebo responses: "Outcome changes that are due to natural history, biases, regression to the mean, and other nonspecific effects."[1]

Expectations: "Constructs that refer to anticipation of outcome that are verbalized and measurable via validated scales."[1]

Expectancy: "A psychophysical predictor that can be present in humans and non-humans without full awareness (implicit expectancies)."[1]

Natural history: "A catch-all term to describe improvement in symptoms of a medical condition that occurs naturally without any interventions."[1]

Regression to the mean: "Regression to the mean refers to the tendency of results that are extreme by chance on first measurement (much higher or lower than average) to move closer to the mean after repeated measurements."[1]

Active control group: "A group assigned to an effective treatment (as opposed to a placebo) as a comparator for the experimental treatment."

Control group: "A group of participants who are randomly assigned to not receive the experimental treatment."

No-treatment group: "A group of participants who are randomly assigned to receive no treatment (lack/absence of treatment)."

False positive errors: "False positive errors, or false positives, indicate that a given condition exists when it does not."

False negative errors: "False negative errors, or false negatives, indicate that a given condition does not exist when it does."

Bias: "Bias is a flaw in the study design or the method of collecting or interpreting information. Biases can lead to incorrect conclusions about the results of a given study or clinical trial. Bias in research in turn, results in deviation from the truth."

Hierarchy model: "A model that structures research giving hierarchies of evidence based on study designs with randomized-clinical trials considered as the highest level of strength and precision in clinical research."

Implications of placebo for the hierarchy model

The above knowledge about what contributes to the placebo response means that the hierarchy model of research quality is based on assumptions that are changing with current mechanistic knowledge related to placebo effects and expectations.[1]

Nearly two-thirds of published clinical research is not replicated.[51] In this regard, Fanelli et al.[52] conducted a meta-analysis (i.e., all areas of scientific research) to assess a set of parameters that are associated with patterns and risk factors for bias and, therefore, lack of replicability. The authors found that small-study effects (i.e., smaller studies reporting larger effect sizes), literature bias (i.e., negative results are less likely to be published), and citation bias are the most common issues. Small-study effects are the most relevant source of bias in meta-analysis.

In addition, failure to incorporate knowledge about placebo responses and effects can become a major factor underlying replication failures. The "decline effect" refers to the observation that the earliest studies often overestimate the magnitude of a given psychological or physiological effect relative to later studies.[53] The decline effect can occur because of a decreasing field-specific publication bias over time or to differences in study design between earlier and later studies.[53] Also, it contributes to replication failures, decreases as more research is done, and usually settles in a much smaller effect sizes than usually claimed in systematic reviews and meta-analyses—the top of the evidence hierarchy. This means that the effect sizes and replicability as approximated by systematic reviews and meta-analyses should start incorporating the main factors (e.g., expectations, cues, and contextual factors) that may trigger placebo responses and effects.

Finally, this variability of clinical effects, even in "proven" treatments, is also influenced by practice delivery and cultural context affecting placebo response and effect size and interactions. Expectations and rituals, the complexity of mindset, and cultural factors also influence variability. This means that efficacy, which is the goal of the research hierarchy, requires evolving for most treatments. Thus, we argue that the hierarchy model might be limited for making decisions about efficacy and effectiveness.

There are many examples that illustrate these points, but let us point out some placebo mechanisms with real-world implications. First, Kirsch and others have shown that the efficacy of US Food and Drug Administration–approved antidepressant medications largely disappears when one considers placebo responses in addition to standard blinding procedure in the research design.[54] The use of an active placebo, which produces side effects designed to mimic the physiological effects of the active treatment, diminishes the antidepressant effects to practically zero. This observation suggests that antidepressant effects may be largely due to nonspecific placebo responses that are not detected in the classical two-group, placebo control design. Moreover, meta-regression approaches showed that the relation of baseline severity and improvement is curvilinear in drug groups with a negative linear pattern in placebo groups.[54]

An excellent three-group study of acupuncture for xerostomia (dry mouth) among patients with head and neck cancer illustrates the impact of culture and context. The study compared sham acupuncture (wrong body points), real acupuncture (right body points), and standard therapy without acupuncture in two locations, one in China and the other in the United States.[55] The results showed significant differences in the effectiveness of sham acupuncture between the US and Chinese samples, reversing the conclusion of whether the real acupuncture effect worked. Thus, context trumped in a direct way the treatment effects. Guidelines would have approved acupuncture based on this study in the Unites States, but not in China, under the standard hierarchy model of good evidence.[56] Thus, the hierarchical model can be appropriate for addressing questions related to efficacy (i.e., regulatory processes) and inadequate for complementary and alternative medicine because of the conflict between internal validity (rigor and the removal of bias) and external validity (generalizability).

Several other models have been proposed, such as the circular model, where multiple methods could provide an estimate of safety and efficacy of an intervention;[57] the medical reversal, referring to the fact that a new clinical trial is superior to prior trials because of more appropriate controls, design, size, or endpoints is in contradiction with current clinical practice; [58,59] and the evidence house model,[60] a model primarily used by primary care. The evidence house model argues that the primary driver for determining what is good evidence is the use of that evidence by specific decision-making populations.[60] The model is organized in 'rooms' and identifies four main decision-makers in health care: (1) regulators and clinical researchers, (2) non-research clinicians, (3) patients, and (4) basic scientists. Each of these decision-makers determines the type of evidence they need for their purposes and then seeks out and finds "good" evidence to support that decision. Briefly, for regulators to determine if an effect from a treatment is due to the purported treatment, results from randomized placebo-controlled trials. However, simple two-group trials are often inadequate to make this determination. More sophisticated designs such as the three-group study on acupuncture and dry mouth[55] are required before declaring the evidence is good and the treatment is effective. This, however, is not sufficient or even necessary for many therapies before their use and reimbursement. That decision needs to be made by clinicians and payers, respectively.

Knowledge about patient-centered outcome research would also need to be incorporated into what constitutes good evidence, especially for the decision-makers.[61] The principles of the Patient-Centered Outcome Research Institute and the 10-step patient engagement framework[62] can overall ensure: (1) Mutual relationships and shared decision-making, where patients and stakeholder partners are involved in discussions that result in decisions related to the study design, study implementation, and findings dissemination. (2) Co-learning, where stakeholder partners guide the interpretation and dissemination of the findings along with the engagement strategies development. (3) Partnership, whereby the researchers create a strong partnership with stakeholder partners. Patient-centered decision-making processes will boost good evidence. As data emerge, stakeholder partners should actively be involved in their assessment and reassessment, and all parties can collaborate to design, implement, and disseminate the study in a manner that ensures translation to patients, their caregivers, and stakeholders.[63] Patients' input is rarely included in the determination of what is good evidence. However, patient-centered outcome research has brought patient perspectives more into the decision-making process around evidence execution but has not sufficiently trained and tapped what patients want when it comes to the type of research information. Patient-centered outcome research does not come from randomized placebo-controlled trials but is a major "room" in the evidence house.[60] The other evidence models listed in this section (e.g., circular, medical reversal) also provide space for incorporating a greater diversity of decision-makers and our current understanding of the complexity of placebo knowledge into determining what is good evidence in placebo-related research (Box 5.4.2).

Conclusions

Our current knowledge about what constitutes and contributes to the placebo effects requires that we redesign the models and methodologies we use to determine what is "good evidence" in placebo research. This redesign will result in improved research practices in which all healthcare-related decision-makers have the type of quality information they require.

Box 5.4.2 Open questions to be addressed

---

1. If a treatment involves a powerful ritual, induces a large effect size, but produces only a small difference from the purported (theoretical) "active" ingredient, should it be accepted mainly on that incremental "real" additional effect?
2. Should relative effects trump overall benefits?
3. How should risk and safety be brought into the equation and when should that override placebo-controlled efficacy?
4. Who should make the decision as to what is acceptable into practice?
5. How should we weigh the opinions of scientists testing their theories; regulators applying their criteria for sales, marketing, and coverage; clinicians trying to sort out what is "evidence-based"; and patients who seek the safest and easiest options with the largest probability for improvement?
6. What influence should these various decision-makers hold on the distinction between "active" and "placebo" components?
7. Scientists look to reduce variability and increase objectivity, but placebo responses are highly variable and affect subjective processes more readily than objective outcomes. Given this, how can we improve the rigor of placebo research?
8. How important is blinding? If placebo effects still occur without blinding, why is blinding needed?
9. How do regulatory agencies drive placebo research for new treatments, and what does that do for what treatments are available?
10. How can the public have more say in what type of research is done and whether placebo comparisons are needed? How can that input be properly included?

Acknowledgments

The authors want to thank Dr. Yavin Shaman for his generous time and insightful comments on the last version of this chapter. This research is supported by National Institute Dental Craniofacial Research, NIDCR (R01 DE025946, LC), and National Institute on Alcohol Abuse and Alcoholism (1R13AA028424, LC). The funding agencies have no role in the study. The views expressed here are the author's own and do not reflect the position or policy of the National Institutes of Health or any other part of the federal government.

References

1. Colloca L. The placebo effect in pain therapies. *Annual Review of Pharmacology and Toxicology.* 2019;59:191–211. http://doi:10.1146/annurev-pharmtox-010818-021542
2. Colloca L, Benedetti F, Porro CA. Experimental designs and brain mapping approaches for studying the placebo analgesic effect. *European Journal of Applied Physiology.* 2008;102(4):371–380. http://doi:10.1007/s00421-007-0593-6
3. Davis CE. Regression to the mean or placebo effect? In: Guess HA, Kleinman A, Kusek JW, Engel LW, eds. *The Science of the Placebo: Toward an Interdisciplinary Research Agenda.* BMJ Books; 2002:158–166.
4. Grimes DA, Schulz KF. Bias and causal associations in observational research. *Lancet.* 2002;359(9302):248–52. http://doi:10.1016/S0140-6736(02)07451-2
5. Allan LG, Siegel S. A signal detection theory analysis of the placebo effect. *Evaluation and the Health Professions.* 2002;25(4):410–20. http://doi:10.1177/0163278702238054
6. Parsons HM. What happened at Hawthorne?: New evidence suggests the Hawthorne effect resulted from operant reinforcement contingencies. *Science.* 1974;183(4128):922–932. http://doi:10.1126/science.183.4128.922
7. Ulmer FC. The Hawthorne effect. *Expanded Function Dental Auxiliary.* 1976;1(2):28.
8. Colloca L, Barsky AJ. Placebo and nocebo effects. *New England Journal of Medicine.* 2020;382(6):554–561. http://doi:10.1056/NEJMra1907805
9. Colloca L, Benedetti F. Placebos and painkillers: Is mind as real as matter? *Nature Reviews Neuroscience.* 2005;6(7):545–52. http://doi:nrn1705[pii]10.1038/nrn1705
10. Ross S, Krugman AD, Lyerly SB, Clyde, J D. Drugs and placebos: A model design. *Psychological Reports.* 1962;10(2):383–392.
11. Kirsch I, Weixel LJ. Double-blind versus deceptive administration of a placebo. *Behavioral Neuroscience.* Apr 1988;102(2):319–323. http://doi:10.1037//0735-7044.102.2.319
12. Colloca L, Lopiano L, Lanotte M, Benedetti F. Overt versus covert treatment for pain, anxiety, and Parkinson's disease. *Lancet Neurology.* 2004;3(11):679–684. http://doi:10.1016/S1474-4422(04)00908-1
13. Benedetti F, Maggi G, Lopiano L, et al. Open versus hidden medical treatments: The patient's knowledge about a therapy affects the therapy outcome. *Prevention & Treatment.* 2003;6:n.p. http://doi:10.1037/1522-3736.6.1.61a
14. Benedetti F, Colloca L, Lanotte M, Bergamasco B, Torre E, Lopiano L. Autonomic and emotional responses to open and hidden stimulations of the human subthalamic region. *Brain Research Bulletin.* 2004;63(3):203–211. http://doi:10.1016/j.brainresbull.2004.01.010
15. Park LC, Covi L. Nonblind placebo trial: An exploration of neurotic patients' responses to placebo when its inert content is disclosed. *Archives of General Psychiatry.* 1965;12:36–45.
16. Kaptchuk TJ, Friedlander E, Kelley JM, et al. Placebos without deception: A randomized controlled trial in irritable bowel syndrome. *PLoS ONE.* 2010;5(12):e15591. http://doi:10.1371/journal.pone.0015591
17. Fava M, Evins AE, Dorer DJ, Schoenfeld DA. The problem of the placebo response in clinical trials for psychiatric disorders: Culprits, possible remedies, and a novel study design approach. *Psychotherapy and Psychosomatics.* 2003;72(3):115–127. http://doi:10.1159/000069738
18. Staud R, Price DD. Role of placebo factors in clinical trials with special focus on enrichment designs. *Pain.* 2008;139(2):479–480. doi:10.1016/j.pain.2008.07.027
19. Marlatt GA, Demming B, Reid JB. Loss of control drinking in alcoholics: An experimental analogue. *Journal of Abnormal Psychology.* 1973;81(3):233–241. http://doi:10.1037/h0034532

20. Epps J, Monk C, Savage S, Marlatt GA. Improving credibility of instructions in the balanced placebo design: A misattribution manipulation. *Addictive Behaviors*. 1998;23(4):427–435.

21. Sutton SR. Great expectations: Some suggestions for applying the balanced placebo design to nicotine and smoking. *British Journal of Addiction*. 1991;86(5):659–662.

22. Mitchell SH, Laurent CL, De Wit H. Interaction of expectancy and the pharmacological effects of d-amphetamine: Subjective effects and self-administration. *Psychopharmacology*. 1996;125(4):371–378.

23. Rohsenow DJ, Bachorowski J-A. Effects of alcohol and expectancies on verbal aggression in men and women. *Journal of Abnormal Psychology*. 1984;93(4):418.

24. Luparello TJ, Leist N, Lourie CH, Sweet P. The interaction of psychologic stimuli and pharmacologic agents on airway reactivity in asthmatic subjects. *Psychosomatic Medicine*. 1970;32(5):509–513. https://doi.org/10.1097/00006842-197009000-00009

25. Wendler D, Miller FG. Deception in the pursuit of science. *Archives of Internal Medicine*. 2004;164(6):597–600. http://doi:10.1001/archinte.164.6.597

26. Pollo A, Amanzio M, Arslanian A, Casadio C, Maggi G, Benedetti F. Response expectancies in placebo analgesia and their clinical relevance. *Pain*. 2001;93(1):77–84.

27. Colloca L, Kisaalita NR, Bizien M, Medeiros M, Sandbrink F, Mullins CD. Veteran engagement in opioid tapering research: A mission to optimize pain management. *Pain Reports*. 2021;6(2):e932. http://doi:10.1097/PR9.0000000000000932

28. Park L; TRIAL CLNP. An exploration of neurotic patients' responses to placebo when its inert content is disclosed. *Archives of General Psychiatry*. 1965;12:36–45.

29. Lembo A, Kelley JM, Nee J, et al. Open-label placebo vs double-blind placebo for irritable bowel syndrome: A randomized clinical trial. *Pain*. 2021;162(9):2428–2435. http://doi:10.1097/j.pain.0000000000002234

30. Nurko S, Saps M, Kossowsky J, et al. Effect of open-label placebo on children and adolescents with functional abdominal pain or irritable bowel syndrome: A randomized clinical trial. *JAMA Pediatrics*. 2022;176(4):349–356. http://doi:10.1001/jamapediatrics.2021.5750

31. Carvalho C, Caetano JM, Cunha L, Rebouta P, Kaptchuk TJ, Kirsch I. Open-label placebo treatment in chronic low back pain: A randomized controlled trial. *Pain*. 2016;157(12):2766–2772. http://doi:10.1097/j.pain.0000000000000700

32. Carvalho C, Pais M, Cunha L, Rebouta P, Kaptchuk TJ, Kirsch I. Open-label placebo for chronic low back pain: A 5-year follow-up. *Pain*. 2021;162(5):1521–1527. http://doi:10.1097/j.pain.0000000000002162

33. Kelley JM, Kaptchuk TJ, Cusin C, Lipkin S, Fava M. Open-label placebo for major depressive disorder: A pilot randomized controlled trial. *Psychotherapy and Psychosomatics*. 2012;81(5):312–4. http://doi:10.1159/000337053

34. Schaefer M, Harke R, Denke C. Open-label placebos improve symptoms in allergic rhinitis: A randomized controlled trial. *Psychotherapy and Psychosomatics*. 2016;85(6):373–374. http://doi:10.1159/000447242

35. Hoenemeyer TW, Kaptchuk TJ, Mehta TS, Fontaine KR. Open-label placebo treatment for cancer-related fatigue: A randomized-controlled clinical trial. *Scientific Reports*. 2018;8(1):2784. http://doi:10.1038/s41598-018-20993-y

36. Pan Y, Meister R, Lowe B, Kaptchuk TJ, Buhling KJ, Nestoriuc Y. Open-label placebos for menopausal hot flushes: A randomized controlled trial. *Scientific Reports*. 2020;10(1):20090. http://doi:10.1038/s41598-020-77255-z

37. Colloca L, Howick J. Placebos without deception: Outcomes, mechanisms, and ethics. *International Review of Neurobiology*. 2018;138:219–240. http://doi:10.1016/bs.irn.2018.01.005

38. Blease C, Colloca L, Kaptchuk TJ. Are open-label placebos ethical? Informed consent and ethical equivocations. *Bioethics*. 2016;30(6):407–414. http://doi:10.1111/bioe.12245

39. Blease CR, Bernstein MH, Locher C. Open-label placebo clinical trials: Is it the rationale, the interaction or the pill? *BMJ Evidence-Based Medicine.* 2020;25(5):159–165. http://doi:10.1136/bmjebm-2019-111209

40. Staud R, Price DD. Importance of measuring placebo factors in complex clinical trials. *Pain.* 2008;138(2):474. http://doi:10.1016/j.pain.2008.07.016

41. Scott AJ, Sharpe L, Quinn V, Colagiuri B. Association of Single-blind placebo run-in periods with the placebo response in randomized clinical trials of antidepressants: A systematic review and meta-analysis. *JAMA Psychiatry.* 2022;79(1):42–49. http://doi:10.1001/jamapsychiatry.2021.3204

42. Coleshill MJ, Sharpe L, Colloca L, Zachariae R, Colagiuri B. Placebo and active treatment additivity in placebo analgesia: Research to date and future directions. *International Review of Neurobiology.* 2018;139:407–441. http://doi:10.1016/bs.irn.2018.07.021

43. Colagiuri B. Participant expectancies in double-blind randomized placebo-controlled trials: Potential limitations to trial validity. *Clinical Trials.* 2010;7(3):246–255. http://doi:10.1177/1740774510367916

44. Schenk LA, Sprenger C, Geuter S, Buchel C. Expectation requires treatment to boost pain relief: An fMRI study. *Pain.* 2014;155(1):150–157. doi:10.1016/j.pain.2013.09.024

45. Hohenschurz-Schmidt D, Draper-Rodi J, Vase L. Dissimilar control interventions in clinical trials undermine interpretability. *JAMA Psychiatry.* 2022;79(3):271–272. http://doi:10.1001/jamapsychiatry.2021.3963

46. Hohenschurz-Schmidt D, Draper-Rodi J, Vase L, et al. Blinding and sham control methods in trials of physical, psychological, and self-management interventions for pain (article II): A meta-analysis relating methods to trial results. *Pain.* 2023;164(3):509–533. doi:10.1097/j.pain.0000000000002730

47. Rosenkjaer S, Lunde SJ, Kirsch I, Vase L. Expectations: How and when do they contribute to placebo analgesia? *Frontiers in Psychiatry.* 2022;13:817179. http://doi:10.3389/fpsyt.2022.817179

48. Younger J, Gandhi V, Hubbard E, Mackey S. Development of the Stanford Expectations of Treatment Scale (SETS): A tool for measuring patient outcome expectancy in clinical trials. *Clinical Trials.* 2012;9(6):767–76. http://doi:10.1177/1740774512465064

49. Colloca L, Akintola T, Haycock NR, et al. Prior Therapeutic Experiences, Not Expectation Ratings, Predict Placebo Effects: An Experimental Study in Chronic Pain and Healthy Participants. *Psychotherapy and Psychosomatics.* 2020;89(6):371–378. http://doi:10.1159/000507400

50. Moerman DE. Cultural variations in the placebo effect: ulcers, anxiety, and blood pressure. *Medical Anthropology Quarterly.* 2000;14(1):51–72. http://doi:10.1525/maq.2000.14.1.51

51. Young NS, Ioannidis JP, Al-Ubaydli O. Why current publication practices may distort science. *PLoS Medicine.* 2008;5(10):e201. http://doi:10.1371/journal.pmed.0050201

52. Fanelli D, Costas R, Ioannidis JP. Meta-assessment of bias in science. *Proceedings of the National Academy of Sciences USA.* 2017;114(14):3714–3719. http://doi:10.1073/pnas.1618569114

53. Schooler J. Unpublished results hide the decline effect. *Nature.* 2011;470(7335):437–437.

54. Kirsch I, Deacon BJ, Huedo-Medina TB, Scoboria A, Moore TJ, Johnson BT. Initial severity and antidepressant benefits: A meta-analysis of data submitted to the Food and Drug Administration. *PLoS Medicine.* 2008;5(2):e45. http://doi:10.1371/journal.pmed.0050045

55. Garcia MK, Meng Z, Rosenthal DI, et al. Effect of true and sham acupuncture on radiation-induced xerostomia among patients with head and neck cancer: A randomized clinical trial. *JAMA Network Open.* 2019;2(12):e1916910. http://doi:10.1001/jamanetworkopen.2019.16910

56. Karst M, Li C. Acupuncture: A question of culture. *JAMA Network Open.* 2019;2(12):e1916929. http://doi:10.1001/jamanetworkopen.2019.16929

57. Walach H, Falkenberg T, Fonnebo V, Lewith G, Jonas WB. Circular instead of hierarchical: Methodological principles for the evaluation of complex interventions. *BMC Medical Research Methodology.* 2006;6:29. http://doi:10.1186/1471-2288-6-29

58. Prasad V, Gall V, Cifu A. The frequency of medical reversal. *Archives of Internal Medicine.* 2011;171(18):1675–1676. http://doi:10.1001/archinternmed.2011.295

59. Prasad V, Ioannidis JP. Evidence-based de-implementation for contradicted, unproven, and aspiring healthcare practices. *Implementation Science.* 2014;9:1. http://doi:10.1186/1748-5908-9-1

60. Jonas WB. The evidence house: How to build an inclusive base for complementary medicine. *Western Journal of Medicine.* 2001;175(2):79–80. http://doi:10.1136/ewjm.175.2.79

61. Sheridan S, Schrandt S, Forsythe L, Hilliard TS, Paez KA. The PCORI engagement rubric: promising practices for partnering in research. *Annals of Family Medicine.* 2017;15(2):165–170.

62. Mullins CD, Abdulhalim AM, Lavallee DC. Continuous patient engagement in comparative effectiveness research. *JAMA.* 2012;307(15):1587–1588.

63. Schanberg LE, Mullins CD. If patients are the true north, patient-centeredness should guide research. *Nature Reviews Rheumatology.* 2019;15(1):5–6.

6

CURRENT AND FUTURE DIRECTIONS

Digital health and health equity

This section sheds light on the integration of placebo effects within evolving healthcare contexts by examining the digital landscape, open access to medical records, and the potential of virtual reality leveraged for improving patient care and outcomes.

Chapter one introduces the person-based approach, demonstrating its use in developing a digital intervention for primary care practitioners based on placebo research findings. It reflects on the potential of this approach to enhance patient care. Chapter two focuses on the practice of providing patients with online access to their medical records, known as "open notes." It examines patients' access to narrative summaries written by clinicians. The chapter highlights the complex impact of open notes on placebo and nocebo effects, particularly with regards to race/ethnicity, justice and equity in clinical care for minority patients.

The transformative role of digital health technologies in healthcare and the patient-provider relationship is acknowledged in Chapter three. The chapter explores the significance of studying placebo and nocebo effects in digital healthcare, and discusses the challenges of isolating and identifying these effects in a digital context. It underscores the need to harness placebo and minimize nocebo effects within the digital health space.

Chapter four explores the role of immersive virtual reality (VR) in medical and nonmedical contexts. The chapter discusses evidence from clinical trials and laboratory studies supporting the use of VR in health care and in education and training for healthcare professionals, allowing realistic and immersive experiences before real-world patient interactions.

6.1

Using the person-based approach to implement placebo research into primary care

Felicity L. Bishop, Jane Vennik, Kirsten A. Smith, Leanne Morrison, and Hazel A. Everitt

Introduction

Placebos have a lengthy history in clinical practice and research.[1-4] Surveys suggest that medical practitioners continue to use placebos and their effects in different ways and to varying degrees in clinical practice.[5,6] However, at least some of these ad hoc uses of placebos and their effects may owe more to the pressures of clinical practice than to an accurate appreciation of the underpinning evidence-base.[7,8] Further, some reported uses of placebos may be inconsistent with evidence-based practice and/or are ethically questionable. In the context of an improved understanding of the neurobiological and psychosocial mechanisms underpinning placebo effects, leading researchers have called for a translational science of placebo effects. This chapter responds to such calls by discussing and reflecting on a systematic approach to implementing placebo research in primary medical care.

How one approaches the implementation of placebo research into clinical practice depends, in no small part, on one's definition of *placebo effects*. Traditional, substance-based, definitions of *placebo effects* hold that they are elicited by the administration of a placebo substance (e.g., the archetypal "sugar pill").[9] From this perspective, implementing placebo research in clinical practice may require the prescription of placebos. And the problem of how to implement placebo research may be approached from a translational science perspective in which the placebo substance is the analogue to the newly discovered drug, ready to be translated through clinical trials and on into clinical practice. One much-discussed complicating factor for this substance-based approach is whether placebos would be prescribed deceptively or openly, along with the ethical issues involved either way.[10-15]

Rather than adopting a substance-based definition, our work is grounded in process-oriented definitions of *placebo effects*, in which they are elicited by the psychosocial context within which treatment occurs including, especially, the patient-clinician interaction.[9] From this perspective, implementing placebo research in clinical practice involves leveraging the psychosocial context that triggers the neurobiological and psychological processes underpinning placebo effects. This approach also aligns with data suggesting that clinicians and patients may be more accepting of harnessing placebo effects through leveraging psychosocial context than through prescribing placebos.[6,9,16] When focusing on the psychosocial context of clinical practice, the problem of how to implement placebo research may be usefully approached by considering how to develop and evaluate complex interventions[17-19] within a broader context of implementation science.[20]

Implementing placebo research as a complex intervention

We have approached the implementation of placebo research into clinical primary care practice as an endeavor requiring the development and evaluation of a complex intervention to change health professionals' behavior. Complex interventions involve multiple interrelated components and may be delivered and/or evaluated on multiple levels including, for example, individual patients, health professionals, clinics, hospitals, and communities. The UK's Medical Research Council (MRC) provides extensive guidance on how to develop and evaluate them,[19] and explicitly includes "interventions directed at health professionals' behavior"[17] as an example of complex interventions. According to this framework, four iterative phases are important: (1) intervention development, based on evidence and theory; (2) feasibility work to test the feasibility and acceptability of both the intervention and the planned evaluation methods; (3) formal evaluation of the intervention's effects; and (4) implementation work to optimize take up in practice and effect.[18,19] The latest iteration of the MRC framework further specifies core elements that cut across all phases: considering context, developing underpinning theory, engaging with stakeholders, identifying uncertainties, refining the intervention, and considering economics.[19]

Complex intervention research is often multidisciplinary, and our work is no exception. The work discussed in this chapter was conducted by a large multidisciplinary team that included people from various disciplines (e.g., primary care clinical academics, psychologists), with diverse research methods expertise (e.g., qualitative, mixed methods, and systematic reviews), and relevant topic expertise (e.g., placebo effects, digital interventions, and behavior change). Working in large multidisciplinary teams brings its own challenges and can require sizable funding. Our clinical collaborators were essential in grounding our work in the realities of clinical practice. And we were motivated not only by a desire to implement promising findings from placebo studies into practice but also by the need to optimize doctor-patient encounters for maximum health benefit in the context of rising demand and over 300 million primary care consultations each year in England.[21,22]

The person-based approach to developing interventions

While the MRC framework highlights key considerations for intervention development, it does not provide detailed practical guidance on how to develop interventions in ways that, for example, reflect the evidence-base, develop underpinning theory, and consider contextual issues. Nor does the MRC framework offer guidance on how to design intervention components so that they are used and engaged with. Multiple approaches to developing interventions have been described[23] and methods aligned to the MRC framework have been elaborated.[24] We adopted the person-based approach (PBA)[25] to develop our intervention. The PBA involves putting intervention users and beneficiaries at the heart of the design and development process, and it uses extensive qualitative research to do this. It aims "to ground the development of behavior change interventions in a profound understanding of the perspective and psychosocial context of the people who will use them, gained through iterative in-depth qualitative research."[25] The PBA thus emphasizes the importance of context and offers systematic ways to explore and address contextual factors.

We decided to use the PBA because:

1. Implementing placebo research in practice has the potential to be controversial. The PBA would help us to put healthcare professionals and patients at the center of our work, and thus to develop an intervention that was not only acceptable but also engaging and persuasive.
2. The PBA's focus on context matched our intended focus on leveraging the psychosocial context of therapeutic encounters.
3. The PBA's focus on context was particularly relevant given that we anticipated important contextual differences between the research laboratory (where much of the evidence-base for placebo effects was generated) and our chosen clinical setting (primary medical care).

4. The PBA has been used successfully to develop engaging and effective behavior change interventions in primary care.[26]
5. The PBA can be integrated with the evidence-based and theory-based approaches required by the MRC framework while putting person-based evidence on an equal footing with quantitative evidence and theory.
6. The PBA offers a systematic means to address some of the MRC framework's core elements in complex intervention development and evaluation, in particular context, engaging with stakeholders, identifying uncertainties, and refining the intervention.
7. The PBA can be integrated with behavioral analyses, and this combination can be helpful for identifying promising techniques for achieving specific behavior changes (contributed by the behavioral analysis) and how best to implement them within the specific context of interest (contributed by the PBA).
8. The PBA provides explicit guidance on how to integrate and use multiple inputs to intervention planning in the form of guiding principles that specify intervention design objectives (i.e., things the intervention should achieve) and associated key features of the intervention (i.e., components that are needed to achieve each objective).

In the following sections, we discuss our use of the PBA alongside evidence- and theory-based approaches and behavioral analyses to develop "Empathico," a brief digital intervention to enable primary care clinicians to better harness placebo effects of communication in consultations. We initially developed Empathico to train clinicians to better communicate clinical empathy and realistic optimism in consultations about osteoarthritis, while expecting it to have much broader relevance to primary care consultations for musculoskeletal and potentially other conditions. Figure 6.1.1 shows how we related the PBA to the broader MRC framework for complex intervention research and summarizes the activities and additional frameworks associated with each phase. A detailed description of our intervention planning and optimization methods has been presented elsewhere.[27] In this chapter, we reflect on our approach and highlight key features of the intervention that emerged from our use of the PBA alongside theory, evidence, and behavioral analyses, within the broader MRC framework. We will not discuss the later phases of feasibility, evaluation, and implementation, but include them in Figure 6.1.1 for a more complete illustration of our use of the PBA for intervention development and evaluation.

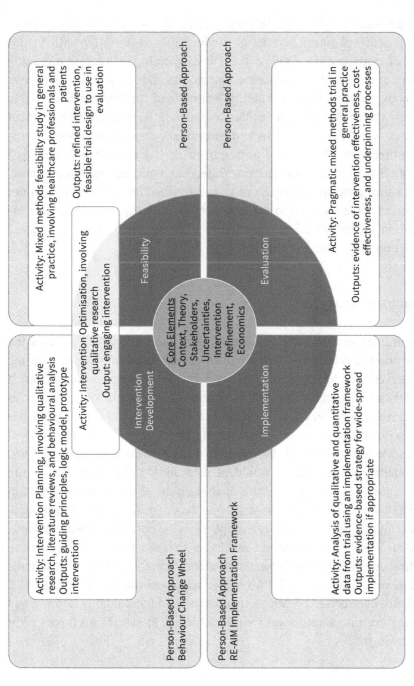

Figure 6.1.1 Illustrating how our activities and outputs (white boxes) relate to the MRC framework for complex intervention research (blue circles) and the PBA and additional frameworks that we used (gray boxes).

Activity: Intervention Planning, involving qualitative research, literature reviews, and behavioural analysis
Outputs: guiding principles, logic model, prototype intervention

Activity: Intervention Optimisation, involving qualitative research
Output: engaging intervention

Activity: Mixed methods feasibility study in general practice, involving healthcare professionals and patients
Outputs: refined intervention, feasible trial design to use in evaluation

Person-Based Approach

Person-Based Approach

Feasibility

Core Elements
Context, Theory, Stakeholders, Uncertainties, Intervention Refinement, Economics

Intervention Development

Evaluation

Activity: Pragmatic mixed methods trial in general practice
Outputs: evidence of intervention effectiveness, cost-effectiveness, and underpinning processes

Person-Based Approach

Implementation

Person-Based Approach
Behaviour Change Wheel

Person-Based Approach
RE-AIM Implementation Framework

Activity: Analysis of qualitative and quantitative data from trial using an implementation framework
Outputs: evidence-based strategy for wide-spread implementation if appropriate

Intervention development: planning and design

The PBA outlines two overlapping phases at the start of intervention development—planning and design—which may also overlap with a third phase of optimization. Within the PBA, planning involves conducting primary and secondary qualitative research to elicit and understand user perspectives on the topic at hand. We combined the PBA with more traditional theory-based and evidence-based intervention development activities—a behavioral analysis and additional systematic reviews of quantitative literature. The insights from our qualitative work, behavioral analysis, and literature reviews were integrated in an overlapping design phase, which culminated in the design of guiding principles for intervention development, a logic model to explain the processes through which key intervention components are expected to elicit specified changes, and the production of an intervention prototype.

Behavioral analysis

A preliminary essential step in developing an intervention is to choose the intervention target(s): what is it that will change as a result of people using the intervention? Multiple processes occur within the psychosocial context of healthcare encounters that might trigger the neuropsychological processes underpinning placebo effects.[28] To help us choose which of these processes to focus on and how to go about enhancing them, we reviewed the evidence-base and used the behavior change wheel to assess which behavior changes, components, and techniques would be most likely to be effective.[29] Figure 6.1.2 summarizes the results of this analysis, parts of which are presented in detail elsewhere[27] and led us to target healthcare professionals' communication of clinical empathy and realistic optimism in consultations with patients. Using the behavior change wheel enabled us to take a systematic approach to selecting our intervention targets, that incorporated qualitative and quantitative evidence and theory. It thus helped us to generate a clear rationale for our choice of intervention targets that was helpful for obtaining funding and ensuring our intervention was well-grounded in literature and theory right from the start.

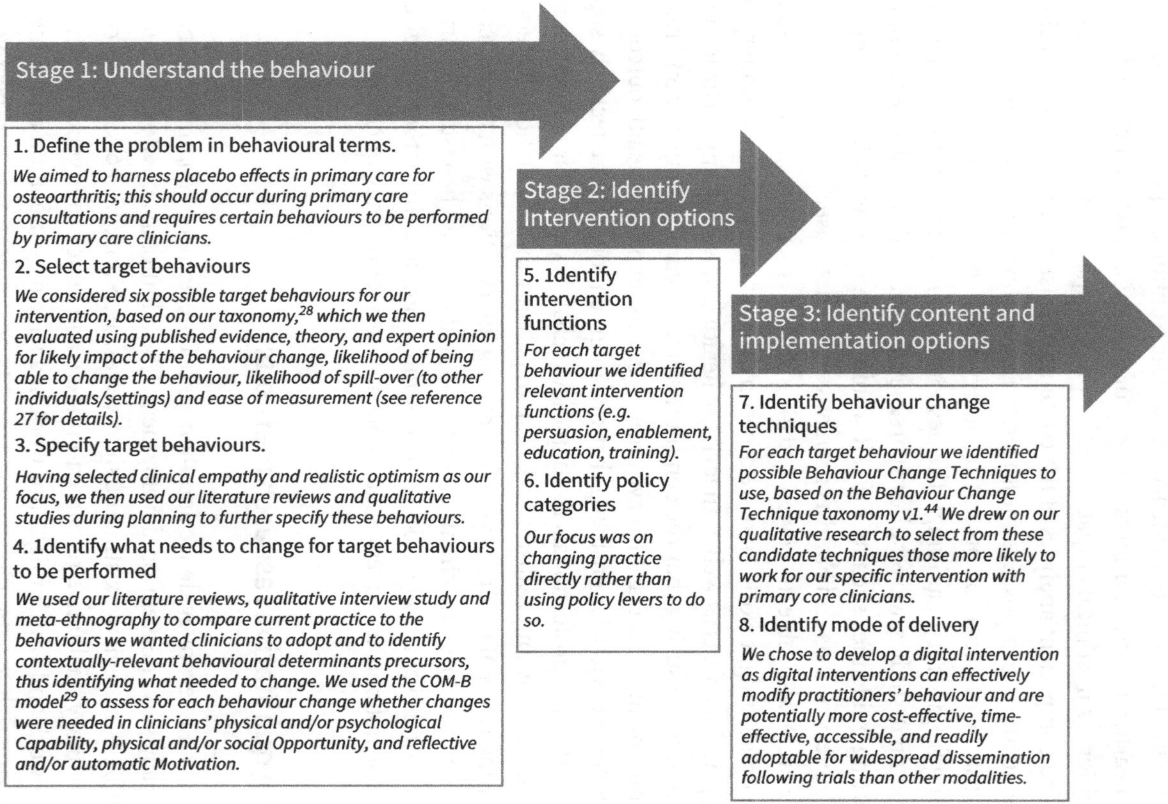

Stage 1: Understand the behaviour

1. Define the problem in behavioural terms.

We aimed to harness placebo effects in primary care for osteoarthritis; this should occur during primary care consultations and requires certain behaviours to be performed by primary care clinicians.

2. Select target behaviours

We considered six possible target behaviours for our intervention, based on our taxonomy,[28] which we then evaluated using published evidence, theory, and expert opinion for likely impact of the behaviour, likelihood of being able to change the behaviour, likelihood of spill-over (to other individuals/settings) and ease of measurement (see reference 27 for details).

3. Specify target behaviours.

Having selected clinical empathy and realistic optimism as our focus, we then used our literature reviews and qualitative studies during planning to further specify these behaviours.

4. Identify what needs to change for target behaviours to be performed

We used our literature reviews, qualitative interview study and meta-ethnography to compare current practice to the behaviours we wanted clinicians to adopt and to identify contextually-relevant behavioural determinants precursors, thus identifying what needed to change. We used the COM-B model[29] to assess for each behaviour change whether changes were needed in clinicians' physical and/or psychological Capability, physical and/or social Opportunity, and reflective and/or automatic Motivation.

Stage 2: Identify Intervention options

5. Identify intervention functions

For each target behaviour we identified relevant intervention functions (e.g. persuasion, enablement, education, training).

6. Identify policy categories

Our focus was on changing practice directly rather than using policy levers to do so.

Stage 3: Identify content and implementation options

7. Identify behaviour change techniques

For each target behaviour we identified possible Behaviour Change Techniques to use, based on the Behaviour Change Technique taxonomy v1.[44] We drew on our qualitative research to select from these candidate techniques those more likely to work for our specific intervention with primary core clinicians.

8. Identify mode of delivery

We chose to develop a digital intervention as digital interventions can effectively modify practitioners' behaviour and are potentially more cost-effective, time-effective, accessible, and readily adoptable for widespread dissemination following trials than other modalities.

Figure 6.1.2 Illustrating how we used the behavior change wheel in the early phases of intervention planning.

Reviewing the evidence-base

By reviewing existing studies, we were able to identify intervention features that had been shown to be effective in laboratory and/or clinical studies. This is vital for creating evidence-based interventions. In our case we drew on an earlier review and meta-analysis of 28 studies that trained healthcare practitioners in clinical empathy and/or positive messages,[30] and carried out detailed component analyses of the contents of existing interventions in clinical empathy[31] and positive messages.[32] This ensured that we were building on existing evidence of promising intervention components, rather than starting from scratch, although the descriptions of interventions in many of the original studies were rather sparse, and increased use of intervention-reporting guidelines such as TIDieR would make it easier to learn from existing interventions and build a cumulative evidence-base.[33]

We were also able to review existing theory to understand how such components might work. Here we drew on theories of mechanisms underpinning placebo effects as well as theories of health behavior change. The former was vital for ensuring that the communication of clinical empathy and realistic optimism could feasibly have positive effects on patient health outcomes. The latter was vital for ensuring that our intervention could effectively support healthcare professionals to adopt new behaviors to better communicate clinical empathy and realistic optimism to patients in consultations. Overall, reviewing relevant theory is vital for creating interventions with theoretically grounded proposed mechanisms of action that can then be tested as part of intervention evaluation work. To successfully complete this activity required expertise not only in placebo studies but also in health behavior change.

Using qualitative research methods

Reviewing relevant evidence and theory are core activities common to many approaches to intervention development. The additional activity specified in the PBA is to review existing qualitative research and, if necessary, to conduct primary qualitative research to understand which intervention features might work and which might not work in a specific population and context. Acquiring rich insight of the needs, priorities and concerns of prospective intervention users can also help developers to consider how to communicate and deliver those intervention features in a way that will be engaging. To plan Empathico, we carried out one systematic review of qualitative studies, one primary interview study, and one primary "think-aloud" interview study.

We conducted a meta-ethnographic review of 26 qualitative studies in which we sought to elucidate and compare primary care patients' and clinicians' perspectives on communication within osteoarthritis consultations.[34] The review findings highlighted that (1) the osteoarthritis section of Empathico needed to convey and address differences between how patients and clinicians view osteoarthritis, and provide information and resources about managing osteoarthritis, and (2) Empathico needed to include practical examples showing how to implement techniques for communicating clinical empathy and realistic optimism in the context of primary care consultations. Without these insights, we might have developed an intervention that engaged clinicians but was not acceptable to patients with osteoarthritis, and we might have provided very brief contextless demonstrations of our techniques that were insufficiently grounded in primary care consultations.

Our combined and comparative focus on patients' and clinicians' perspectives, epitomized by our meta-ethnography but also present in other aspects of our work, was essential for developing an intervention in which both patients and clinicians could be considered stakeholders. We needed to design Empathico such that it would engage clinicians and support them in making evidence-based and theory-based changes to how they communicate clinical empathy and realistic optimism. But we also needed to ensure that such changes in clinician communication would be accepted and ideally well-received by patients (otherwise we risked disrupting trusting therapeutic relationships and creating negative feedback for clinicians that would discourage sustained behavior change). This dual focus on patients and clinicians may also be helpful in other interventions to implement placebo effects by leveraging the psychosocial context of healthcare interactions.

We also conducted a primary qualitative study where we interviewed 20 primary care clinicians, exploring their perspectives on communication skills training, clinical empathy, and realistic optimism, within the context of primary care.[35] Thematic analysis of the transcripts showed that our intervention needed to (1) address clinicians' concerns that incorporating new communication skills in consultations would increase consultation duration, which would create additional unwanted stress given current high workloads in primary care is at a premium, and increasing expressions of empathy might increase their risk of burn-out, and (2) address misunderstandings that conveying optimism might involve creating false hope and that clinical empathy cannot be communicated authentically without over-investment of emotional capital. These findings fed into the guiding principles and behavioral analysis and thus informed how we presented the intervention content. Without this study, we may have developed an intervention that did not explain sufficiently clearly how clinical empathy and realistic optimism differ from everyday empathy and optimism and such an intervention would have been misinterpreted by some clinicians and implemented inappropriately or not at all. We might also have failed to ensure and communicate that implementing our suggested communication techniques would not increase consultation duration, which would probably have led to clinicians disengaging from the intervention at an early stage.

Our third piece of qualitative work was the think-aloud study. Box 6.1.1 describes the think-aloud method as it is used within the PBA. We asked seven primary care clinicians to work through a promising existing intervention, identified within our evidence review, that we had selected as the basis for Empathico, speaking their thoughts out loud and answering open-ended questions about their experiences. This study was important because it told

---

BOX 6.1.1 Think-aloud interviews for intervention development and optimization

Think-aloud interviews require participants to verbalize their thoughts by speaking to them out loud in the presence of a researcher (or sometimes just a recording device). This real-time verbal data provides insight into what is being attended to[39] and how it is being interpreted.[40] The PBA advocates using think-aloud interviews as a qualitative approach during intervention development to "elicit, observe and analyze user reactions to every intervention element" and optimize the intervention accordingly.[25] This involves having research participants drawn from the population of target users, work through sections of the intervention while speaking their thoughts out loud in the presence of a researcher who also asks additional probing and follow-up questions to elicit a more complete picture of how the intervention is being used and interpreted. A key objective is to identify features of the intervention that are engaging and interpreted as intended (which should be retained), and features of the intervention that are off-putting and/or misunderstood (which should be removed or adapted). The data may be analyzed thematically[41] and/or using the Table of Changes method (Box 6.1.2). And, typically, think-aloud studies would be carried out iteratively, making changes to the intervention after each batch of interviews to test out how those changes are responded to by other users. With multimodule digital interventions like Empathico, it can be desirable to do some think-aloud interviews focused in depth on individual modules (or even individual pages) of the intervention, although it is also important to obtain data from target intervention-users on intervention sections used within the context of the whole intervention.

us how to improve the existing intervention to better engage clinicians. For example, the data showed that we needed to improve the structure and coherence of the material, to add and reframe content so that participants felt they were learning new skills, and to be more convincing that implementing our suggestions would not increase consultation durations. The latter point encouraged us to produce professionally acted consultations demonstrating the use of Empathico in the context of a whole consultation in under 10 minutes.

In summary, by using primary and secondary qualitative research when planning our intervention, we were able to identify psychosocial factors that needed to be addressed for it to be engaging and potentially effective in routine clinical practice settings. Our intervention planning was also enhanced by ensuring we attended to both clinicians and patients in this phase and thus addressed both perspectives in our initial intervention design.

Intervention development: optimization

Toward the end of the initial planning and design phases, after a prototype intervention has been planned and constructed, the optimization phase of intervention development can be said to begin. At this point, the focus moves from planning and initially drafting the intervention to optimizing the contents, organization, and other features of the intervention. The aim is to iteratively refine the intervention, using qualitative methods to ensure that it is optimally engaging and feasible to use. The nature and mechanisms of optimal or "effective" engagement are dynamic and multifaceted; intervention users need to sufficiently engage with both the intervention itself and the behaviors that we wanted them to adopt. This engagement can be behavioral (e.g., logging in, practicing target behaviors) and experiential (e.g., interest, perceived utility, relevance, and practicality) and can be shaped by contextual factors such as social support and organizational culture.[36,37]

Within the PBA, work to optimize the intervention to achieve effective engagement importantly still refers to and may iteratively refine other products of intervention planning, such as the guiding principles for intervention development and the logic model of how the intervention is thought to work. The optimization phase may overlap with both intervention development and feasibility phases of the MRC framework; optimization studies precede feasibility studies, which then, in turn, also contribute to further intervention optimization. Within the PBA, key activities include capturing user responses to all intervention components and iteratively modifying the intervention accordingly and carrying out longitudinal case studies of independent intervention use. We followed this approach but supplemented it with an additional study focused on patients to maintain our dual focus on clinicians as intervention users and patients as intervention recipients or beneficiaries, as appropriate for an intervention to implement placebo research by modifying clinician communication within consultations.

In our main optimization work preceding our feasibility study we carried out three primary qualitative studies to capture the broad range of contextual issues that might affect engagement with and ultimate effectiveness of Empathico. Maintaining our dual focus on patients and clinicians, one qualitative study focused on patients and two focused on clinicians. We interviewed 33 primary care patients to identify barriers and areas for improvement in the behaviors that Empathico encourages clinicians to adopt. To enable them to comment on these behaviors, we showed patients vignettes and films demonstrating model Empathico behaviors within a primary care consultation. This "vignette" approach is commonly used in communication studies and was very helpful for eliciting patients' perspectives in a timely manner such that they could contribute to the intervention optimization before the intervention was ready for clinicians to implement in an actual consultation. For example, findings from this study led us to ensure that Empathico conveyed the importance of clinicians having prior knowledge of their patients and their (long-term) condition.

The first of our studies with clinicians involved conducting qualitative think-aloud interviews with 15 primary care clinicians, ensuring all components of the intervention were worked through at least once and making iterative changes after every few interviews. The second study with clinicians involved having five clinicians work through the entire intervention in their own time before being interviewed about their experiences retrospectively. The think-aloud study provided insights into specific pages and contents and was complemented by the retrospective interview study which provided additional insights into the intervention flow, coherence, and feasibility in its entirety. We optimized the intervention as a consequence of this feedback and reached a point of saturation, where minimal barriers to implementation were identified in subsequent interviews.

One challenge of the PBA intervention development is the sheer volume of data that can be generated through qualitative studies. PBA researchers have developed a "Table of Changes" method to address this challenge, and this is summarized in Box 6.1.2.[38] This method proved invaluable in organizing and analyzing the data from all our optimization studies, and prioritizing which changes needed to be made to the intervention. It also provided an incredibly

BOX 6.1.2 Table of changes method for intervention optimization

The Table of Changes is a rapid method of analysis that tabulates and codes comments as broadly positive or negative and maps them against each intervention page, section, or feature. For example, this can be implemented in Excel. The table also has space for researchers to suggest possible changes to the intervention that would address the comment, for example, by removing a barrier to engagement or clarifying confusing content that has been misinterpreted. These possible changes need to be consistent with the intervention's guiding principles and ideally discussed as a team. Typically, more possible changes are identified through this process than can feasibly be implemented, and so they need to be prioritized. To help prioritize, PBA researchers have used MoSCoW criteria ("must have this," "should have this," "could have this," and "won't have this")[42] in discussion with relevant experts in the project team.[43]

detailed and searchable audit trail, enabling us to view new data within the context of earlier comments and the rationale for previous changes; this was invaluable given the iterative nature of intervention optimization.

Summary and future directions

We have used the PBA alongside behavioral analyses and theory-based and evidence-based approaches to intervention development. We framed this within the broader context of the MRC's framework for the design and evaluation of complex interventions. This may appear to be an excessive number of frameworks that required a considerable multistudy project to develop an intervention to implement placebo research in primary care. The complexity and resource-intensive nature of such involved careful and detailed work was indeed challenging and could not have been undertaken without sufficient funding for a multidisciplinary team of collaborators and researchers. However, we feel that the challenges of implementing placebo research in primary care require a systematic and involved process of intervention development. The PBA has now been used quite extensively in the planning, optimization, and feasibility testing of digital health interventions. We hope that, as it has done for others, using this approach has helped us to produce an engaging intervention that will effectively encourage and train primary care clinicians to communicate more clinical empathy and realistic optimism to their patients and, thus, to improve patient outcomes through placebo-like mechanisms.

References

1. Booth C. The rod of Aesculapios: John Haygarth (1740–1827) and Perkins' metallic tractors. *Journal of Medical Biography*. 2005;13(3):155–161. http://doi:10.1177/096777200501300310
2. Czerniak E, Davidson M. Placebo, a historical perspective. *European Neuropsychopharmacology*. 2012;22(11):770–774. http://doi:10.1016/j.euroneuro.2012.04.003
3. Jutte R. The early history of the placebo. *Complementary Therapies in Medicine*. 2013;21(2):94–97. http://doi:10.1016/j.ctim.2012.06.002
4. Kaptchuk TJ. Powerful placebo: The dark side of the randomised controlled trial. *Lancet*. 1998;351:1722–1775.
5. Howick J, Bishop FL, Heneghan C, et al. Placebo use in the United Kingdom: Results from a national survey of primary care practitioners. *PLoS ONE*. 2013;8(3):e58247. http://doi:10.1371/journal.pone.0058247
6. Linde K, Atmann O, Meissner K, et al. How often do general practitioners use placebos and non-specific interventions? Systematic review and meta-analysis of surveys. *PLoS ONE*. 2018;13(8):e0202211. http://doi:10.1371/journal.pone.0202211
7. Comaroff J. A bitter pill to swallow: Placebo therapy in general practice. *Sociological Review*. 1976;24(1):79–96.
8. Bishop FL, Howick J, Heneghan C, et al. Placebo use in the United Kingdom: A qualitative study exploring GPs' views on placebo effects in clinical practice. *Family Practice*. 2014 Jun;31(3):357–363. http://doi:10.1093/fampra/cmu016
9. Hardman DI, Geraghty AW, Lewith G, et al. From substance to process: A meta-ethnographic review of how healthcare professionals and patients understand placebos and their effects in primary care. *Health (London)*. 2018 May;24(3):315–340. http://doi: 10.1177/1363459318800169
10. Blease C, Colloca L, Kaptchuk TJ. Are open-label placebos ethical? Informed Consent and ethical equivocations. *Bioethics*. 2016;30(6):407–414. http://doi:10.1111/bioe.12245
11. Bok S. The ethics of giving placebos. *Scientific American*. 1974;231(5):17–23.
12. Brody H. The lie that heals: The ethics of giving placebos. *Annals of Internal Medicine*. 1982;97:112–118.
13. Lichtenberg P, Heresco-Levy U, Nitzan U. The ethics of the placebo in clinical practice. *Journal of Medical Ethics*. 2004;30:551–554.
14. Louhiala P. The ethics of the placebo in clinical practice revisited. *Journal of Medical Ethics*. 2009;35(7):407–409.
15. Miller FG, Colloca L. The legitimacy of placebo treatments in clinical practice: Evidence and ethics. *AJOB*. 2009;9(12):39–47. http://doi:10.1080/15265160903316263
16. Ratnapalan M, Coghlan B, Tan M, et al. Placebos in primary care? A nominal group study explicating UK GP and patient views of six theoretically plausible models of placebo practice. *BMJ Open*. 2020;10(2):e032524. http://doi:10.1136/bmjopen-2019-032524
17. Campbell M, Fitzpatrick R, Haines A, et al. Framework for design and evaluation of complex interventions to improve health. *British Medical Journal (Clinical Research Ed)*. 2000;321(7262):694–696. http://doi:10.1136/bmj.321.7262.694
18. Craig P, Dieppe P, Macintyre S, et al. Developing and evaluating complex interventions: The new Medical Research Council guidance. *British Medical Journal*. 2008;337:a1655.

19. Skivington K, Matthews L, Simpson SA, et al. A new framework for developing and evaluating complex interventions: Update of Medical Research Council guidance. *British Medical Journal.* 2021;374:n2061. http://doi:10.1136/bmj.n2061

20. Bauer MS, Damschroder L, Hagedorn H, et al. An introduction to implementation science for the non-specialist. *BMC Psychology.* 2015;3(1):32. http://doi:10.1186/s40 359-015-0089-9

21. Digital N. *Appointments in General Practice.* October 2018. Accessed August 1, 2019. https://digital.nhs.uk/data-and-information/publications/statistical/appointments-in-general-practice/oct-2018

22. Baird B, Charles A, Honeyman M, Maguire D, Das P. Understanding pressures in general practice [Internet]. London, UK: The King's Fund; 2016 [cited 2023 Jul 7]. Available from: https://www.kingsfund.org.uk/sites/default/files/field/field_publication_file/Under standing-GP-pressures-Kings-Fund-May-2016.pdf

23. O'Cathain A, Croot L, Sworn K, et al. Taxonomy of approaches to developing interventions to improve health: A systematic methods overview. *Pilot and Feasibility Studies.* 2019;5(1):41. http://doi:10.1186/s40814-019-0425-6

24. O'Cathain A, Croot L, Duncan E, et al. Guidance on how to develop complex interventions to improve health and healthcare. *BMJ Open.* 2019;9(8):e029954. http://doi:10.1136/bmjo pen-2019-029954

25. Yardley L, Morrison L, Bradbury K, et al. The person-based approach to intervention development: Application to digital health-related behavior change interventions. *Journal of Medical Internet Research.* 2015 Jan30:17(1):e30. doi:10.2196/jmir.4055.

26. Little P, Stuart B, Hobbs FDR, et al. An internet-based intervention with brief nurse support to manage obesity in primary care (POWeR+): A pragmatic, parallel-group, randomised controlled trial. *Lancet Diabetes & Endocrinology.* 2016;4(10):821–828. http://dx.doi.org/ 10.1016/S2213-8587(16)30099-7

27. Smith KA, Vennik J, Morrison L, et al. Harnessing placebo effects in primary care: Using the person-based approach to develop an online intervention to enhance practitioners' communication of clinical empathy and realistic optimism during consultations. *Frontiers in Pain Research.* 2021Aug24;2: 721222. doi:10.3389/fpain.2021.721222.

28. Bishop FL, Coghlan B, Geraghty AW, et al. What techniques might be used to harness placebo effects in non-malignant pain? A literature review and survey to develop a taxonomy. *BMJ Open.* 2017;7(6):e015516. http://doi:10.1136/bmjopen-2016-015516

29. Michie S, van Stralen MM, West R. The behaviour change wheel: A new method for characterising and designing behaviour change interventions. *Implementation Science.* 2011;6(1):42. http://doi:10.1186/1748-5908-6-42

30. Howick J, Moscrop A, Mebius A, et al. Effects of empathic and positive communication in healthcare consultations: A systematic review and meta-analysis. *Journal of the Royal Society of Medicine.* 2018;111(7):240–252. http://doi:10.1177/0141076818769477

31. Smith KA, Bishop FL, Dambha-Miller H, et al. Improving empathy in healthcare consultations: A secondary analysis of interventions. *Journal of General Internal Medicine.* 2020;35(10):3007–3014. http://doi:10.1007/s11606-020-05994-w

32. Howick J, Lyness E, Albury C, et al. Anatomy of positive messages in healthcare consultations: Component analysis of messages within 22 randomised trials. *European Journal for Person Centered Healthcare.* 2019;7(4):656–664.

33. Hoffmann TC, Glasziou PP, Boutron I, et al. Better reporting of interventions: Template for intervention description and replication (TIDieR) checklist and guide. *British Medical Journal.* 2014;348:g1687. doi:10.1136/bmj.g1687.

34. Vennik J, Hughes S, Smith KA, et al. Patient and practitioner priorities and concerns about primary healthcare interactions for osteoarthritis: A meta-ethnography. *Patient Education and Counseling.* 2022 July;105(7):1865–1877. doi:10.1016/j.pec.2022.01.009.

35. Hughes SV, Smith, J, Bostock, K, et al. Exploring primary care practitioner views about the use of optimistic and empathic communication in consultations. *BJGP Open.* 2022 Sep 28;6(3):BJGPO.2021.0221. doi:10.3399/BJGPO.2021.0221.

36. Yardley L, Spring BJ, Riper H, et al. Understanding and promoting effective engagement with digital behavior change interventions. *American Journal of Preventive Medicine.* 2016;51(5):833–842. http://dx.doi.org/10.1016/j.amepre.2016.06.015

37. Perski O, Blandford A, West R, et al. Conceptualising engagement with digital behaviour change interventions: A systematic review using principles from critical interpretive synthesis. *Translational Behavioral Medicine.* 2017;7(2):254–267. http://doi: 10.1007/s13142-016-0453-1

38. Bradbury K, Morton K, Band R, et al. Using the person-based approach to optimise a digital intervention for the management of hypertension. *PLoS ONE.* 2018;13(5):e0196868. http://doi:10.1371/journal.pone.0196868

39. Ericsson KA, Simon HA. Verbal reports as data. *Psychological Review.* 1980;87(3):215–251. http://doi:10.1037/0033-295X.87.3.215

40. Tourangeau R, Rips LJ, Rasinski K. *The Psychology of Survey Response.* Cambridge University Press; 2000.

41. Yardley L, Morrison L, Andreou P, et al. Understanding reactions to an internet-delivered health-care intervention: Accommodating user preferences for information provision. *BMC Medical Informatics and Decision Making.* 2010;10:52. doi:10.1186/1472-6947-10-52.

42. Clegg D, Barker R. *Case Method Fast-Track: A RAD Approach.* Addison-Wesley; 1994.

43. Payne L, Ghio D, Grey E, et al. Optimising an intervention to support home-living older adults at risk of malnutrition: a qualitative study. *BMC Family Practice.* 2021;22(1):219. http://doi:10.1186/s12875-021-01572-z

44. Michie S, Richardson M, Johnston M, et al. The behavior change technique taxonomy (v1) of 93 hierarchically clustered techniques: Building an international consensus for the reporting of behavior change interventions. *Annals of Behavioral Medicine.* 2013;46(1):81–95.

6.2

Sharing online clinical notes with patients

Implications for placebo and nocebo effects and racial health equity

Charlotte Blease

Introduction

Clinicians, in around 20 countries worldwide, offer patients online access to their clinical records. Full record access includes problems lists, test results, medications, allergies, vaccinations, hospital referral letters, and even the narrative reports written by doctors and other providers. Often referred to as "open notes," the practice is slowly growing, and in some countries, is advanced.[1,2] For example, by 2018 in Sweden, most patients were offered open notes via *Journalen*, the nationwide patient portal. In the United States, in 2021, a new federal ruling enacted as part of the Bipartisan 21st Century Cures Act[3,4] mandated that, with few exceptions, all health providers must share immediate access to patients' full electronic medical records. The rule did not come in a vacuum; by 2021, 50 million people already had online access to their records. However, uptake of the practice is still limited including in other wealthy Western countries and, in Canada and Germany, open notes are available to some patients but not yet offered universally. Meanwhile, in the UK, it was announced that from April 2022, patients who sign up for an online health service, such as the NHS App,[5] will soon be able to access their primary care health record, including the narrative consultation notes written by their GPs;[6] roll out has now been postponed until the end of 2022.

When patients access their online records, communication between clinicians and patients is no longer merely restricted to dialogue arising in real-time, during face-to-face or telemedicine visits. Encouragingly, now in multiple surveys, the majority of patients who access their online clinical notes report benefits including strengthened trust in clinicians, greater understanding about their treatments, better recall about treatment plans, greater engagement in their care, and enhanced understanding about the rationale for prescribed treatments and interventions.[7-10] Currently, it is not known whether patient access to online clinical notes might also influence placebo or nocebo effects. Nonetheless, considering what is known about mechanisms of placebo and nocebo effects, it would be surprising if this new digital communication tool did not play a role in influencing health changes according to placebo and nocebo mechanisms.

In this chapter, I outline why Placebo Studies should focus on open notes, particularly when it comes to the potential distribution of placebo and nocebo effects. Building on previous work, I begin by briefly describing the potential ways in which open notes might elicit placebo and nocebo effects via the tone and content of clinician communication. Then, taking a deeper look at race/ethnicity dimensions of patient surveys and analyses of clinical notes, I mount preliminary evidence suggesting we might also expect to see differences in how placebo and nocebo effects are experienced along the lines of patient race/ethnicity. The ethical implications of this nascent area of research will be considered.

Placebo and nocebo effects in clinic communication

Placebo studies have burgeoned in recent years.[11] A growing body of multidisciplinary research shows that placebo effects are genuine psychobiological events that elicit beneficial physiological responses. A number of commonly reported symptoms and conditions appear to be particularly susceptible to placebo effects, including pain, depression and anxiety, and fatigue.[12,13] In 2018, a Delphi Poll of experts in Placebo Studies recommended clinicians should strive to harness placebo effects in clinical contexts.[14] Research in Placebo Studies has focused on "response expectancies" (p. 198) as a core mechanism of placebo effects[15] (p. 198). Most of these studies focus on augmentation of patients' consciously or subconsciously held beliefs that treatments will be beneficial. Expectancies can be influenced by learning processes including classical conditioning,[16-21] and verbal instructions.[22-24] For example, Locher and colleagues reported that placebos administered with a plausible rationale elicited significantly higher levels of pain relief via placebo effects than placebos given without a rationale.[22]

Perceptions about clinicians' competence and empathy may also influence outcome expectancies, and have been demonstrated to strengthen placebo

effects.[25,26] For example, Howe et al. found that after inducing an allergic reaction in participants, those who had both positive expectations of allergy relief and interacted with a provider who demonstrated high warmth and high
competence, displayed the largest reduction in their allergic reaction as measured by the size of the weal, compared with participants allocated to providers
in low warmth, low competence conditions.[25] Howe memorably characterized the influence of placebo effects as facilitated by perceptions that, "the
clinician gets me" (warmth) via displays of compassion, support, and personalized engagement, and "the clinician gets it" (competence) via displays of expertise, knowledge, and skill.[27]

Nocebo effects are often characterized as the "evil twin" of placebo effects
and understood to be mediated by patients' negative expectations about
an intervention or prognosis giving rise in turn, to adverse health effects.[28]
Compared with studies into placebo effects, to date, considerably less research
has explored nocebo effects. However, studies show that negative expectancies
about interventions may lead to adverse effects including experiencing greater
side effects of treatments.[28-30] For example, in a study of beta blockers for cardiac disease and hypertension, disclosing to patients that side effects may include erectile dysfunction led to a doubling of this reported problem among
informed participants compared with those not informed.[31] A study led by
Benedetti investigated what would happen when morphine administration
was interrupted during postoperative pain.[23] One group received information that morphine administration was interrupted; in another group morphine administration was terminated without participants being informed.
Knowing morphine administration was interrupted caused patients to experience more intense pain with more than twice as many patients requesting
further pain medication when they knew that morphine administration was
interrupted compared with those who were unaware of the interruption.

Connecting "open notes" with placebo studies

Might open notes also be a forum with the potential to influence placebo and
nocebo effects?[32] In previous work, my colleagues and I proposed that patient
access to the very narrative summaries written by their clinicians might indeed present a novel platform for eliciting placebo and nocebo effects under
certain conditions.[33] Bridging research in Placebo Studies with open notes,
three hypotheses were proffered, describing the specific conditions under
which patients might experience placebo effects:

"Hypothesis 1: Clinical notes convey positive expectations about the success of the treatment, and/or the patient's progress/prognosis; and/or

Hypothesis 2: Patients perceive the clinical notes to convey a persuasive rationale for treatment(s); and/or

Hypothesis 3: Patients perceive clinicians to be competent (e.g., the notes demonstrate complete and accurate information about the patients' conditions, and proposed treatments), and warm (e.g., the notes provide a high level of personal support, encouragement, and empathy for the patient's circumstances)."

In addition, we advanced a fourth hypothesis that patients might experience nocebo effects if:

"Hypothesis 4: Clinical notes convey negative expectations about the success of the treatment, including potential negative side effects."

We examined how a wide range of mixed methods survey research into patients' and clinicians' experiences with open notes offered tantalizing, preliminary evidence to motivate deeper research into whether the very words written by doctors might influence these placebo and nocebo effects.[33] Our goal was to build hypothesis, rather than to offer concrete evidence of health effects. In short, we proposed that inviting patients to read their clinical notes may be viewed as a treatment tool that could be used to maximize the therapeutic benefits of placebo effects by communicating positive expectations to patients via clinical notes, including via cues of clinician warmth and competency. In contrast, we cautioned that nocebo effects might be inadvertently elevated if patients access information about their treatment plan that leads them to infer negative expectancies about interventions and treatment plans.

Health disparities and placebo and nocebo effects: a new research agendum

The question about whether well-documented health disparities can be driven by placebo and nocebo effects is both timely and important, though for many years, it was an overlooked agendum in Placebo Studies. Recently, however, a range of conceptual, ethical and empirical papers have begun to consider closely whether some patient populations may be less susceptible to placebo effects, or more at risk of experiencing nocebo effects in patient-clinician visits.[34-37] For example, in Friesen and Blease, drawing on evidence of inequalities in clinical encounters relating to race/ethnicity, income, and even health diagnoses,[38] we proposed that differences in expressions of clinician warmth and empathy, and perceived support, may reduce experienced placebo effects among some already at-risk populations.[34] Extending this line of reasoning, in 2021, Yetman and colleagues also proposed that, since expectation in the clinical setting is strongly influenced by the attitude, affect, and communication style of the healthcare provider, differences in quality of care in the clinical setting for non-White patients—including inferior patient-clinician communication, medical mistrust, and perceived discrimination—may yield systematically lower placebo effects and/or yield increased nocebo effects.[35]

Fascinating empirical studies have also begun to explore the connection between nonclinical factors related to identity, and the expression of placebo effects. For example, in 2020, Okusogu et al. investigated placebo effects in healthy, and chronic pain participants with a diagnosis of temporomandibular disorder, who self-identified as either African American/Black or White.[36] Investigators found White participants reported greater conditioning effects, reinforced relief expectations, and placebo effects when compared with their African American/Black counterparts. In secondary analyses on the effect of experimenter-participant race and sex concordance, same experimenter-participant race induced greater placebo hypoalgesia in patients with temporomandibular disorder, while different sex dyads induced greater placebo hypoalgesia in healthy participants. Investigating racial/ethnicity differences and the influence on placebo effects, Letzen et al. found that, compared with non-Hispanic White participants, non-Hispanic Black participants experienced lower rates of placebo effects following administration of a placebo with the ambiguous verbal suggestion that, "the substance would either increase pain sensation, decrease it, or leave it unchanged."[37] Although this study did not explore causal explanations, as the authors noted, a legacy of perceived/anticipated discrimination and provider mistrust, exacerbated by historic medical abuses, may have influenced the trajectory of higher pain ratings among Black participants.

Preliminary evidence for racial/ethnic differences with open notes

If open notes do indeed influence placebo and nocebo effects, and if some patient populations are exposed to systematic differences in the tone or content of their documentation, or (alternatively) derive systematically more positive benefits from accessing their notes, it is reasonable to postulate that systemic differences in the expression of placebo or nocebo effects might also arise. In short, it is worthwhile to consider whether the notes housed in electronic medical records potentially transmit distinctive expressions of clinician warmth, empathy, support, and expectancies about treatments that may in turn affect patient health. Further, while considerable research has focused on disparities arising in face-to-face patient-doctor communication, considering increasing attention to disparities research in placebo/nocebo effects, I argue it is imperative to consider the potential of open notes to—quite literally— influence health effects.[39]

In what follows, I draw on a range of empirical studies to explore patient race/ethnicity to reveal interesting preliminary evidence supporting only Hypotheses 2–4 (as outlined, above) which, I argue, now warrant further directive scrutiny.

Preliminary evidence for provision of a treatment rationale

As conveyed, in Hypothesis 2, patients may experience enhanced placebo effects if they perceive their clinical notes to convey a persuasive rationale for treatments. Survey analyses suggest many patients with experience of the practice report better understanding of treatment rationales as a result of accessing their online clinical notes.[9,10,40] This might provide a novel pathway to elicit placebo effects. For example, Walker at al. conducted a large US survey across three health systems with over 22,000 respondents who had read at least one visit note in the previous year, in which the majority of patients reported that reading their notes was very important for taking care of their health (73%, 16 354/22 520), feeling more in control of their healthcare (70%, 15 726/ 22 515), and remembering their treatment plan (66%, 14 821/22 516); only a small minority—3% and 5%—of patients reported being very confused or more anxious by what they read.[7] Moreover, authors found that less-educated, non-White, older, and Hispanic patients, and individuals who usually did not speak English at home, were most likely to report major benefits from note reading. In 2018, in a study at an urban medical center, Gerard et al. reported that 70.7% (130/184) of Black patients and 69.9% (153/219) of Hispanic/ Latino patients reported that notes are extremely important to feel informed about their care.[41] Similarly, in 2021, a survey by Bell involving over 10,000 patients and their families reported differences for race/ethnicity with respect to understanding the reasons for tests: 81% ($n = 214$) of Asian patients, 79% ($n = 143$) of Black patients, and 81% ($n = 203$) of Hispanic/Latino patients, compared with 74% ($n = 3743$) of White patients, reported understanding the reason for tests "quite a bit" or "very much" after reading their online clinical notes (< 0.001). Although only preliminary, these findings suggest open notes might especially offer patients from minority backgrounds important opportunities to enhance response expectancies, thereby facilitating placebo effects.[42]

Preliminary evidence for perceptions of clinician competence and warmth

To enhance positive expectancies via the competence/warmth pathway (Hypothesis 3), open notes might enhance patient readers' perceptions of clinician competence ("the clinician 'gets 'it'") and/or perceptions of clinician warmth ("the clinician 'gets me'").[27] Again, evidence from closed-ended patient surveys suggests open notes might be a forum where differences in patient experiences do arise along race/ethnicity lines. For example in the survey by Bell involving over 10,000 patients and their families, patients who were non-White or less educated reported more benefits from accessing their online clinical notes than their counterparts: while the numbers are small, 48% (121/253) of Black patients and 53% (188/354) of Hispanic patients trusted their provider more after reading their notes, compared with 42% (2826/6763) of White patients (the majority of the remainder reported no change).[43] Similarly, 47% (120/253) of Black patients and 54% (190/354) of Hispanic patients reported strengthened goal alignment with their clinician after reading their clinical notes, compared with 39% (2611/6763) of White patients. Gerard et al. reported that, compared with White patients, non-White patients were more than twice as likely to report that accessing their notes was extremely important for engaging in their care.[41] Although it is unclear whether patients perceived clinicians to be more competent or warmer, these findings do suggest strengthened relational benefits from access that might facilitate placebo effects.

Preliminary evidence for nocebo effects

Open notes might also be a forum for inducing negative expectancies via nocebo effects (Hypothesis 4), and evidence suggests that persons from racial or ethnic minorities may be more vulnerable. Although few surveys have explored negative patient experiences with open notes along the lines of race or ethnicity, Fernández et al. found that 11% ($n = 2411$) of patients who accessed their notes in the three-centered US study felt judged or offended by what they read, which included forms of labeling and disrespectful language.[44] In their qualitative analysis, patients who (a) described their race as other, (b) rated their health fair or poor, (c) reported being unable to work, or (d) reported having read four or more notes were more likely than their counterparts to feel judged or offended.

Multiple studies have also begun to analyze linguistic features of documentation in the electronic medical record, revealing stigmatizing language to be more common in visit note summaries written about Black or minority patients compared with White patients. Although it is unclear from such studies whether patients who accessed their notes experience negative expectancies about their treatment or clinicians, thereby eliciting nocebo effects, the findings offer tangible preliminary evidence about the potential for health disparities to arise via access. For example, a study by Beach and colleagues found similar patterns of stigmatizing linguistic features, such as the use of quotations (e.g., "patient had a 'reaction' to the medication"), judgment words (e.g., "patient insists," "patient claims") or use of "evidentials," that is, a sentence construction in which patients' symptoms or experiences are reported as hearsay.[45] Their sample of 9,251 notes written by 165 physicians about 3,374 unique patients, found that notes written about Black patients had higher odds of containing at least one quote and at least one judgment word, and used more evidentials compared to notes about White patients (e.g., "the patient reports the headache started yesterday"). Further evidence comes from a study conducted by Sun et al., which analyzed a sample of 40,113 history and physical notes (January 2019–October 2020) from 18,459 patients in an urban medical center.[46] Specifically, investigators searched for sentences containing a negative descriptor (e.g., "patient is noncompliant," "patient is nonadherent," and "patient is uncooperative") of the patient or the patient's behavior. Controlling for sociodemographic and health characteristics, the study found that compared with White patients, Black patients had 2.54 times the odds of having at least one negative descriptor in their online history and physical notes. Finally, Himmelstein et al. undertook a cross-sectional study of admission notes using natural language processing on 48,651 admission notes written (January to December 2018) about 29,783 unique patients by 1,932 clinicians at a large, urban academic medical center.[47] Their findings revealed clinical visit notes about non-Hispanic Black patients compared with non-Hispanic White patients had a 0.67 (95% CI 0.15–1.18) percentage points greater probability of containing stigmatizing language.

Discussion

Survey research and findings from electronic health record analyses offer an invaluable starting point for exploring the possibility that patients might experience placebo and nocebo effects after accessing their clinical notes, and further, that these experiences might differ along the lines of patient race/ethnicity. On the strength of preliminary data, a mixed picture emerges—open notes might facilitate both placebo effects and nocebo effects among minority patients. With regard to the former, especially if notes are devoid of negative biases or offensive descriptors, open notes could offer new opportunities to extend the visit, thereby elongating and strengthening patient-clinical interactions by promoting understanding about treatment rationales, and by enhancing perceptions of clinician warmth and competence. This online elongation of the visit might mitigate the higher rates of communication breakdowns that can arise when patients perceive or anticipate negative biases during health interactions: with access to their clinical notes, patients may thereby be afforded opportunities to read and understand their health information away from the pressures of face-to-face consultations where anxiety or negative emotions may arise.[42] Hence, the findings that non-White patients experience greater benefits associated with empowerment, understanding, and trust in clinicians after reading their notes, might lead to a boost in placebo effects via novel routes. However, documentation analyses demonstrate that patients from Black and other minority backgrounds may also be more vulnerable to negative stereotyping and stigmatizing language. If they read such notes, patients might be at greater risk of experiencing negative expectancies, which may render them more vulnerable to nocebo effects compared with White patients. Future studies are needed to understand how race and/or ethnicity about the patient reading the notes would trigger a different reaction to a note written by a Black physician versus a White physician.

Potential disparities in the distribution of placebo and nocebo effects with open notes invite challenging ethical considerations. If minority patients appear to benefit from placebo effects online this might be because of continued systemic biasing within face-to-face or telemedicine clinical consultations. In short, even if patients do derive potential advantages from reading their clinical notes online, this may be because of persistent experienced or anticipated negative biases arising during their visits. Another concern is the digital divide in healthcare: patients who may benefit from a boost in placebo effects may be the least likely to use health portals and to read their clinical notes. Lack of broadband access can be a barrier for minorities,[48] and in the United States, the likelihood of receiving an access code to activate health portals is significantly lower for Black, Hispanic patients, older persons, and those with a lower income.[49] Understandably, many medical researchers have raised concerns about how the digital divide may increase inequalities. Notably, survey findings show that patients who access their clinical notes report better understanding about the side effects of medications.[8,9] If, owing to digital divides, Black or other minority patients access their clinical notes at a lower rate, they may be forgoing exposure to potential nocebo effects that could arise from greater awareness about medication side effects. However, by inadvertently avoiding nocebo effects they may also risk avoiding the multiple benefits patients derive from reading their clinical notes. Another vulnerability may arise when patients from racial or ethnic minorities do go online to access their clinical notes. Exposed to a greater risk of reading negative or stigmatizing language than White patients, they may thereby be exposed to a higher risk of nocebo effects.

Greater awareness and training among clinicians about how to write notes that patients will read, including how to avoid stigmatizing phrases or linguistic constructions especially when documenting the health of already disadvantaged patient populations, will be imperative to avoid risks. In addition, wider questions remain about how to resolve the potential dilemma associated with greater transparency in relation to treatment side effects, which may prompt greater risk of nocebo effects, when patients access their clinical notes. One possibility is that by embedding clever eHealth design techniques such as the use of tooltips (boxes of information that pop out, when the cursor hovers over it), health portals, and electronic health records could hide detailed information about treatment side effects with the disclaimer that patient awareness might prompt negative effects; however, transparency could also be fully offered to patients, should they wish to access it, by allowing patients to actively click or select for more information using their online portal.

There are several limitations with the data used in this chapter. Most surveys of patients' experiences with open notes are restricted to a few medical centers, restricting generalizability. In addition, it is unclear whether responses were biased by patients more engaged with their portal, or who were already more positive or negative about open notes. Finally, sample sizes for patients from minority backgrounds were small. Linguistic analysis of documentation, while illuminating, does not yet provide clear evidence about patients' experiences with reading their notes.

To better connect open notes with placebo research with the possibility of inequities in the distribution of placebo and nocebo effects, researchers will need to embark on novel experimental designs. In Blease et al. (2022), I elaborated on a variety of approaches that might be adopted to explore the relationship between open notes and placebo and nocebo effects.[33] However, these approaches should now be innovatively adapted by experienced placebo researcher experimentalists to devise new ways to explore the potential for racial differences.

Conclusions

Patient access to open notes is here to stay. Inviting patients to read their clinical notes online might lead to genuinely beneficial or adverse health outcomes by facilitating placebo or nocebo effects. However, the distribution of placebo or nocebo effects via open notes might be demographically uneven. While preliminary evidence suggests that disparities relating to the delivery of care in face-to-face visits may differ like patient race and ethnicity, emerging findings suggest open notes can also be a forum where negative biases are either not detected because they are not documented or where stereotyping biases are also transmitted and potentially perceived. Therefore, depending on what the patient reads in their online documentation, persons from Black or other minority backgrounds may, counterintuitively, both be more likely to experience placebo effects and nocebo effects via access. If the hypotheses outlined in this paper are supported, it will be imperative for medical educators to train clinicians to adopt communication and writing styles that maximize placebo effects and minimize the harms of nocebo effects, especially among already disadvantaged patient populations.

References

1. Salmi L, Brudnicki S, Isono M, et al. Six countries, six individuals: Resourceful patients navigating medical records in Australia, Canada, Chile, Japan, Sweden and the USA. *BMJ Open*. 2020;10(9):e037016.
2. Salmi L, Blease C, Hägglund M, Walker J, DesRoches CM. *US Policy Requires Immediate Release of Records to Patients*. British Medical Journal Publishing Group; 2021.
3. Health and Human Services Department, USA. *21st Century Cures Act: Interoperability, Information Blocking, and the ONC Health IT Certification Program*. 2020. Accessed July 15, 2020. https://www.govinfo.gov/content/pkg/FR-2020-05-01/pdf/2020-07419.pdf
4. Blease C, Walker J, DesRoches CM, Delbanco T. New US Law Mandates Access to Clinical Notes: Implications for Patients and Clinicians. *Annals of Internal Medicine*. 2021 Jan;174(1):101–102. doi:10.7326/M20-5370.
5. NHS. *NHS App*. 2022. Accessed February 14, 2022. https://www.nhs.uk/nhs-app/
6. NHS Digital. *Accelerating Patient Access to Their Record*. 2021. Accessed October 28, 2021. https://digital.nhs.uk/services/nhs-app/nhs-app-guidance-for-gp-practices/accelerating-patient-access-to-their-record

7. Walker J, Leveille S, Bell S, et al. OpenNotes after 7 years: Patient experiences with ongoing access to their clinicians' outpatient visit notes. *Journal of Medical Internet Research.* 2019;21(5):e13876.

8. DesRoches CM, Bell SK, Dong Z, et al. Patients managing medications and reading their visit notes: A survey of OpenNotes participants. *Annals of Internal Medicine.* 2019;171(1):69–71.

9. Blease C, Dong Z, Torous J, Walker J, Hägglund M, DesRoches CM. Association of patients reading clinical notes with perception of medication adherence among persons with serious mental illness. *JAMA Network Open.* 2021;4(3):e212823–e212823.

10. Moll J, Rexhepi H, Cajander A, et al. Patients' experiences of accessing their electronic health records: National patient survey in Sweden. *Journal of Medical Internet Research.* 2018;20(11):e278.

11. Blease C. Consensus in placebo studies: Lessons from the philosophy of science. *Perspectives in Biology and Medicine.* 2018;61(3):412–429.

12. Kaptchuk TJ, Miller FG. Placebo effects in medicine. *New England Journal of Medicine.* 2015;373(1):8–9.

13. Sugarman MA, Loree AM, Baltes BB, Grekin ER, Kirsch I. The efficacy of paroxetine and placebo in treating anxiety and depression: A meta-analysis of change on the Hamilton Rating Scales. *PLoS ONE.* 2014;9(8):e106337.

14. Evers AW, Colloca L, Blease C, et al. Implications of placebo and nocebo effects for clinical practice: Expert consensus. *Psychotherapy and Psychosomatics.* 2018;87(4):204–210.

15. Kirsch I. Response expectancy and the placebo effect. *International Review of Neurobiology.* 2018;138:81–93. doi:10.1016/bs.irn.2018.01.003.

16. Rescorla RA. Pavlovian conditioning: It's not what you think it is. *American Psychologist.* 1988;43(3):151.

17. Kirsch I, Lynn SJ, Vigorito M, Miller RR. The role of cognition in classical and operant conditioning. *Journal of Clinical Psychology.* 2004;60(4):369–392.

18. Amanzio M, Benedetti F. Neuropharmacological dissection of placebo analgesia: Expectation-activated opioid systems versus conditioning-activated specific subsystems. *Journal of Neuroscience.* 1999;19(1):484–494.

19. Colloca L, Benedetti F, Pollo A. Repeatability of autonomic responses to pain anticipation and pain stimulation. *European Journal of Pain.* 2006;10(7):659–665.

20. Colloca L, Tinazzi M, Recchia S, et al. Learning potentiates neurophysiological and behavioral placebo analgesic responses. *Pain.* 2008;139(2):306–314.

21. Colloca L, Benedetti F. Placebo analgesia induced by social observational learning. *Pain.* 2009;144(1–2):28–34.

22. Locher C, Nascimento AF, Kirsch I, Kossowsky J, Meyer A, Gaab J. Is the rationale more important than deception? A randomized controlled trial of open-label placebo analgesia. *Pain.* 2017;158(12):2320–2328.

23. Benedetti F, Maggi G, Lopiano L, et al. Open versus hidden medical treatments: The patient's knowledge about a therapy affects the therapy outcome. *Prevention & Treatment.* 2003;6(1):1a.

24. Tondorf T, Kaufmann LK, Degel A, et al. Employing open/hidden administration in psychotherapy research: A randomized-controlled trial of expressive writing. *PLoS ONE.* 2017;12(11):e0187400.

25. Howe LC, Goyer JP, Crum AJ. Harnessing the placebo effect: Exploring the influence of physician characteristics on placebo response. *Health Psychology.* 2017;36(11):1074.

26. Howe LC, Leibowitz KA, Perry MA, et al. Changing patient mindsets about non-life-threatening symptoms during oral immunotherapy: A randomized clinical trial. *Journal of Allergy and Clinical Immunology: In Practice.* 2019 May-Jun;7(5):1550–1559. doi:10.1016/j.jaip.2019.01.022.

27. Howe LC, Leibowitz KA, Crum AJ. When your doctor "gets it" and "gets you": The critical role of competence and warmth in the patient-provider interaction. *Frontiers in Psychiatry*. 2019;10:475.

28. Colloca L, Barsky AJ. Placebo and nocebo effects. *New England Journal of Medicine*. 2020;382(6):554–561.

29. Benedetti F, Lanotte M, Lopiano L, Colloca L. When words are painful: Unraveling the mechanisms of the nocebo effect. *Neuroscience*. 2007;147(2):260–271.

30. Colloca L, Benedetti F. Nocebo hyperalgesia: how anxiety is turned into pain. *Current Opinion in Anesthesiology*. 2007;20(5):435–439.

31. Silvestri A, Galetta P, Cerquetani E, et al. Report of erectile dysfunction after therapy with beta-blockers is related to patient knowledge of side effects and is reversed by placebo. *European Heart Journal*. 2003;24(21):1928–1932.

32. Blease C, DesRoches CM. Open notes in patient care: Confining deceptive placebos to the past? *Journal of Medical Ethics*. 2021Aug;48(8):572–574. doi:10.1136/medethics-2021-107746.

33. Blease CR, Delbanco T, Torous J, et al. Sharing clinical notes, and placebo and nocebo effects: Can documentation affect patient health? *Journal of Health Psychology*. 2022;27(1):135–146.

34. Friesen P, Blease C. Placebo effects and racial and ethnic health disparities: An unjust and underexplored connection. *Journal of Medical Ethics*. 2018;44(11):774–781.

35. Yetman HE, Cox N, Adler SR, Hall KT, Stone VE. What do placebo and nocebo effects have to do with health equity? The hidden toll of nocebo effects on racial and ethnic minority patients in clinical care. *Frontiers in Psychology*. 2021 Dec23;12:788230. doi:10.3389/fpsyg.2021.788230.

36. Okusogu C, Wang Y, Akintola T, et al. Placebo hypoalgesia: Racial differences. *Pain*. 2020;161(8):1872.

37. Letzen JE, Dildine TC, Mun CJ, Colloca L, Bruehl S, Campbell CM. Ethnic differences in experimental pain responses following a paired verbal suggestion with saline infusion: A quasiexperimental study. *Annals of Behavioral Medicine*. 2021;55(1):55–64.

38. FitzGerald C, Hurst S. Implicit bias in healthcare professionals: A systematic review. *BMC Medical Ethics*. 2017;18(1):19.

39. Blease C, Salmi L, Rexhepi H, Hägglund M, DesRoches CM. Patients, clinicians and open notes: Information blocking as a case of epistemic injustice. *Journal of Medical Ethics*. 2021 May 14;48(10):785–793. doi:10.1136/medethics-2021-107275.

40. Rexhepi H, Ahlfeldt RM, Cajander A, Huvila I. Cancer patients' attitudes and experiences of online access to their electronic medical records: A qualitative study. *Health Informatics Journal*. 2018;24(2):115–124.

41. Gerard M, Chimowitz H, Fossa A, Bourgeois F, Fernandez L, Bell SK. The importance of visit notes on patient portals for engaging less educated or nonwhite patients: Survey study. *Journal of Medical Internet Research*. 2018;20(5):e191. doi:10.2196/jmir.9196.

42. Blease C, Fernandez L, Bell SK, Delbanco T, DesRoches C. Empowering patients and reducing inequities: Is there potential in sharing clinical notes? *BMJ Quality & Safety*. 2020;29(10):1–2.

43. Bell SK, Folcarelli P, Fossa A, et al. Tackling ambulatory safety risks through patient engagement: What 10,000 patients and families say about safety-related knowledge, behaviors, and attitudes after reading visit notes. *Journal of Patient Safety*. 2021 Dec1;17(8):e791–e799. doi:10.1097/PTS.0000000000000494.

44. Fernandez A, Schillinger D, Warton EM, et al. Language barriers, physician-patient language concordance, and glycemic control among insured Latinos with diabetes: The Diabetes Study of Northern California (DISTANCE). *Journal of General Internal Medicine*. 2011;26(2):170–176.

45. Beach MC, Saha S, Park J, et al. Testimonial injustice: Linguistic bias in the medical records of black patients and women. *Journal of General Internal Medicine*. 2021;36(6):1708–1714.

46. Sun M, Oliwa T, Peek ME, Tung EL. Negative patient descriptors: Documenting racial bias in the electronic health record. *Health Affairs*. 2022 Feb;41(2):203–211. doi:10.1377/hlthaff.2021.01423.

47. Himmelstein G, Bates D, Zhou L. Examination of stigmatizing language in the electronic health record. *JAMA Network Open*. 2022;5(1):e2144967–e2144967.

48. Rodriguez JA, Lipsitz SR, Lyles CR, Samal L. Association between patient portal use and broadband access: A national evaluation. *Journal of General Internal Medicine*. 2020 Dec;35(12):3719–3720. doi:10.1007/s11606-020-05633-4.

49. Ancker JS, Barrón Y, Rockoff ML, et al. Use of an electronic patient portal among disadvantaged populations. *Journal of General Internal Medicine*. 2011;26(10):1117–1123.

6.3
The rise of digital health and digital medicine

How digital technologies will change or affect placebo and nocebo effects

Ellenor Brown, Susan Persky, Patricia D. Franklin, Chamindi Seneviratne, Jason Noel, and Luana Colloca

Introduction

The global COVID-19 pandemic limited or prevented traditional in-person interactions with healthcare providers, placing greater emphasis on remote solutions. This crisis came in the midst of the already increasing development of digital health technologies that have transformed healthcare and the patient-provider relationship. The new digitally enhanced landscape of healthcare will undoubtedly present new considerations for patient care, including processes related to placebo effects. Placebo effects are positive outcomes that are attributable to the psychosocial aspects of care rather than the direct action of a medication or treatment.[1] When outcomes are negative, these are called nocebo effects.[2–4]

Placebo effects are multifactorial and potent influences on patient outcomes. These effects have been considered in a multitude of contexts, although considerations have typically centered on traditional clinical models. As digital therapeutics grew rapidly in development and adoption, some consideration has been given to these effects in digital healthcare. However, in comparison to the massive proliferation of digital health technologies, the literature is sparse. Therefore, there is a growing need to understand, identify, and harness placebo effects in the digital health space as these technologies become an ever-present part of our daily living.

Applying existing knowledge to digital contexts

Placebo and nocebo effects arise from various sources along the health and wellness continuum. Even before patients seek treatment, their thoughts, emotions, personal or observed experiences, exposure to media messaging, disease experience, and related expectations are key components in determining clinical outcomes and patient satisfaction.[5] Traditional placebo research has identified many features of the patient experience that come into play, such as the type and appearance of the treatment setting (e.g., home vs hospital, physical layout), characteristics of the treatment itself (e.g., pill color and taste, perceived cost), provider perceptions and attitudes toward the treatment and patient, and the quality of the patient-provider relationship (e.g., rapport, empathy, trust).[5-7] This last feature—the patient-provider relationship—has proven to be particularly important in traditional settings. Verbal and nonverbal cues from providers, expressing focused attention, compassion, empathy, positivity, and hope, for example, have been shown to enhance patient outcomes and minimize the occurrence of adverse side effects.[5,7-9] Providing positive expectations for the intervention or potential side effects of the intervention[10,11] can reduce incidence and severity of side effects or increase tolerance.[12,13] Unfortunately, the inverse is also true: negative framing can induce, exacerbate, or increase incidence of negative or nocebo effects.[14]

In the movement toward digital therapeutics, many of these same principles apply, but need to be reexamined in their new contexts. Several facets of digital medicine such as telemedicine and patient monitoring technologies will likely retain elements of the patient-provider interaction and relationship. However, communication channels will not look the same (e.g., reduced nonverbal cues in telemedicine, asynchronous communication related to monitoring data). As such, it will be necessary to examine how our understanding and expectations for placebo and nocebo effects may also need to change.

Digital health technologies

The US Food and Drug Administration identifies the following categories within the scope of digital health: (1) mobile health, (2) health information technology, (3) wearable devices, (4) telehealth and telemedicine, and (5) personalized medicine.[15] This encompasses applications from online systems that support real-time interaction between patient and provider, to online portals, digital medication reminders, and mindfulness apps, to virtual reality-based exposure therapy to treat phobias, to remote cardiac and glucose monitors and to activity trackers. Examples of digital health technologies are listed in Box 6.3.1.

Reasons for the broad and rapid adoption of digital health and healthcare tools relate to the wide variety of benefits they can provide as an adjunct or replacement for traditional healthcare approaches. For example, digital health tools can provide increased access to healthcare providers and continuity of care, increased opportunities for medical data collection in daily living environments with health data feedback provided to the patient, and opportunities to provide enhanced experiences such as gamification and personalization. Such benefits must be weighed against significant risks, such as breach of confidentiality and disparity in access across populations.

Box 6.3.1 Digital health applications (selected list)

Smartphone Apps
Medication adherence reminders
Relaxation training
Biometric trackers, e.g., for blood glucose, menstrual cycles

Informatics
Electronic Medical Records
Online triage and appointment booking
Online health promotion and information resources

Wearables
Fitness/activity trackers
Continuous glucose monitoring sensors
Ambulatory cardiac monitors

Telehealth
Videoconferencing
Remote monitoring
Remote medication dispensing

Healthcare Mixed Reality
Controlled virtual environments
Teleoperated surgical procedures
Expert and robot training

It is not possible to generalize as to the efficacy and effectiveness of digital therapeutics; there are many examples of digital approaches that have been found to be as effective, more effective, or less effective than their analog counterparts. Design features of a given digital approach or given study that at first might seem minor, upon further study can prove to be very influential. As an example, consider the complexity of factors influencing the effectiveness of telemedicine applications for depression treatment. Research has compared computerized cognitive behavioral therapy (cCBT) to standard care. cCBT as an adjunct to standard care and supplemented by weekly phone calls from, in this case, trained technical support staff,[16,17] as well as the feasibility of unguided stand-alone cCBT in the management of mild to moderate depressive symptoms.[18] Although cognitive behavioral therapy (CBT) is a proven treatment for depression and developer-led cCBT studies have reported improved outcomes relative to standard care, the results of this early independent study of cCBT showed no significant differences from usual care. In this case, it was argued that participants lacked external sources of clinical support that are often present but undervalued in similar studies, which negatively affected outcomes. In contrast, studies conducted under supervision by healthcare providers or trained therapists as support staff demonstrate moderate effect sizes comparable to in-person therapy,[19] and increasing levels of support produce better outcomes.[20] Another example is the difficulty with engagement and retention that has plagued studies of digital mental health applications in the past. These issues compromise reliability and interpretation of study data and highlight potential challenges for widespread, long-term use.[16] Participants cite issues such as difficulty with logging in regularly, lack of clinical support, feelings of isolation and loneliness, and lack of accountability.[16,17] These and other studies highlight the complex relationship between patient engagement, treatment effectiveness, and the many venues for potential placebo effects. Digital therapeutics cannot be considered wholly outside of the interpersonal social context simply because they are technologically mediated.

Placebo and nocebo considerations in digital medicine

Given the importance of placebo and nocebo effects for digital health technologies, it is remarkable that there is a dearth of articles that explicitly address the topic. In translating knowledge from traditional interventions to fit a new situation, we can consider possible differential placebo and nocebo effects in light of several key differences between traditional and digital health interventions, and in terms of common beliefs about the tech-based platforms that underlie them.

The digital placebo effect

Torous and Firth comment on placebo effects of mobile apps for mental health, highlighting several considerations for "the digital placebo effect."[21] This effect hinges on beliefs and emotions about the relevant technology itself, such as perceived changes in the strength of technologically mediated patient-provider interactions, design features of the technology, and information provided to patients.[21] Digital technologies such as push-notifications, dynamic personalization, and data feedback loops, by their nature, readily integrate features not often seen in traditional interventions, any of which may contribute to placebo effects. A patient's existing emotions, expectations, and beliefs about the technology will likely influence patient engagement and may influence expectancies as well. For example, on the positive side, the phenomenon of "phone separation," or anxiety induced by inability to attend to one's phone[22] could improve the effectiveness of phone notifications as reminders or means to convey encouragement. Similarly, the feeling that an intervention is "high tech" could engender positive expectations about its efficacy.[23] On the other hand, digital platforms could infuse the patient's daily life with an additional source of anxiety and disruption. Attending to one's health data on a regular basis can provide continual reminders of symptoms or the need to monitor for poor health or side effects, which has been associated with possible nocebo effects in previous work.[24] Distrust or discomfort with technologies or digital surveillance, on the other hand, could color patients' feelings about the interventions they support, and perhaps even the healthcare providers involved in such interventions. Such associations have implications for compliance or adherence, clinical outcomes, and reporting of side effects, and are broadly applicable across the spectrum of digital health technology.[21] For digital therapeutics, treatment effects are hard to disentangle from placebo effects based solely on perceptions of the technology.

Consistent with the concept of a placebo, applications that seemingly provide no therapeutic intervention may still initiate a chain of therapeutic outcomes simply because of their ubiquity in daily life. Kauer et al. evaluated the use of smartphone apps for self-monitoring in early-stage depression in teenagers.[25] One arm of the study involved regular reporting of mood, stress, and daily activities. The other was an "attention comparison" protocol, recording only daily activities. Both arms increased emotional self-awareness and decreased depression scores through simple increases in self-awareness and, thus, led to improved outcomes.[21]

Digital interpersonal interaction

The traditional in-person consultation provides a varied and complex set of stimuli, some of which are altered or absent in a telemedicine context. Unsurprisingly, studies have demonstrated that some treatments that are effective in traditional settings are less so in digital form. For example, rallying social support from family and friends is a proven strategy for smoking cessation programs but was ineffective in a smoking cessation app where social support was provided via text, email, or social media.[26]

Benedetti et al.[5] describe several nonverbal elements of communication and therapeutic experience that have implications for the placebo effect. Among these, facial expressions, eye contact, and tactile stimulus are especially likely to be unavailable in the telemedical context. Facial expressions and gaze direction may be distorted by poor video connectivity, lower fidelity if avatars are used, or may be absent altogether. The importance of these cues may explain correlations between patient satisfaction and use of video during remote consultations.[27] Tactile stimulus within the healthcare context is not only the physical tasks of palpation, manipulation, and examination of the patient's body. It is also part of nonverbal communication, where touch is a means to convey emotion and build connection.[28] Feelings of trust, compassion, kindness, and confidence could be conveyed through a handshake or in the placement of the doctor's hand on the patient's body. The loss of these communication channels, and related benefits of placebo effect, could reduce effectiveness of digital technologies. Interestingly, however, it is reported that in many in-person clinical interactions, physicians often spend much of the visit looking at their computer while taking notes in the office.[29] Researchers have observed that when this factor is considered, physicians may be perceived to spend much more time looking at the patient during telemedicine consultations, either because the computer contains the camera that transmits to the patient, or because physicians view a phone or other mediating device more often because of increased attentional needs or to gain more information in the remote context.[30] This increased perception of attention, eye contact, and visibility of facial expressions may have, in turn, improved patient satisfaction despite the lack of verbal cues. In some ways, then, these more advanced digital interventions can improve upon the communication problems introduced by electronic medical records and other digital innovations of the past.

In addition, some of the challenges of digital interaction for the patient-provider interaction may be mitigated by having an existing relationship with the provider with whom a patient later engages through telemedicine.[27] When a digital tool replaces or supplements the healthcare provider's role, emotions, expectations, and trust usually invested in the provider may instead be applied to the technology and social interactions mediated by the technology.[31] Such possibilities may further reduce deficits of interpersonal interaction introduced by digital mediation.

Despite what may be lost through use of digital technology, research has demonstrated that providers are able to perform many critical tasks and provide adequate care across various uses and patient populations.[32-34] Patients, moreover, report high satisfaction with remote sessions and the convenience they offer.[35] On the provider end, several studies have highlighted a low provider satisfaction and expectations for telemedicine, or a disconnect in satisfaction between patient and provider.[36,37] Beyond the inability of providers to use all their senses for clinical observation, an aspect of digital health is the additional work required to integrate, process, and form conclusions from new data sources. Certainly, these provider attitudes and emotional states can have important implications for their own treatment expectations, which feed into placebo effects that stem from interaction.

Digital health monitoring

When digital monitoring data are accessible by the patient, such data affect patients' understanding of their health, and can further influence expectancies of how an intervention may affect health outcomes in the future.[38] Studies have shown that patients who believe that self-monitoring provides better knowledge about their bodies feel more in control of their health. When data are within acceptable ranges, patients feel more secure, reassured, and encouraged.[39,40] However, data that suggest poor health or conflicts with patients' own subjective assessment of their health can be upsetting, provoking fear, anxiety, shame, frustration, and helplessness.[39,40] While some level of discomfort may be motivational, regular exposure could be demoralizing, causing treatment nonadherence and avoidance. Similarly, patients who become too attached to the data and feel empowered by the technology may begin to avoid healthcare providers, as they perceive less need for regular contact.

These perceptions are greatly influenced by the choices made in developing data tools and dashboards. For example, whether a patient's biomarker data are compared to the general public, versus patients with similar health conditions, patients of similar age, and so-on, provides the context used to understand the self and one's progress.[41] In other ways, data that feel objective may leave patients less room to apply an experiential lens to understand their day-to-day health and, thus, less likelihood for placebo effects. For example, if patients can see the hills and valleys of their blood pressure readings over time, they may be less likely to take comfort in the self-perception that it is stable or on a downward trajectory.

Again, individual differences in patients' beliefs and attitudes can influence response to monitoring data and their influence on placebo and nocebo. Monitoring requires more presence of health and illness in daily life, as noted above.[31] Development of routines and expertise to assess some physiological markers may be perceived as empowerment or as obligation.[31] Oudshoorn and colleagues reported that some heart patients resisted monitoring technologies because they resented the constant reminders of illness, the tasks of monitoring, and turning their homes into clinics.[42] Patients may also feel that they are losing their personal autonomy to suit the needs of self-care healthcare. Others may feel that digital therapeutics provide independence, safety, and security.

Addressing placebo effects in trials of digital therapeutics

The controls used in trials of digital therapeutics are often similar or the same as those for traditional ones. However, alternative or adjunctive approaches have been developed to address new issues that arise with digital technology. Looking at the body of work on smartphone app-based interventions, one can see the variety of approaches that researchers have taken to address placebo and nocebo effects. Familiar approaches, common in trials of digital therapeutics, include the use of attention placebos (i.e., control conditions in which the time and attention received by the intervention group is mimicked), treatment as usual, waiting list arms, and active comparators.[43,44] An approach that may be particularly helpful in digital settings is use of psychological placebo (i.e., control conditions where an inactive element is perceived as active by participants). For example, Chittaro and colleagues[45] compared a biofeedback-based game for relaxation training with sham biofeedback generated during a prior game session. As such, the purported active element was isolated in study design.

Other approaches adapted from traditional research compare effects of the focal digital media with another, usually less intensive, media source or one that addresses fewer communication channels. For example, one could compare the focal smartphone-based app with an audio-only application that has similar look and functionality. Placebo apps as controls fits into this condition wherein participants are assigned the active app versus one not designed to treat the focal conditions.[43,46,47] Another example is the use of sham virtual reality controls in which the intervention is compared to a 2-D video viewed in the same type of headset. This approach aims to control potential expectancy effects associated with the virtual reality hardware.[48] To effectively use a sham or inactive comparison, however, it is important to be aware of the effects of the "placebo app." For example, Flett and colleagues[46] compared two mental health apps to an inactive control—the notetaking app Evernote. The Evernote group was designed to account for digital placebo and treatment expectancies. Participants were asked to record memories for the week prior, termed *organizational reminiscing*. Participants in the control group reported poorer mental health outcomes with more frequent use. It was posited that excessive "organizational reminiscing" caused rumination or "an awareness of unmet goals," translating into negative emotion. Essentially, the more people use an ineffective tool, the worse they feel. These possibilities cannot be disentangled in study design, but it appears that the content of the inactive control actually functioned as nocebo and thus created validity issues for the trial.

Digital applications are also frequently compared with print media, static information provision, and other related controls that provide elements of an app's content without the digital elements (e.g., interactive features). For example, Wegner and colleagues[49] compared internet-delivered CBT for bulimia nervosa to a conventional self-help manual based in the same therapy approach. These approaches focus more on the added value of the digital format and capabilities as opposed to looking for effects over and above these features. In some ways, this approach is the opposite of those that aim to hold constant influence of the digital device. This design may become less popular as digital interfaces continue to supplant traditional ones in many aspects of daily life. However, the fact that both digital sham controls and nondigital active controls are valid, useful comparators in clinical trials underscores the ultimate fact that the elements present in controls should depend upon the purported mechanism of action for the digital application and the potential claims that one wishes to make based on study results.

Certainly, other evaluation approaches beyond the traditional randomized clinical trial can be useful in the context of digital interventions. For example, Hrynyschyn and colleagues[50] reviewed alternative trial designs and found a few examples of factorial designs, sequential multiple assignment randomized trials, and other "alternative" approaches. These designs can be a good fit given the complexity and flexibility of digital health interventions, as well as address potential sources of placebo and nocebo effects to the extent that features that underlie these effects are represented across the multiple comparator groups. Such alternative approaches may become increasingly popular as the complexity and scope of digital interventions continues to grow.

Challenges and future directions

As noted in the previous section, the evolution of digital therapeutics is constant, and the pace of development is quick. The traditional randomized control trial may not keep pace with ever-increasing complexity, flexibility, responsiveness, and personalization made possible by digital intervention platforms. In recent years, such applications have begun to integrate more just-in-time elements, experienced by only some users under particular situations, artificial intelligence aspects that personalize interventions to individuals, machine learning algorithms to process and provide user health data, and virtual reality settings for interventions that can take users out of their own reality. The ability to identify the scope of the intervention that is experienced, including content exposures, dose, and so-on, becomes a moving target. In conjunction, it will likely become more difficult to design control conditions that match or approximate all active features of digital interventions such that they can be used broadly across participants. In step with this, the amount of data underpinning many digital interventions, as well as the data collected by the intervention, has become far larger than ever before. New design, documentation, and evaluation approaches have begun to evolve, relying on similar technologies (e.g., flexible algorithms, Artificial Intelligence, and machine learning) to power them.[51,52] As these tools emerge, they create new potential for placebo and nocebo effects that should be considered. For some, an AI-powered health intervention may feel particularly promising while others may approach with trepidation.[23] New technology also brings new questions. For example, can an AI internalize and recapitulate treatment expectancies? These are the types of questions we will have to consider as technology advances.

Conclusions

The scope of digital therapeutics is wide, and the potential variations in influence of placebo effects is understudied. Evaluations tend to compare these interventions to usual treatment, waitlist, and sometimes no comparator at all rather than including control conditions that can squarely assess and address placebo and nocebo effects. As such, much more work is needed to understand these potential sources of bias in digital medicine. As technology grows, these challenges will grow. There is, therefore, a pressing need to develop strategies to evaluate and address placebo and nocebo effects in trials of the future, as well as finding ways to harness them for therapeutic benefit as part of the new wave of sprawling, complex, adaptive digital therapeutics.

References

1. Colloca L, Benedetti F. Placebos and painkillers: Is mind as real as matter. *Nature Reviews Neuroscience*. 2005;6(7):545–552.
2. Colloca L. Tell me the truth and I will not be harmed: Informed consents and nocebo effects. *American Journal of Bioethics*. 2017;17(6):46–48.
3. Colloca L, Barsky AJ. Placebo and nocebo effects. *New England Journal of Medicine*. 2020;382(6):554–561.
4. Klinger R, Blasini M, Schmitz J, Colloca L. Nocebo effects in clinical studies: Hints for pain therapy. *Pain Reports*. 2017 Mar-Apr;2(2):e586. doi:10.1097/PR9.0000000000000586.
5. Benedetti F. Placebo and the new physiology of the doctor-patient relationship. *Physiological Reviews*. 2013;93(3):1207–1246.
6. Di Blasi Z, Harkness E, Ernst E, Georgiou A, Kleijnen J. Influence of context effects on health outcomes: A systematic review. *Lancet*. 2001;357(9258):757–762.
7. Chavarria V, Vian J, Pereira C, et al. The placebo and nocebo phenomena: Their clinical management and impact on treatment outcomes. *Clinical Therapeutics*. 2017;39(3):477–486.
8. Del Canale S, Louis DZ, Maio V, et al. The relationship between physician empathy and disease complications: An empirical study of primary care physicians and their diabetic patients in Parma, Italy. *Academic Medicine*. 2012;87(9):1243–1249.
9. Pollo A, Amanzio M, Arslanian A, Casadio C, Maggi G, Benedetti F. Response expectancies in placebo analgesia and their clinical relevance. *Pain Reports*. 2001;93(1):77–84.
10. Benedetti F. How the doctor's words affect the patient's brain. *Evaluation & the Health Professions*. 2002;25(4):369–386.
11. Benedetti F. Mechanisms of placebo and placebo-related effects across diseases and treatment. *Annual Review of Pharmacology and Toxicology*. 2008;48:33–60.
12. O'Connor AM, Pennie RA, Dales RE. Framing effects on expectations, decisions, and side effects experienced: The case of influenza immunization. *Journal of Clinical Epidemiology*. 1996;49(11):1271–1276.
13. Glare P, Fridman I, Ashton-James CE. Choose your words wisely: The impact of message framing on patients' responses to treatment advice. *International Review of Neurobiology*. 2018;139:159–190.

14. Colloca L, Sigaudo M, Benedetti F. The role of learning in nocebo and placebo effects. *Pain.* 2008;136(1): 211–218.

15. US Food and Drug Administration. *What Is Digital Health.* 2020. Accessed September 9, 2022.   https://www.fda.gov/medical-devices/digital-health-center-excellence/what-digital-health

16. Gilbody S, Littlewood E, Hewitt C, et al. Computerised cognitive behaviour therapy (ccbt) as treatment for depression in primary care (Reeact Trial): Large scale pragmatic randomised controlled trial. *British Medical Journal.* 2015;351:h5627.

17. Knowles SE, Lovell K, Bower P, Gilbody S, Littlewood E, Lester H. Patient experience of computerised therapy for depression in primary care. *BMJ Open.* 2015;5(11):e008581.

18. Stearns-Yoder KA, Ryan AT, Smith AA, Forster JE, Barnes SM, Brenner LA. Computerized cognitive behavioral therapy intervention for depression among veterans: acceptability and feasibility study. *JMIR Formative Research.* 2022 Apr 25;6(4):e31835. doi:10.2196/31835.

19. Andersson G, Cuijpers P, Carlbring P, Riper H, Hedman E. Guided internet-based vs. face-to-face cognitive behavior therapy for psychiatric and somatic disorders: A systematic review and meta-analysis. *World Psychiatry.* 2014;13(3):288–295.

20. Johansson R, Andersson G. Internet-based psychological treatments for depression. *Expert Review of Neurotherapeutics.* 2012;12(7):861–870.

21. Torous J, Firth J. The digital placebo effect: Mobile mental health meets clinical psychiatry. *Lancet Psychiatry.* 2016;3(2):100–102.

22. Clayton RB, Leshner G, Almond A. The extended Iself: The impact of Iphone separation on cognition, emotion, and physiology. *Journal of Computer-Mediated Communication.* 2015;20(2):119–135.

23. Gao S, He L, Chen Y, et al. Public perception of artificial intelligence in medical care: Content analysis of social media. *Journal of Medical Internet Research.* 2020;22(7):e16649.

24. Faurholt-Jepsen M, Frost M, Ritz C, et al. Daily electronic self-monitoring in bipolar disorder using smartphone—the MONARCA I Trial: A randomized, placebo-controlled, single-blind, parallel group trial. *Psychological Medicine.* 2015;45(13):2691–2704.

25. Kauer SD, Reid SC, Crooke AHD, et al. Self-monitoring using mobile phones in the early stages of adolescent depression: Randomized controlled trial. *Journal of Medical Internet Research.* 2012;14(3):e1858.

26. Heffner JL, Vilardaga R, Mercer LD, Kientz JA, Bricker JB. Feature-level analysis of a novel smartphone application for smoking cessation. *American Journal of Drug and Alcohol Abuse.* 2015;41(1):68–73.

27. Omari AM, Antytonacci CL, Zaifman J, et al. Patient satisfaction with orthopedic telemedicine health visits during the Covid-19 pandemic. *Telemedicine Journal and E-Health.* 2022 Jun;28(6):806–814. doi:10.1089/tmj.2021.0170.

28. Kelly M, Svrcek C, King N, Scherpbier A, Dornan T. Embodying empathy: A phenomenological study of physician touch. *Medical Education.* 2020 May;54(5):400–407. doi:10.1111/medu.14040.

29. Overhage JM, McCallie D Jr. Physician time spent using the electronic health record during outpatient encounters: A descriptive Study. *Annals of Internal Medicine.* 2020 Feb 4;172(3):169–174. doi:10.7326/M18-3684. Erratum in: *Annals of Internal Medicine.* 2020 Oct 6;173(7):596.

30. Liu X, Sawada Y, Takizawa T, et al. Doctor-patient communication: A comparison between telemedicine consultation and face-to-face consultation. *Internal Medicine.* 2007;46(5):227–232.

31. Lupton D. The digitally engaged patient: Self-monitoring and self-care in the digital health era. *Social Theory & Health.* 2013;11(3):256–270.

32. Morland LA, Mackintosh MA, Rosen CS, et al. Telemedicine versus in-person delivery of cognitive processing therapy for women with posttraumatic stress disorder: A randomized noninferiority trial. *Depression and Anxiety*. 2015;32(11):811–820.

33. Timpel P, Oswald S, Schwarz PEH, Harst L. Mapping the evidence on the effectiveness of telemedicine interventions in diabetes, dyslipidemia, and hypertension: An umbrella review of systematic reviews and meta-analyses. *Journal of Medical Internet Research*. 2020;22(3):e16791.

34. Hormaza-Jaramillo A, Arredondo A, Forero E, et al. Effectiveness of telemedicine compared with standard care for patients with rheumatic diseases: A systematic review. *Telemedicine Journal and e-Health*. 2022;28(12):1852–1860. doi:10.1089/tmj.2022.0098

35. Wehrle CJ, Lee SW, Devarakonda AK, Arora TK. Patient and physician attitudes toward telemedicine in cancer clinics following the COVID-19 pandemic. *JCO Clinical Cancer Informatics*. 2021 Apr;5:394–400. doi:10.1200/CCI.20.00183.

36. Buvik A, Bugge E, Knutsen G, Småbrekke A, Wilsgaard T. Quality of care for remote orthopaedic consultations using telemedicine: A randomised controlled trial. *BMC Health Services Research*. 2016;16(1):1–11.

37. Wongworawat MD, Capistrant G, Stephenson JM. The opportunity awaits to lead orthopaedic telehealth innovation: AOA critical issues. *JBJS*. 2017;99(17):e93.

38. Choudhury A, Asan O. Impact of using wearable devices on psychological distress: Analysis of the Health Information National Trends survey. *International Journal of Medical Informatics*. 2021;156:104612.

39. Hortensius J, Kars MC, Wierenga WS, Kleefstra N, Bilo HJ, Van Der Bijl JJ. Perspectives of patients with type 1 or insulin-treated type 2 diabetes on self-monitoring of blood glucose: A qualitative study. *BMC Public Health*. 2012;12(1):1–11.

40. Huniche L, Dinesen B, Nielsen C, Grann O, Toft E. Patients' use of self-monitored readings for managing everyday life with COPD: A qualitative study. *Telemedicine and e-Health*. 2013;19(5):396–402.

41. Arigo D, Brown MM, Pasko K, Suls J. Social comparison features in physical activity promotion apps: Scoping meta-review. *Journal of Medical Internet Research*. 2020;22(3):e15642.

42. Oudshoorn N. Resistance and boundary work. In: Telecare Technologies and the Transformation of Healthcare. 2011; Springer: 68–88.

43. Torous J, Lipschitz J, Ng M, Firth J. Dropout rates in clinical trials of smartphone apps for depressive symptoms: A systematic review and meta-analysis. *Journal of Affective Disorders*. 2020;263:413–419.

44. Thabrew H, Stasiak K, Hetrick SE Wong, S, Huss JH, Merry SN. E-health interventions for anxiety and depression in children and adolescents with long-term physical conditions. *Cochrane Database of Systematic Reviews*. 2018 Aug 15;8(8):CD012489. doi:10.1002/14651858.CD012489.pub2.

45. Chittaro L, Sioni R. Affective computing vs. affective placebo: Study of a biofeedback-controlled game for relaxation training. *International Journal of Human-Computer Studies*. 2014;72(9):663–673.

46. Flett JA, Hayne H, Riordan BC, Thompson LM, Conner TS. Mobile mindfulness meditation: A randomised controlled trial of the effect of two popular apps on mental health. *Mindfulness*. 2019;10(5):863–876.

47. Arean PA, Hallgren KA, Jordan JT, et al. The use and effectiveness of mobile apps for depression: Results from a fully remote clinical trial. *Journal of Medical Internet Research*. 2016;18(12):e6482.

48. Garcia LM, Birckhead BJ, Krishnamurthy P, et al. An 8-week self-administered at-home behavioral skills-based virtual reality program for chronic low back pain: Double-blind, randomized, placebo-controlled trial conducted during Covid-19. *Journal of Medical Internet Research*. 2021;23(2):e26292.

49. Wagner G, Penelo E, Nobis G, et al. Predictors for good therapeutic outcome and drop-out in technology assisted guided self-help in the treatment of bulimia nervosa and bulimia like phenotype. *European Eating Disorders Review*. 2015;23(2):163–169.

50. Hrynyschyn R, Prediger C, Stock C, Helmer SM. Evaluation methods applied to digital health interventions: What is being used beyond randomised controlled trials? A scoping review. *International Journal of Environmental Research and Public Health*. 2022;19(9):5221.

51. Guo C, Ashrafian H, Ghafur S, Fontana G, Gardner C, Prime M. Challenges for the evaluation of digital health solutions-A call for innovative evidence generation approaches. *NPJ Digit Medicine*. 2020 Aug 27;3:110. doi:10.1038/s41746-020-00314-2.

52. Cruz Rivera S, Liu X, Chan AW, et al. Guidelines for clinical trial protocols for interventions involving artificial intelligence: The SPIRIT-AI extension. *Lancet Digital Health*. 2020;2(10):e549–e560.

6.4

A glimpse of the multiple applications of virtual reality

Analgesia, embodiment and rehabilitation, interactive education, and communication

Yang Wang, Rachel Massalee, Kris Beebe, William Latham, Lance Putnam, Janine Westendorp, Andrea Evers, Marco Testa, Denise Silber, Zina Trost, Giancarlo Colloca, and Luana Colloca

Introduction

Virtual reality (VR) is an artificial environment that aims to create an experience of presence and immersion via 360-degree sight, sound, and vibration stimuli. When head-mounted display (HMD) and head-tracking systems were first introduced around the 1960s, VR was primarily used in the military to view hazardous conditions remotely.[1,2] In recent years, VR has reached a level of precision and affordability such that it can be considered a reliable and accessible tool in the clinical field.[3] During the past few decades, VR technologies have been increasingly incorporated into clinical, empirical, and educational approaches, especially serving as a potential adjuvant in treating clinical acute pain. However, much needs to be understood on the mechanisms, efficacy, and effectiveness of VR in medicine.

As of May 1, 2022, 1,395 VR-based (completed and ongoing) trials conducted in the United States have been registered to ClinicalTrials.gov, reflecting 739 conditions. Of these, 322 trial listings included the word *pain*; 224 included the word *rehabilitation*; 193 included the term *anxiety*; 37 included the term *depression*; and 31 included the term *schizophrenia*. Colloca and colleagues recently published a systematic review of the literature for VR and experimental, acute, and chronic pain,[4] in which they found 288 VR articles and identified 58 data-based articles[4] directly investigating the relationship between VR and pain in both healthy and pain-afflicted populations, using objective and subjective measures of pain as the primary outcomes

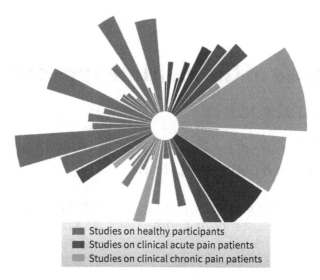

Studies on healthy participants
Studies on clinical acute pain patients
Studies on clinical chronic pain patients

Figure 6.4.1 Studies to identify the role of VR in pain reduction.
During the past few decades, studies have been conducted to identify the role of VR in pain reduction, with most of the research studying healthy participants (marked in green) and acute clinical pain (marked in blue). Fewer studies have focused on VR-related analgesia in chronic pain population (marked in yellow). The larger area indicates the larger sample size of the study.

(Figure 6.4.1). The authors identified three significant gaps in knowledge regarding the action mechanisms of VR-induced pain reduction, particularly in chronic pain. First, they found a general lack of heuristic models, with only a few exceptions[4–6] for understanding the mechanisms underlying VR-induced pain reduction.[4] Second, the majority of studies have been conducted for acute pain (experimental and clinical acute pain), therefore limiting the translatability of this knowledge to chronic pain populations. Third, they identified a lack of rigor in methodological aspects, such as using appropriate controls for evaluating VR efficacy (i.e., sham VR, control VR, versus no-intervention).

Theories related to virtual reality

Several theories have proposed how VR may alleviate symptoms in various conditions, such as posttraumatic stress disorders[7–10] and pain.[11–14] Exposure to immersive VR contexts and distraction attributes symptom improvement to the competing engagement of pathways for memory or emotions that detract from those devoted to stress and pain signaling and allow for improved stress and pain control.[15,16] Specifically, if attention is allocated to the VR environment, less attention could be available for pain processing, resulting in reduced pain perception.[17]

Trost and colleagues recently advanced a heuristic model of understanding VR effects on pain, suggesting four central dimensions of VR as core parameters that can contribute to benefits such as pain reduction.[18] These four central dimensions of VR included presence, immersion, interactivity, and embodiment. *Presence* refers to the state of *being* in one environment (i.e., the extent to which individuals feel they are *part of the* virtual world ("you are there")). Unlike Presence, the immersion dimension emphasizes the subjective experience of being *absorbed* or *caught-up* in one environment. *Immersiveness* has also been used to characterize the 2D versus 360-degree nature of VR visual displays. Interactivity refers to how people can *interact* with the VR environment via body or eye movements tracked through sensors implemented in the HMD. *Embodiment* is the *sense of having the body of oneself* in the VR environment. Although embodiment can be facilitated via input to several senses (e.g., auditory, kinesthetic), thus far, embodiment has primarily relied on the colocation of the physical and virtual body (i.e., a "virtual" body that mimics the same gesture following an individual's movement). Embodiment manipulations can prompt the brain to consider the "virtual" body as part of the real body; thus, embodiment has been applied to interventions for phantom limb pain,[19] complex regional pain syndrome,[20] and spinal cord injury pain and rehabilitation,[21,22] which can require visual "illusory" input of normal function, akin to mirror therapy. In the attempt to apply VR technologies as a nonpharmacological intervention for pain and other symptoms treatment, an increasing number of studies have examined these distinct VR dimensions and their analgesic effect in both experimental and clinical settings.

Virtual reality in laboratory settings

Most of the experimental studies examining VR mechanisms for pain reductions have focused on the presence and immersion dimensions of VR.[4,23–26] An early functional magnetic resonance imaging study[27] examined a small cohort of healthy participants undergoing both VR and in-take opioids while having experimental heat pain. This study used a virtual environment, SnowWorld (www.vrpain.com, Seattle, WA). Participants interacted with the virtual environment in this VR context by "shooting" a virtual snowball with a remote button. The authors found that VR-related analgesia and opioid-induced pain reduction had similar brain activation patterns, including attenuations of pain-related neural activity in the insula, anterior cingulate cortex and primary and secondary somatosensory cortex.[27] Albeit the small sample size and healthy participant cohort, this result highlighted the critical translational value of VR in clinical applications. More importantly, the shared brain representations between VR- and opioid- analgesic effects suggested the potential involvement of the endogenous opioid system in VR mechanisms in evoking pain reductions.

Recently, research on mechanisms of VR analgesia has also focused on the role of descending pain modulation.[28,29] One study used conditioned pain modulation (CPM) as a measure of descending pain modulation to be compared with VR-induced analgesic effects to capsaicin-induced secondary hyperalgesia. CPM is the reduction of pain perception after applying a conditioned stimulus to a remote part of the body.[30] In this study, Hughes and Colleagues[29] employed a passive viewing VR displaying Polar Obsession (National Geographic) via the Oculus Rift VR headset. The authors found that baseline CPM levels strongly positively correlated with the levels of VR-induced pain reductions.[28] In fact, their findings showed that more than 60% variance of VR-related analgesia was shared with CPM effects, suggesting possible overlapping mechanisms between VR-related pain reductions and endogenous pain inhibition pathways.

Colloca and colleagues conducted a well-controlled, within-subjects design study in healthy participants.[31] The authors used a commercial VR context theBlu (Wevr, Inc.) that demonstrated underwater scenes together with ambient music. They measured the objective assessment of thermal pain tolerance limits,[32,33] as well as affective and evaluative processes associated with experiencing experimental heat pain related outcomes including mood, situational anxiety, and pain unpleasantness when participants were exposed to the VR context.[31] They used Skin Sympathetic Response (SSR)[34–38] as physiological measurements for body responses to experimental nociceptive stimuli and showed that participants reacted to VR with higher levels of SSR when higher levels of pain were tolerated as compared to control conditions. During the VR intervention, an increase of parasympathetic activity concurrent to the increase in SSR was also observed, suggesting a state of relaxation despite participants higher-tolerated heat painful stimulations.[31] These findings indicated that immersive VR may foster a net gain in experimentally induced and painful heat tolerance limits that were paralleled by autonomic body responses. By employing a distraction task ("2-back working memory") as a control condition, the authors revealed that the distraction mechanism could not fully explain the VR-induced analgesia. Instead, the concurrent activation of parasympathetic response highlighted the critical role of body relaxation as a physiological basis for immersive VR-induced analgesic effects, providing evidence that VR might work throughout a multisensorial stimulation resulting in reduction of pain-related outcomes. In addition, the degree of enjoyment of the VR was positively associated with the increase in pain tolerance limits, indicating that VR contexts would need to be perceived as enjoyable to elicit emotional and sensorial changes in association to pain.

Virtual Reality in clinical settings and practices

Although the fundamental mechanisms of VR analgesia are still unclear, the efficacy and effectiveness of VR on clinical pain reductions have already been examined in a variety of clinical conditions, including burn wound-care pain,[39–41] dental procedures,[42–44] vaccination,[45–47] and chronic pain.[48–51]

A recent meta-analysis summarizing VR-induced effects in treating acute pain in adults indicates a significant moderate analgesic effect size (Cohen's d = 0.66).[52] Currently, there are three trials related to the use of VR in childbirth registered to ClinicalTrials.gov. Childbirth is of potentially great interest due to current childbirth protocols, including the concomitant use of anesthetics which holds potential risks. VR may represent an alternative to anesthetics and find applications for labor pain. In fact, Wong, Spiegel, and Gregory, in "Virtual Reality Reduces Pain in Laboring Women: A Randomized Controlled Trial," introduced a VR labor protocol visualization that was designed by Applied VR. The labor protocol contains relaxant natural scenes along with meditation auditory guidance specifically for laboring. They reported that the nulliparous women in the VR arm of the study experienced a 52% decrease in pain and a lower heart rate post intervention.[53]

With regards to VR applications in chronic pain management, Jones and colleagues used a 5-minute VR intervention named Cool! (DeepStream VR, Inc.) for a group of various chronic pain patients, including, for example, cervical pain, lumbar spine pain, hip pain, and shoulder pain. They found substantial pain rating reductions *during* the VR session as compared to the pre-VR session.[54] However, because of limited research, the long-term benefits of VR remain to be addressed.[55] Evidence from a randomized controlled trial with a 21-day VR program developed by Applied VR in at-home settings, demonstrated that VR benefits in chronic pain-related outcomes started to strengthen only after 2 weeks of intervention in patients with nonmalignant low back pain or fibromyalgia.[48]

Another follow-up trial established posttreatment efficacy for chronic low back pain patients in an 8-week home-based therapeutic VR (EaseVRx), randomized 1:1 to one of two 56-day VR programs. The intervention includes a VR pain relief skills VR program that incorporates cognitive behavioral therapy (CBT), relaxation response exercise, breathing training, mindfulness training, cognition and emotion regulation, and pain neuroscience education versus a sham VR program that was comprised of 2D nature scenery with neutral music within an identical commercial VR headset. Immediate post-VR intervention results demonstrated a significant reduction for therapeutic VR compared to sham VR for pain intensity, interference (i.e., activity, mood, and stress but not sleep), physical function, and sleep disturbance. Intention-to-treat analyses indicated superiority for therapeutic VR for pain intensity and activity, including stress with a durability over a 3-month posttreatment period.[49] Longer follow-ups and larger studies are needed to identify the dose-response of VR on chronic pain and prove efficacy of VR over controls.

On November 16, 2021, the US Food and Drug Administration (FDA) authorized the marketing of the first prescription-use immersive VR system designed for chronic pain management: the above-mentioned EaseVRx (https://www.fda.gov/news-events/press-announcements/fda-authorizes-marketing-virtual-reality-system-chronic-pain-reduction). EaseVRx uses multifaceted pain relief skill training programs that incorporate CBT principles, relaxation skills, mindfulness trainings, and pain educations, as well as other behavioral therapy techniques including biofeedback to reduce pain and pain interference. The EaseVRx program embeds a psychophysiological feedback system that can capture the exhalation and, thus, is able to provide biofeedback for relaxation training. Moreover, the pain distraction game modules reflected the interactivity components of VR. The prescription VR device for at-home treatment includes a VR headset, a controller, and a breathing amplifier for self-use deep breathing exercises. EaseVRx VR is a skills-based treatment program that teaches patients techniques such as deep relaxation, attention/distraction shifting, interoceptive awareness and perspective-taking, healthy movements, acceptance, and pain rehabilitation. It consists of 56 VR sessions, each 2–16 minutes, designed to be used at home daily for 8 weeks.

Based on a clinical trial with 179 chronic low back pain patients, more than 60% of chronic pain patients using EaseVRx reported higher than 30% pain reductions, in comparison with about 41% of chronic pain participants who were using control VR devices that did not utilize EaseVRx trainings and feedback. This FDA approval in marketing VR is no doubt a breakthrough for

VR clinical applications as an alternative or adjuvant for common pharmacological pain therapeutics.

Methodological limitations

To obtain future FDA clearances and approvals, adequate VR controls are necessary. It is crucial to understand to what extent VR analgesic effects contribute to placebo effects. We identified a lack of rigor in methodological aspects, such as the use of appropriate groups for evaluating VR efficacy (i.e., sham VR, control VR, versus no-intervention).[4] For example, including a sham VR condition *and* a no-intervention or no-treatment control condition permits isolating placebo effects. Namely, a sham VR condition consists of watching a video on an HMD. The sham HMD is stereoscopic but does not contain a 360-degree visual input and does not track head movements. Therefore, a sham VR will be able to isolate the component of immersion and engagement features from an immersive VR. This selection of controls aligns with the recent recommendation for studying VR efficacy in clinical trials.[56] This sham procedure is different from simply watching a 2D video on a tablet (or monitor), which is not an adequate sham. Tablet display of the identical context of VR has also been used to isolate the presence and immersion components from visual and auditory stimuli input.[57] Patients may indeed improve by merely wearing VR goggles. Adequate controls allow us to understand whether VR works by placebo effects, further moving the field forward.

VR embodiment and rehabilitation

Because of its intrinsic characteristics, VR technology simulates a physical experience and transcends its limits through modulating individuals' sense of place and noninvasively alternating their body representations.[58] From this point of view, VR is a multifaceted intervention that has shown effects on multiple sensorial pathways connected to mood and the sense of pleasure.[26]

Several principles of body mechanics and treatment underpin the use of VR in rehabilitation. The context in which body movement plays a crucial role in influencing motor planning through an internal inferential process (i.e., Predictive Processing theory) that integrates sensory-motor, emotional, and cognitive inputs.[59,60] This theoretical framework minimizes the predictive error on the incoming external and internal stimuli by comparing an expected state with the afferent multisensory stimulations. Under this hypothesis, prediction errors can be reduced using two opposite strategies: an action or learning.[60,61] *Action* refers to the "Active Inference" model, which focuses on an individual's prior predictions and acts by modulating the incoming information to match the expectations. *Learning* refers to the "Perceptual Inference" model, which relates to the multisensory inputs used to update the individual's expectations accounting for a posteriori information.

These same principles are adopted in the rehabilitation field to broaden the understanding of pain. In the pathogenesis of chronic pain, false narrations about the self in context and expectations about pain perceptions are factors that can lead to fear-avoidance and kinesiophobia.[62] Fear and maladaptive expectations may worsen motor performance and increase pain perception. In the specific case of chronic low back pain, patients in the acute phase may reduce their movements to protect their bodies from further injuries. However, the perpetration of these responses could generate unconscious maladaptive learning mechanisms, as well as reinforce fearful cognitions, which brings the pain process to its chronic phase.[62] The previous experience of pain can induce the expectation that lumbar movements are dangerous, changing the idea of self in context and generating a series of responses like increases in muscle tone, reduction in pain threshold, and restriction in spine flexion.[63] Conversely, owing to a positive context such as the presence of a health professional or positive feedback about their clinical state, the hypothesis about the state of the body can be updated following the Perceptual Inference model. This will succeed in moving toward an interpretation of the internal stimulus as "not dangerous" and favoring pain relief.

In this context, VR represents an ideal approach that taps into the predictive processing theory by modifying the temporal and spatial context in a way that is not predictable by a person immersed in the virtual simulation, and ultimately modulating their expectations. [64] In their recent study, Manoni, and colleagues explored VR technology to investigate the effect of positive expectations induced by verbal and visual-haptic stimuli.[65] Thirty-six healthy participants were assigned to three intervention groups that received the same sham physiotherapy maneuver and were asked to perform an anterior trunk flexion under different conditions in IVR: (i) a verbal-induced neutral expectation group; (ii) a verbal-induced positive expectation group; and (iii) a verbal-induced positive expectation group reinforced by the visual-haptic illusion of being able to touch the floor in VR. A significant difference in trunk flexion was found for the latter group, highlighting the potential role of VR in modifying the performance of trunk flexion as well as expanding its use for future investigations on individuals with low back pain. The virtual immersive gaming to optimize recovery (VIGOR) trial[66] is another example of

VR applications for rehabilitation. In this RCT, France and Thomas aimed to address the kinematic factors associated with pain-related fear via 9 weeks of VR game treatment in participants with chronic low back pain. The VR game treatment is designed with an increasing challenge to lumbar spine motion.

In a pragmatic trial, Karuna Labs created a VR training program, KarunaHOME, for participants with ongoing pain. The program is an immersive digital therapeutic that uses VR to address movement-related chronic pain conditions. It uses a combination of visual feedback, graded movements, and simulated activities of daily living in a safe and calming environment. By employing a virtual avatar that mimics the movement of the user, a VR user can adjust the movement to fit the virtual avatar. In this way, it is possible to facilitate movement and reduce pain. The visual experience of seeing the body moving in VR is employed to challenge the brain's expectations of what the body can do. It also helps recreate the association between movement and pain through visual enhancements and tricks. Patients are expected to create weekly goals and action steps in order to achieve them. They must also complete weekly VR exercises and other skills and activities that are decided on. A clinical trial on the effectiveness of the intervention is ongoing but high engagement and satisfaction have supported the feasibility of this longitudinal multifaced VR program.

VR educational programs, interactivity, and patient-provider communications

Along with rapid technological development, new directions of VR applications have emerged in the educational and medical fields. Focusing on the interactivity dimension of VR, VR training tools can be developed for teachers, students, and healthcare professionals to develop educational programs for learners ranging from preschoolers to medical students (e.g., anatomy classes)[67–74] to healthcare professionals. These tools can optimize patient-clinician communication and placebo effects while also minimizing nocebo effects in clinical practices.

Among experts and clinicians in Placebo Research, there is consensus that all groups of healthcare providers should be trained to utilize expectancy effects in patients' treatments.[75] Provider-patient communication is the most promising avenue for enhancing expectancy effects. For example, healthcare providers could enhance treatment outcomes if they clearly outline the treatment mechanisms and expected benefits. Providers could also prevent side effects by fine-tuning the information they give patients. Virtual training tools can be developed based on the most recent scientific insights and expert consensus, which Delphi methodology has investigated systematically during two expert-based conferences.[76]

Specifically, VR training can be developed to familiarize healthcare professionals with state-of-the-art theoretical knowledge on placebo and nocebo effects. In addition to raising awareness about the role of placebo and nocebo effects in everyday clinical practice, training can also help providers obtain skills to optimize placebo effects and minimize nocebo effects in clinical practice through VR communications. This training tool could include theoretical background and hands-on practice, and most importantly, communication with simulated virtual patients. A virtual training tool can allow healthcare providers to interact with computer-simulated patients (i.e., an avatar) in various scenarios, providing a naturalistic learning environment that teaches patients how to maximize positive expectancies and minimize negative expectancies in provider-patient communication in an ethical and evidence-based approach. To facilitate feasibility and user convenience, all developmental phases of virtual tools should include structurally ensured cooperation with end-users and experts in user-centered designs. Future research projects could investigate the effects of the virtual training tool for healthcare professionals on patients' satisfaction and treatment outcomes as well as Delphi surveys.

Future directions

The advances in VR technologies include group-level VR-accessible programs (Figure 6.4.2). For instance, VR group therapy was designed to relieve stress and anxiety in college students.[77] Moreover, using VR-based avatar programs allows therapists to minimize the influences of the potential biases and stigma caused by mental illnesses, sex, racial ethnicity, and socioeconomic disparities, while keeping the strengths of group therapy and in-person visits.[78–80] Applying the technology of VR group counseling to the education field, the concept of a "VR class" has also been introduced where the education materials are implemented in a VR environment.[81] The VR class allows students to be more engaged in the education processes and minimize external inputs. Nonetheless, it should be noted that technical issues and simulator sickness needs to be reduced for VR counseling and VR class. Having the advantages of providing a well-controlled experiment setup, researchers have been working on combining VR and eye tracking to maximize the ecological validity of the experiment as well as achieving in-depth behavior

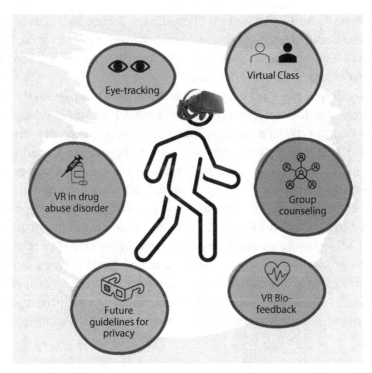

Figure 6.4.2 Future directions of VR.
Future directions of VR include VR-combined eye-tracking technology, VR group counseling and class, VR accommodations with biofeedback, and the application of VR in drug abuse disorder. Policymakers should consider up-to-date regulations to achieve the balance between protecting user privacy and maximizing VR benefits.

monitoring.[82] A recent study employed a VR combined eye-tracking system to study attentional vigilance to socially threatening information,[83] providing preliminary evidence supporting VR together with eye tracking as an innovative tool to investigate *bias* in a realistic environment. Given that drug desires critically rely on specific visual, auditorial, and sensory stimuli, VR can be an ideal tool to fight against addiction[84] through the mimicking of triggers for drug desire and cravings. Through repeated practice, individuals with drug abuse can overcome cravings for the drug.[84,85] As a proof-of-concept study, Tsai and colleagues[86] integrated multimodel sensors, such as electrocardiogram (ECG), SSR and eye tracking, together with a VR context that simulates a drug consumption scenario. Their findings, that patients with methamphetamine use disorder demonstrated higher arousal than healthy controls when exposed to the virtual drug consumption environment, provided evidence for the validation of VR as a tool for inducing drug cravings within drug misusers in mechanistic studies. In the field of psychiatry, accommodations of VR and brain connector hubs or wearable sensors have been employed to facilitate biofeedback,[87] albeit the effectiveness of VR biofeedback needs to be confirmed in a broader range of clinical samples.[88]

Finally, despite rapid advances in VR technology, challenges exist that must be addressed by the rapidly evolving field. First, VR technology coupled with sensors that can collect a variety of biomedical information may create new issues for user privacy and confidentiality. Policymakers should consider examining and reforming the current regulatory landscape of data privacy in the context of this new technology. Second, health care professionals need to protect at-risk patients from physical and psychological distress potentially triggered by ill-adapted VR programs; the potential risks of (particularly prolonged) VR exposure are still being elaborated in research. In a related vein, practical deployment remains a challenge in real-world settings, as headsets are typically sent to hospitals locked with only one accessible user application. Finally, we are in the early stages of financial modeling and distribution of VR applications, with many open questions despite recent FDA approval.

References

1. Maeda T, Arai H, Tachi S. Design and evaluation of binocular head-mounted displays. *Journal of the Robotics Society of Japan*. 1992;10(5):655–665.
2. Sutherland I. *The Ultimate Display*. Proceedings of IFIP Congress; 1965:506–508. https://my.eng.utah.edu/~cs6360/Readings/UltimateDisplay.pdf.
3. Sansone LG, Stanzani R, Job M, Battista S, Signori A, Testa M. Robustness and static-positional accuracy of the SteamVR 1.0 virtual reality tracking system. *Virtual Reality*. 2022;26:903–924. https://doi.org/10.1007/s10055-021-00584-5
4. Honzel E, Murthi S, Brawn-Cinani B, et al. Virtual reality, music, and pain: Developing the premise for an interdisciplinary approach to pain management. *Pain*. 2019;160(9):1909–1919.
5. Trost Z, France C, Anam M, Shum C. Virtual reality approaches to pain: Toward a state of the science. *Pain*. 2021 Feb 1;162(2):325–331. doi:10.1097/j.pain.0000000000002060.
6. Matamala-Gomez M, Donegan T, Bottiroli S, Sandrini G, Sanchez-Vives MV, Tassorelli C. Immersive virtual reality and virtual embodiment for pain relief. *Frontiers in Human Neuroscience*. 2019;13:279.
7. Miyahira SD, Folen RA, Hoffman HG, Garcia-Palacios A, Spira JL, Kawasaki M. The effectiveness of VR exposure therapy for PTSD in returning warfighters. *Studies in Health Technology and Informatics*. 2012;181:128–132.
8. Miyahira SD, Folen RA, Hoffman HG, Garcia-Palacios A, Schaper KM. Effectiveness of brief VR treatment for PTSD in war-fighters: A case study. *Studies in Health Technology and Informatics*. 2010;154:214–219.
9. Rizzo AA, Difede J, Rothbaum BO, et al. VR PTSD exposure therapy results with active duty OIF/OEF combatants. *Studies in Health Technology and Informatics*. 2009;142:277–282.

10. Rizzo AA, Graap K, Perlman K, et al. Virtual Iraq: Initial results from a VR exposure therapy application for combat-related PTSD. *Studies in Health Technology and Informatics.* 2008;132:420–425.

11. Scapin S, Echevarria-Guanilo ME, Boeira Fuculo Junior PR, Goncalves N, Rocha PK, Coimbra R. Virtual reality in the treatment of burn patients: A systematic review. *Burns.* 2018 Sep;44(6):1403–1416. doi:10.1016/j.burns.2017.11.002.

12. Li A, Montano Z, Chen VJ, Gold JI. Virtual reality and pain management: Current trends and future directions. *Pain Management.* 2011;1(2):147–157.

13. Wiederhold BK, Soomro A, Riva G, Wiederhold MD. Future directions: Advances and implications of virtual environments designed for pain management. *Cyberpsychology, Behavior, and Social Networking.* 2014;17(6):414–422.

14. Hoffman HG, Richards TL, Coda B, et al. Modulation of thermal pain-related brain activity with virtual reality: Evidence from fMRI. *Neuroreport.* 2004;15(8):1245–1248.

15. Loreto-Quijada D, Gutierrez-Maldonado J, Nieto R, et al. Differential effects of two virtual reality interventions: Distraction versus pain control. *Cyberpsychology, Behavior, and Social Networking.* 2014;17(6):353–358.

16. Gold JI, Belmont KA, Thomas DA. The neurobiology of virtual reality pain attenuation. *Cyberpsychology, Behavior, and Social Networking.* 2007;10(4):536–544.

17. Keefe FJ, Huling DA, Coggins MJ, et al. Virtual reality for persistent pain: A new direction for behavioral pain management. *Pain.* 2012;153(11):2163.

18. Trost Z, France C, Anam M, Shum C. Virtual reality approaches to pain: Toward a state of the science. *Pain.* 2021;162(2):325–331.

19. Lenggenhager B, Arnold CA, Giummarra MJ. Phantom limbs: Pain, embodiment, and scientific advances in integrative therapies. *Wiley Interdisciplinary Reviews: Cognitive Science.* 2014;5(2):221–231.

20. Chau B, Phelan I, Ta P, et al. Immersive virtual reality for pain relief in upper limb complex regional pain syndrome: A pilot study. *Innovations in Clinical Neuroscience.* 2020;17(4-6):47–52.

21. Pozeg P, Palluel E, Ronchi R, et al. Virtual reality improves embodiment and neuropathic pain caused by spinal cord injury. *Neurology.* 2017;89(18):1894–1903.

22. Trost Z, Anam M, Seward J, et al. Immersive interactive virtual walking reduces neuropathic pain in spinal cord injury: Findings from a preliminary investigation of feasibility and clinical efficacy. *Pain.* 2022;163(2):350–361.

23. Hoffman HG, Sharar SR, Coda B, et al. Manipulating presence influences the magnitude of virtual reality analgesia. *Pain.* 2004;111(1-2):162–168.

24. Hoffman HG, Seibel EJ, Richards TL, Furness TA, Patterson DR, Sharar SR. Virtual reality helmet display quality influences the magnitude of virtual reality analgesia. *Journal of Pain.* 2006;7(11):843–850.

25. Hoffman HG, Richards TL, Bills AR, et al. Using fMRI to study the neural correlates of virtual reality analgesia. *CNS Spectrums.* 2006;11(1):45–51.

26. Colloca L, Raghuraman N, Wang Y, et al. Virtual reality: Physiological and behavioral mechanisms to increase individual pain tolerance limits. *Pain.* 2020;161(9):2010–2021.

27. Hoffman HG, Richards TL, Van Oostrom T, et al. The analgesic effects of opioids and immersive virtual reality distraction: Evidence from subjective and functional brain imaging assessments. *Anesthesia & Analgesia.* 2007;105(6):1776–1783.

28. Demeter N, Josman N, Eisenberg E, Pud D. Who can benefit from virtual reality to reduce experimental pain? A crossover study in healthy subjects. *European Journal of Pain.* 2015;19(10):1467–1475.

29. Hughes SW, Zhao H, Auvinet EJ, Strutton PH. Attenuation of capsaicin-induced ongoing pain and secondary hyperalgesia during exposure to an immersive virtual reality environment. *Pain Reports.* 2019;4(6):e790. doi:10.1097/PR9.0000000000000790.

30. Ramaswamy S, Wodehouse T. Conditioned pain modulation—A comprehensive review. *Neurophysiologie Clinique*. 2021;51(3):197–208.

31. Colloca L, Raghuraman N, Wang Y, et al. Virtual reality: Physiological and behavioral mechanisms to increase individual pain tolerance limits. *Pain*. 2020 Sep 1;161(9):2010–2021. doi:10.1097/j.pain.0000000000001900.

32. Fruhstorfer H, Lindblom U, Schmidt WC. Method for quantitative estimation of thermal thresholds in patients. *Journal of Neurology, Neurosurgery, and Psychiatry*. 1976;39(11):1071–1075.

33. Nielsen CS, Price DD, Vassend O, Stubhaug A, Harris JR. Characterizing individual differences in heat-pain sensitivity. *Pain*. 2005;119(1-3):65–74.

34. Dube AA, Duquette M, Roy M, Lepore F, Duncan G, Rainville P. Brain activity associated with the electrodermal reactivity to acute heat pain. *Neuroimage*. 2009;45(1):169–180.

35. Eriksson M, Storm H, Fremming A, Schollin J. Skin conductance compared to a combined behavioural and physiological pain measure in newborn infants. *Acta Paediatrica*. 2008;97(1):27–30.

36. Fujita T, Fujii Y, Okada SF, Miyauchi A, Takagi Y. Fall of skin impedance and bone and joint pain. *Journal of Bone and Mineral Metabolism*. 2001;19(3):175–179.

37. Harrison D, Boyce S, Loughnan P, Dargaville P, Storm H, Johnston L. Skin conductance as a measure of pain and stress in hospitalised infants. *Early Human Development*. 2006;82(9):603–608.

38. Schestatsky P, Valls-Sole J, Costa J, Leon L, Veciana M, Chaves ML. Skin autonomic reactivity to thermoalgesic stimuli. *Clinical Autonomic Research*. 2007;17(6):349–355.

39. Hoffman HG, Chambers GT, Meyer III WJ, et al. Virtual reality as an adjunctive non-pharmacologic analgesic for acute burn pain during medical procedures. *Annals of Behavioral Medicine*. 2011;41(2):183–191.

40. Smith V, Warty RR, Sursas JA, et al. The effectiveness of virtual reality in managing acute pain and anxiety for medical inpatients: Systematic review. *Journal of Medical Internet Research*. 2020;22(11):e17980.

41. Scapin S, Echevarría-Guanilo ME, Junior PRBF, Gonçalves N, Rocha PK, Coimbra R. Virtual reality in the treatment of burn patients: A systematic review. *Burns*. 2018;44(6):1403–1416.

42. Joda T, Gallucci G, Wismeijer D, Zitzmann N. Augmented and virtual reality in dental medicine: A systematic review. *Computers in Biology and Medicine*. 2019;108:93–100.

43. Sullivan C, Schneider PE, Musselman RJ, Dummett Jr C, Gardiner D. The effect of virtual reality during dental treatment on child anxiety and behavior. *ASDC Journal of Dentistry for Children*. 2000;67(3):193–196, 160.

44. Huang T-K, Yang C-H, Hsieh Y-H, Wang J-C, Hung C-C. Augmented reality (AR) and virtual reality (VR) applied in dentistry. *Kaohsiung Journal of Medical Sciences*. 2018;34(4):243–248.

45. Althumairi A, Sahwan M, Alsaleh S, Alabduljobar Z, Aljabri D. Virtual reality: Is it helping children cope with fear and pain during vaccination? *Journal of Multidisciplinary Healthcare*. 2021;14:2625.

46. Vandeweerdt C, Luong T, Atchapero M, et al. Virtual reality reduces COVID-19 vaccine hesitancy in the wild: A randomized trial. *Scientific Reports*. 2022;12(1):1–7.

47. Real FJ, DeBlasio D, Beck AF, et al. A virtual reality curriculum for pediatric residents decreases rates of influenza vaccine refusal. *Academic pediatrics*. 2017;17(4):431–435.

48. Darnall BD, Krishnamurthy P, Tsuei J, Minor JD. Self-administered skills-based virtual reality intervention for chronic pain: Randomized controlled pilot study. *JMIR Formative Research*. 2020;4(7):e17293.

49. Garcia LM, Birckhead BJ, Krishnamurthy P, et al. Three-month follow-up results of a double-blind, randomized placebo-controlled trial of 8-week self-administered at-home

behavioral skills-based virtual reality (VR) for chronic low back pain. *Journal of Pain*. 2022;23(5):822–840.

50. Garcia LM, Birckhead BJ, Krishnamurthy P, et al. An 8-week self-administered at-home behavioral skills-based virtual reality program for chronic low back pain: Double-blind, randomized, placebo-controlled trial conducted during COVID-19. *Journal of Medical Internet Research*. 2021;23(2):e26292.

51. Garcia LM, Darnall BD, Krishnamurthy P, et al. Self-administered behavioral skills-based at-home virtual reality therapy for chronic low back pain: Protocol for a randomized controlled trial. *JMIR Research Protocols*. 2021;10(1):e25291.

52. Mallari B, Spaeth EK, Goh H, Boyd BS. Virtual reality as an analgesic for acute and chronic pain in adults: A systematic review and meta-analysis. *Journal of Pain Research*. 2019;12:2053.

53. Wong MS, Spiegel BMR, Gregory KD. Virtual reality reduces pain in laboring women: A randomized controlled trial. *American Journal of Perinatology*. 2021;38(S 01):e167–e172.

54. Jones T, Moore T, Choo J. The impact of virtual reality on chronic pain. *PLoS ONE*. 2016;11(12):e0167523.

55. Ahmadpour N, Randall H, Choksi H, Gao A, Vaughan C, Poronnik P. Virtual reality interventions for acute and chronic pain management. *International Journal of Biochemistry and Cell Biology*. 2019;114:105568.

56. Birckhead B, Khalil C, Liu X, et al. Recommendations for methodology of virtual reality clinical trials in health care by an international working group: Iterative study. *Journal of Medical Internet Research*. 2019;6(1):e11973.

57. Felix RB, Rao A, Khalid M, et al. Adjunctive virtual reality pain relief following traumatic injury: Protocol for a randomised within-subjects clinical trial. *BMJ Open*. 2021;11(11):e056030.

58. Slater M. Place illusion and plausibility can lead to realistic behaviour in immersive virtual environments. *Philosophical Transactions of the Royal Society B: Biological Sciences*. 2009;364(1535):3549–3557.

59. de Bruin L, Michael J. Prediction error minimization: Implications for embodied cognition and the extended mind hypothesis. *Brain and Cognition*. 2017;112:58–63.

60. Gadsby S, Hohwy J. *Predictive Processing and Body Representation*. Routledge; 2021. Accessed on: 11 May 2023, https://www.routledgehandbooks.com/doi/10.4324/978042 9321542-16

61. Seth AK, Friston KJ. Active interoceptive inference and the emotional brain. *Philosophical Transactions of the Royal Society B: Biological Sciences*. 2016;371(1708):20160007.

62. Crombez G, Eccleston C, Van Damme S, Vlaeyen JW, Karoly P. Fear-avoidance model of chronic pain: The next generation. *Clinical Journal of Pain*. 2012;28(6):475–483.

63. Vlaeyen JWS, Linton SJ. Fear-avoidance and its consequences in chronic musculoskeletal pain: A state of the art. *Pain*. 2000;85(3):317–332.

64. Nishigami T, Wand BM, Newport R, et al. Embodying the illusion of a strong, fit back in people with chronic low back pain: A pilot proof-of-concept study. *Musculoskeletal Science and Practice*. 2019;39:178–183.

65. Mattia Manoni SB, Job M, Sansone LG, Viceconti A, Testa M. Positive expectations lead to motor improvement: An immersive virtual reality pilot study. *Psychological Research*. 2022;in review.

66. France CR, Thomas JS. Virtual immersive gaming to optimize recovery (VIGOR) in low back pain: A phase II randomized controlled trial. *Contemporary Clinical Trials*. 2018;69:83–91.

67. Zhao X, Li X. Comparison of standard training to virtual reality training in nuclear radiation emergency medical rescue education. *Disaster Medicine and Public Health Preparedness*. 2022;17:e197. doi:10.1017/dmp.2022.65.

68. Yildiz H, Demiray A. Virtual reality in nursing education 3D intravenous catheterization E-learning: A randomized controlled trial. *Contemporary Nurse.* 2022 Feb-Apr;58(2-3):125–137. doi:10.1080/10376178.2022.2051573.

69. Williams M. Virtual reality in ophthalmology education: Simulating pupil examination. *Eye (Lond).* 2022 Nov;36(11):2084–2085. doi:10.1038/s41433-022-02078-3.

70. Wang N, Abdul Rahman MN, Lim BH. Teaching and curriculum of the preschool physical education major direction in colleges and universities under virtual reality technology. *Computational Intelligence and Neuroscience.* 2022;2022:3250986.

71. van der Kruk SR, Zielinski R, MacDougall H, Hughes-Barton D, Gunn KM. Virtual reality as a patient education tool in healthcare: A scoping review. *Patient Education and Counseling.* 2022 Jul;105(7):1928–1942. doi:10.1016/j.pec.2022.02.005.

72. Turso-Finnich T, Jensen RO, Jensen LX, Konge L, Thinggaard E. Virtual reality head-mounted displays in medical education: A systematic review. *Simulation in Healthcare.* 2023 Feb 1;18(1):42–50. doi:10.1097/SIH.0000000000000636.

73. Nakai K, Terada S, Takahara A, Hage D, Tubbs RS, Iwanaga J. Anatomy education for medical students in a virtual reality workspace: A pilot study. *Clinical Anatomy.* 2022;35(1):40–44.

74. Liaw SY, Ooi SL, Mildon R, Ang ENK, Lau TC, Chua WL. Translation of an evidence-based virtual reality simulation-based interprofessional education into health education curriculums: An implementation science method. *Nurse Education Today.* 2022;110:105262.

75. Evers AW, Colloca L, Blease C, et al. What should clinicians tell patients about placebo and nocebo effects? Practical considerations based on expert consensus. *Psychotherapy and Psychosomatics.* 2021;90(1):49–56.

76. Evers AW, Colloca L, Blease C, et al. Implications of placebo and nocebo effects for clinical practice: Expert consensus. *Psychotherapy and Psychosomatics.* 2018;87(4):204–210.

77. Lin AP, Trappey CV, Luan C-C, Trappey AJ, Tu KL. A test platform for managing school stress using a virtual reality group chatbot counseling system. *Applied Sciences.* 2021;11(19):9071.

78. Lem WG, Kohyama-Koganeya A, Saito T, Oyama H. Effect of a virtual reality contact-based educational intervention on the public stigma of depression: Randomized controlled pilot study. *JMIR Formative Research.* 2022;6(5):e28072.

79. Yuen ASY, Mak WWS. The effects of immersive virtual reality in reducing public stigma of mental illness in the university population of Hong Kong: Randomized controlled trial. *Journal of Medical Internet Research.* 2021;23(7):e23683.

80. van Bennekom MJ, de Koning PP. Reducing the stigma on posttraumatic stress disorder in militaries through virtual reality. *Mhealth.* 2018;4:5.

81. Yoshimura A, Borst CW. Remote instruction in virtual reality: A study of students attending class remotely from home with VR headsets. *Mensch und Computer 2020-Workshopband.* 2020. doi:10.18420/muc2020-ws122-355. https://vrlab.cmix.louisiana.edu/papers/Yoshimura_Borst_RemoteInstructionInVirtualReality_MuC2020.pdf

82. Clay V, König P, König S. Eye tracking in virtual reality. *Journal of Eye Movement Research.* 2019 Apr 5;12(1):10.16910/jemr.12.1.3. doi:10.16910/jemr.12.1.3.

83. Reichenberger J, Pfaller M, Mühlberger A. Gaze behavior in social fear conditioning: An eye-tracking study in virtual reality. *Frontiers in Psychology.* 2020; :35.

84. Gupta S, Chadha B. *Virtual Reality Against Addiction.* Paper presented at the International Conference on Computing, Communication & Automation. 2015.

85. Christofi M, Michael-Grigoriou D, Kyrlitsias C. A virtual reality simulation of drug users' everyday life: The effect of supported sensorimotor contingencies on empathy. *Frontiers in Psychology.* 2020;11:1242.

86. Tsai M-C, Chung C-R, Chen C-C, et al. An intelligent virtual-reality system with multi-model sensing for cue-elicited craving in patients with methamphetamine use disorder. *IEEE Transactions on Biomedical Engineering*. 2021;68(7):2270–2280.

87. Luddecke R, Felnhofer A. Virtual reality biofeedback in health: A scoping review. *Applied Psychophysiology and Biofeedback*. 2022;47(1):1–15.

88. Kothgassner OD, Goreis A, Bauda I, Ziegenaus A, Glenk LM, Felnhofer A. Virtual reality biofeedback interventions for treating anxiety: A systematic review, meta-analysis and future perspective. *Wiener klinische Wochenschrift*. 2022;134(Suppl 1):49–59.

Index